Principles of Immunopharmacology

Edited by:

F.P. Nijkamp
M.J. Parnham

Birkhäuser Verlag
Basel · Boston · Berlin

Editors:

Prof. Dr. Frans P. Nijkamp
Professor of Pharmacology and Toxicology
Faculteit der Farmacie
Universiteit te Utrecht
Sorbonnelaan 16
NL-3584 CA Utrecht
The Netherlands

Prof. Dr. Michael J. Parnham
Director of Pharmacology and Toxicology
PLIVA d.d.
Research Institute
Prilaz baruna Filipovica 25
HR-10000 Zagreb
Croatia

And

Professor of Pharmacology and Toxicology
Pharmacological Institute for Life Scientists
J.W. Goethe University
Biocentre
Marie-Curie-Str. 9
D-60439 Frankfurt a.M.
Germany

Library of Congress, Cataloging-in-Publication Data
Principles of immunopharmacology / edited by: F.P. Nijkamp; M.J.
    Parnham.
        p. cm.
    Includes bibliographical references and index.
    ISBN 3-7643-5780-0 (soft cover : alk. paper). – ISBN
0-8176-5780-0 (soft cover: alk. paper)
        1. Immunopharmacology 2. Immunotoxicology. 3. Immunodiagnosis.
    4. Immune system–Effect of drugs on. I. Nijkamp, Franciscus
    Petrus, 1947– . II. Parnham, Michael J., 1951–
        [DNLM: 1. Immunity-drug effects. 2. Immunity, Cellular-
    physiology. 3. Adjuvants, Immunologic–pharmacology.
    4. Immunosuppressive Agents–pharmacology. 5. Immunotherapy.
    6. Immunologic Tests. QW 540 P957 1999]
    RM370.P75 1999
        616.07'9–dc21
DNLM/DLC
for Library of Congress

Deutsche Bibliothek Cataloging-in-Publication Data
Principles of immunopharmacology / ed. by: F.P. Nijkamp; M.J.
Parnham. – Basel ; Boston ; Berlin : Birkhäuser, 1999
        ISBN 3-7643-5780-0 (Basel…)
        ISBN 0-8176-5780-0 (Boston)

© 1999 Birkhäuser Verlag, PO Box 133, CH-4010 Basel, Switzerland
Printed on acid-free paper produced from chlorine-free pulp. TCF ∞
Cover design: Markus Etterich, Basel
Printed in Germany
ISBN 3-7643-5780-0
ISBN 0-8176-5780-0
9 8 7 6 5 4 3 2 1

Table of contents

D Immunotoxicology

Preface

The rapid developments in immunology in recent years have dramatically expanded our knowledge of mammalian host defence mechanisms. The molecular mechanisms of cellular interactions during immune responses have been unravelled, the intracellular responses involved in signal transduction delineated and an ever increasing number of soluble mediators of immune and inflammatory reponses have been discovered.

The initial result of this explosion of knowledge has been to provide the researcher and the clinician with an arsenal of diagnostic tools with which the immunological bases of disease processes can be investigated. This has made disease diagnosis much more precise, enabling the physician to tailor therapy much more closely to the individual patient's needs. However, better understanding of disease processes only provides a gradual improvement in therapy. This is because the new molecular targets that have been uncovered must first be tested as potential bases for immunomodulatory drug actions, and then the new compounds must be subject to extensive development studies. As a result of the molecular unravelling of the immune system, we now understand more precisely the mechanisms of action of some established therapies, such as antiallergic and antiasthma agents, including the corticosteroids. New rational treatments based on molecular mechanisms are also now entering clinical practice and are making their mark on cancer, infectious and autoimmune disease therapy.

Concomitantly with these advances in understanding of molecular mechanisms of immunity, immunodiagnosis and immunotherapy, it has become possible to test more accurately the way in which a variety of drug classes interact with the immune system. It is of particular importance to regulatory authorities that the toxic side-effects of immunomodulatory drugs can be distinguished from their beneficial therapeutic effects.

Currently, it is only possible to obtain an overview of these various aspects of immunopharmacology by reading a range of immunological, pharmacological, diagnostic and toxicological literature. Good immunological textbooks are available, while immunopharmacology is covered mainly in terms of the inflammatory response. *Principles of Immunopharmacology* is intended to provide for the first time in a single volume a basic understanding of immunological mechanisms, a review of important immunodiagnostic tools and a description of the main pharmacological agents which modify the immune response, together with an introduction to immunotoxicology. As such we hope that it will be useful as a reference text for physicians, researchers and students with a rudimentary knowledge of immunology.

We, the editors, are grateful to all the authors who have invested their time and effort into this volume. We have received continuous help and encouragement from Petra Gerlach and Katrin Serries of Birkhäuser Verlag and particular thanks are due to Dinij van der Pal for administrative assistance.

Frans P. Nijkamp
Michael J. Parnham   March, 1999

List of contributors

Ruud Albers, Research Institute of Toxicology, Utrecht University, P.O. Box 80176, NL-3508 TD Utrecht, The Netherlands

Sergey G. Apasov, Laboratory of Immunology, National Institute of Allergy and Infectious Diseases, National Institutes of Health, Bethesda, MD 20892, USA

Clarissa Bachmeier, Departments of Rheumatology and Clinical Pharmacology, St Vincent's Hospital, Victoria Street, Darlinghurst NSW 2010, Sydney, Australia

Peter J. Barnes, Department of Thoracic Medicine, National Heart and Lung Institute, Imperial College, Dovehouse St, London SW3 6LY, UK
E-mail: p.j.barnes@ic.ac.uk

J. Edwin Blalock, Department of Physiology and Biophysics, University of Alabama at Birmingham, 1918 University Blvd., McCallum Building, Birmingham, AL 35294-0005, USA
E-mail: Blalock@uab.edu

Reinder L.H. Bolhuis, Department of Clinical and Tumor Immunology, Daniel den Hoed Kliniek, P.O. Box 5201, NL-3008 AE Rotterdam, The Netherlands

Peter M. Brooks, Departments of Rheumatology and Clinical Pharmacology, St Vincent's Hospital, Victoria Street, Darlinghurst NSW 2010, Sydney, Australia

Julia C. Buckingham, Department of Neuroendocrinology, Division of Neuroscience and Psychological Medicine, Imperial College School of Medicine, Charing Cross Hospital, Fulham Palace Road, London W6 8RF, UK,
E-mail: j.buckingham.ic.ac.uk

Phillip G. Conaghan, Departments of Rheumatology and Clinical Pharmacology, St Vincent's Hospital, Victoria Street, Darlinghurst NSW 2010, Sydney, Australia

Richard O. Day, Departments of Rheumatology and Clinical Pharmacology, St Vincent's Hospital, Victoria Street, Darlinghurst NSW 2010, Sydney, Australia
E-mail: R.Day@unsw.edu.au

Eric J. De Waal, Laboratory for Medicines and Medical Devices, National Institute of Public Health and the Environment, P.O. Box 1, NL-3720 BA Bilthoven, The Netherlands

Gerhard Dickneite, Centeon Pharma GmbH, Postfach 12 30, D-35002 Marburg, Germany

Rod J. Flower, Department of Biochemical Pharmacology, St Bartholomew's and the Royal London School of Medicine and Dentistry at Queen Mary and Westfield College, Charterhouse Square, London EC1M 6BQ, UK
E-mail: r.j.flower@qmw.ac.uk

Nick J. Goulding, Department of Biochemical Pharmacology, St Bartholomews and the Royal London School of Medicine and Dentistry at Queen Mary and Westfield College, Charterhouse Square, London EC1M 6BQ, UK
E-mail: n.j.goulding@mds.qmw.ac.uk

Garry G. Graham, Schools of Physiology and Pharmacology and Medicine, Faculty of Medicine, University of New South Wales, Sydney, Australia
E-mail: g.graham@unsw.edu.au

Jan W. Gratama, Department of Clinical and Tumor Immunology, Daniel den Hoed Kliniek, P.O. Box 5201, NL-3008 AE Rotterdam, The Netherlands
E-mail: gratama@immh.azr.nl

Peter Gronski, Centeon Pharma GmbH, Postfach 12 30, D-35002 Marburg, Germany
E-mail: Gronski@msmbwmd.hoechst.com

Richard J. Gryglewski, Department of Pharmacology, Medical College of Jagiellonian University, 16 Grzegorzecka, 31-531 Krakow, Poland

C. Erik Hack, Central Laboratory of the Netherlands Red Cross Blood Transfusion Service and Laboratory for Experimental and Clinical Immunology, Academic Medical Center, University of Amsterdam, Plesmanlaan 125, NL-1066 CX Amsterdam, The Netherlands
E-mail: C_Hack@CLB.nl

Malcolm L. Handel, Departments of Rheumatology and Clinical Pharmacology, St Vincent's Hospital, Victoria Street, Darlinghurst NSW 2010, Sydney, Australia

Peter S. Heeger, Cleveland VA Medical Center, Division of Nephrology, Department of Medicine, 111K(W), 10701 East Blvd., Cleveland, OH 44106, USA
E-mail: heeger.peter@cleveland.va.gov

Klaus Hermann, Klinische Kooperationsgruppe Umweltdermatologie und Allergologie GSF/TUM, Gebäude 34, Halle Süd 2, Ingolstädter Landstr.1, D-85764 Neuherberg, Germany
E-mail: Hermann@GSF.de

Stephen T. Holgate, Southampton General Hospital, Tremona Road, Southampton SO16 6YD, UK
E-mail:sth@soton.ac.uk

Imran R. Hussain, Southampton General Hospital, Tremona Road, Southampton SO16 6YD, UK
E-mail:irh@soton.ac.uk

Wim Jiskoot, Department of Pharmaceutics, University of Utrecht, P.O. Box 80082, NL-3508 TB Utrecht, The Netherlands
E-mail: w.jiskoot@pharm.uu.nl

Ernst-Jürgen Kanzy, Centeon Pharma GmbH, Postfach 12 30, D-35002 Marburg, Germany

Richard Korbut, Department of Pharmacology, Medical College of Jagiellonian University, 16 Grzegorzecka, 31-531 Krakow, Poland
E-mail: mfkorbut@kinga.cyf_kr.pl

K. Noel Masihi, Robert Koch Institute, Nordufer 20, D-13353 Berlin, Germany
E-Mail: MasihiK@rki.de

Kees Nooter, Department of Medical Oncology, Rotterdam Cancer Institute (Daniel den Hoed Kliniek) and University Hospital, NL-3008 AE Rotterdam, The Netherlands

Michael J. O'Sullivan, Fluorescence Assay Technology Department, Amersham Pharmacia Biotech Ltd., Cardiff Laboratories, Whitchurch, Cardiff CF4 7YT, Wales, UK
E-mail: michael.o'sullivan@eu.apbiotech.com

Michael J. Parnham, PLIVA, Research Institute, Prilaz baruna filipovica 25, HR-10000 Zagreb, Croatia
E-mail: michael.parnham@pliva.hr

Zdenek Pelikan, Department of Allergology & Immunology, Institute of Medical Sciences "De Klokkenberg", Galderseweg 81, NL-4836 AE Breda, The Netherlands

Raymond H.H. Pieters, Research Institute of Toxicology, Utrecht University, P.O. Box 80176, NL-3508 TD Utrecht, The Netherlands

Valerie F.J. Quesniaux, Transplantation Research, Building S.386/155A, Novartis Pharma Inc, P.O. Box, CH-4002 Basel, Switzerland
E-mail: Valerie.Quesniaux@pharma.novartis.com

Klaus Resch, Institut für Molekularpharmakologie, Medizinische Hochschule Hannover, Carl-Neuberg-Straße 1, D-30625 Hannover, Germany

Ger T. Rijkers, Dept. of Immunology, University Hospital for Children and Youth, The Wilhelmina Children's Hospital, Lundlaan 6, NL-3512 Utrecht, The Netherlands
E-mail: grijkers@wkz.azu.nl

Johannes Ring, Klinische Kooperationsgruppe Umweltdermatologie und Allergologie GSF/TUM, Gebäude 34, Halle Süd 2, Ingolstädter Landstr.1, D-85764 Neuherberg, Germany

Dirk Roos, Central Laboratory of the Netherlands Red Cross Blood Transfusion Service and Laboratory for Experimental and Clinical Immunology, Academic Medical Center, University of Amsterdam, Plesmanlaan 125, NL-1066 CX Amsterdam, The Netherlands
E-mail: D_Roos@CLB.nl

Marcella Sarzotti, Department of Immunology, Duke University Medical Center, Jones Bldg., Box 3010, Durham, NC 27710, USA
E-mail: msarzott@duke.edu

Max H. Schreier, Transplantation Research, Building S.386.1040, Novartis Pharma Inc, P.O. Box, CH-4002 Basel, Switzerland
E-mail: max.schreier@pharma.novartis.com

Henk-Jan Schuurman, Transplantation Research, Building S.386.516, Novartis Pharma AG, PO Box, CH-4002 Basel, Switzerland
E-mail: henk.schuurman@pharma.novartis.com

Friedrich R. Seiler, Oberer Eichweg 10, D-35001 Marburg, Germany

Michail V. Sitkovsky, Laboratory of Immunology, National Institute of Allergy and Infectious Diseases, National Institutes of Health, Building 10, Room 11N311, Bethesda, MD 20892, USA
E-mail m_sitkovsky@nih.gov

Harm Snippe, Eijkman-Winkler Institute dor Microbiology, Infectious Diseases and Inflammation, Utrecht University Hospital, Room G04.614, PO Box 85.500, NL-3508 GA Utrecht, The Netherlands
E-mail: H.Snippe@lab.azu.nl

Hergen Spits, Netherlands Cancer Institute, Plesmanlaan 121, NL-1066 CX Amsterdam, The Netherlands
E-mail: hergen@nki.nl

James E. Talmadge, University of Nebraska Medical Center, 600 South 42nd Street, Omaha, NE 68198-5660, USA
E-mail: jtalmadg@unmc.edu

C. Ellen van der Schoot, Central Laboratory of the Blood Transfusion Service, Plesmanlaan 125 1066 CX Amsterdam, The Netherlands
E-mail: schoot@clb.nl

Henk van Loveren, Laboratory for Pathology and Immunobiology, National Institute of Public Health and the Environment, P.O. Box 1, NL-3720 BA Bilthoven, The Netherlands

Jan Verhoef, Eijkman-Winkler Institute for Microbiology, Infectious Diseases and Inflammation, Utrecht University Hospital, Room G04.614, PO Box 85.500, NL-3508 GA Utrecht, The Netherlands

Joseph G. Vos, Laboratory for Pathology and Immonology, National Institute of Public Health and the Environment, P.O. Box 1, NL-3720 BA Bilthoven, The Netherlands
E-mail: j.vos@rivm.nl

Douglas A. Weigent, University of Alabama at Birmingham, 1918 University Blvd., MCLM 894, McCallum Building, Birmingham, AL 35294-0005, USA
E-mail: weigent@uab.edu

Donald M. Weir, Department of Medical Microbiology, University of Edinburgh Medical School, Edinburgh, EH8 9AG, UK
E-mail: dmweir@ed.ac.uk

Kenneth M. Williams, Departments of Rheumatology and Clinical Pharmacology, St Vincent's Hospital, Victoria Street, Darlinghurst NSW 2010, Sydney, Australia

Gerhard Zenke, Transplantation Research, Building S.386.127, Novartis, PO Box, CH-4002 Basel, Switzerland
E-mail: gerhard.zenke@pharma.novartis.com

A   Mechanisms of immunity

Specificity of the immune system: structure and generation of diversity

Donald M. Weir

Antigens

An antigen is any material capable of provoking the lymphoid tissues of an animal to respond by generating an immune reaction specifically directed at the inducing agent and not at other unrelated substances. Complex structures, like bacteria and viruses, as well as single molecules can act as antigens, but the response is not to the entire structure but to individual chemical groups that have a specific three-dimensional shape. The specificity of the response for these antigenic determinants or epitopes is an important characteristic of immune responses. The immunological reaction of an animal to contact with antigen, called the acquired immune response, takes two forms: (1) the humoral or circulating antibody response and (2) the cell-mediated response. An antibody directed against an epitope of a particular molecule will react only with this determinant or other very similar structures. Even minor chemical changes in the conformation of the epitope will markedly reduce the ability of the original antibody to react with the altered material.

antigenic determinants
epitopes
acquired response

Antibody binds directly to structures on the surface of an antigen that have a three-dimensional shape complementary to the binding site of the antibody. Cell-mediated reactions are also directed against sites within antigens. The main effector cells in this type of response, T-lymphocytes, possess a receptor (known as the T-cell receptor) that will bind to a complementary shape generated from an antigen. T-cells are stimulated by fragments of foreign material presented to them by molecules present on the surface of host cells. The T-cell receptor recognizes both the antigen fragment and the self-structure to which it is bound. Therefore, T-lymphocytes recognize small pieces of foreign material attached to host-cell surface molecules.

complementary shape

Antigens are divided into (1) substances which are able to generate an immune response by themselves and are termed immunogens and (2) molecules which are able to react with antibodies but are unable to stim-

immunogens

Principles of Immunopharmacology, ed. by F. P. Nijkamp and M. J. Parnham
©1999 Birkhäuser Verlag Basel/Switzerland

haptene

carriers

ulate their production directly. The latter substances are often low molecular weight chemicals, termed haptens, that will react with preformed antibodies but only become immunogenic when attached to large molecules, called carriers.

General properties

A substance that acts as an antigen in one species of animal may not do so in another because it is represented in the tissues or fluids of the second species. This underlines the requirement that the antigen must be a foreign substance to elicit an immune response. For example, egg albumin, whilst an excellent antigen in rabbits, fails to induce an antibody response in fowls. The more foreign, evolutionarily distant, a substance is to a particular species, the more likely it is to be a powerful antigen. A widely recognized requirement for a substance to be antigenic in its own right, without having to be attached to a carrier molecule, is that it should have a molecular weight in excess of 5000. Some low molecular weight chemical substances appear to contradict the requirement that an anti-

**low MW
chemicals**

gen be large. Among these are included picryl chloride, formaldehyde and drugs in wide clinical use such as aspirin, penicillin and sulphonamides. These substances are highly antigenic particularly if applied to the skin. This is due to the ability of such materials to form complexes by means of covalent bonds with tissue proteins. The complex of these substances,

**hapten carrier
complexes**

acting as haptens, with a tissue protein, acting as a carrier, forms a complete antigen. These products can lead to the development of various types of unhelpful immunological responses known as hypersensitivity reactions (sometimes referred to as allergies, see Chapters A1, A9, B1).

Epitopes and paratopes

The immune system does not recognize an infectious agent or foreign molecule as a whole but as we have seen reacts to structurally distinct areas – antigenic determinants or epitopes. Thus exposure to a microorganism will generate an immune response to many different epitopes The antiserum produced will contain different antibodies reactive with each determinant. This will ensure that an individual will be protected from the microorganism by producing a response to at least a few of the possible determinants.

A response to antigen involves the specific interaction of components of the immune system, antibodies and lymphocytes, with epitopes on the antigen. The lymphocytes have receptors on their surface that function as the recognition units – on B-lymphocytes cell-bound immunoglobulin acts as receptors and on T-lymphocytes the recognition unit is the T-cell receptor. The interaction between an antibody (or cell-bound receptor) and antigen is governed by the complementarity of the electron cloud surrounding the determinants. The overall configuration of the outer electrons, not the chemical nature of the constituent residues, determines the shape of the epitope and its complementary paratope (part of antibody or T-cell receptor that interacts with the epitope).

paratope

Antigenic epitopes may be present within a single segment of the primary sequence or made up of residues far apart in the primary sequence but brought together on the surface by the folding of the molecule into its native conformation. The former are known as sequential epitopes and those formed from distant residues are conformational epitopes.

sequential epitopes
conformational epitopes

Immunoglobulins

Towards the end of the nineteenth century Von Behring and Kitasato in Berlin found that the blood serum of an appropriately immunized animal contained specific neutralizing substances or antitoxins. This was the first demonstration of the activity of what are now known as antibodies or immunoglobulins. Antibodies are glycoproteins that bind specifically to the antigen that induced their formation. They are produced when immunogenic molecules are recognised and responded to by the host's lymphoid system and are present in the serum body, fluids and attached to the surface of certain cell types. The terms antibody and immunoglobulin are interchangeable.

antitoxins

The liquid collected from blood that has been allowed to clot is known as serum. It contains a number of molecules but no cells or clotting factors. If serum is prepared from an animal that has been exposed to an antigen, it is known as an antiserum since it will contain antibodies of varying specificity reactive with the inducing antigen. When the components of serum are separated electrophoretically due to differences in their charge, the heterogeneity of the immunoglobulins can be seen, i.e. they appear as broad bands.

serum

There are five distinct classes or isotypes of immunoglobulins, namely IgG, IgA, IgM, IgD and IgE. They differ from each other in size, charge, carbohydrate content and, of course, amino acid composition (Table 1). Within certain classes there are subclasses that show slight differences in structure and function from other members of the class. These classes and

isotypes

Table 1 *Physicochemical properties of human immunoglobulins*

Characteristic	IgA	IgD	IgE	IgG	IgM[#] (pentamer)
Mean serum concentration (mg/dl)[*]	300	5	0.005	1400	150
Molecular weight (kDa)	160	184	188	160	970
Carbohydrate (%)	7–11	9–14	12	2–3	12
Half-life (days)	6	3	2	21	5
Heavy-chains	α	δ	ε	γ	μ

The immunoglobulin serotype is determined by the type of heavy-chain present. Different functional characteristics (e.g. complement activation) are also controlled by the heavy-chain. Variation within a class gives rise to subclasses.
[#]*Data for IgM as a pentamer;* [*]*dl, 100 ml.*

subclasses can be separated from each other serologically, i.e. using antibody. This is achieved by injecting immunoglobulins into a different species (e.g. human immunoglobulin into a sheep). This will induce the sheep to make anti-human immunoglobulin antibodies that can be used to differentiate between the different isotypes (see also Chapter C2).

Antibody structure

light chains
heavy chains

Antibody molecules all have the same basic four-chain structure composed of two light-chains and two heavy-chains (Fig. 1A). The light-chains (mol wt 25 000) are one of two types designated kappa (κ) and lambda (λ), and only one type is found in a single antibody. The heavy-chains vary in molecular weight from 50 to 75 kDa, and it is these chains that determine the isotype. The chains are held together by disulphide bridges and noncovalent interactions.

domains

Individual light-chains are composed of two distinct areas or domains of approximately 110 amino acids. One end of the chain is identical in all members of the same isotype and is termed the constant domain of the light-chain, C_L. The other end shows considerable sequence variation and is known as the variable domain, V_L. The heavy-chains are also split into domains of approximately the same size, the number varying between the five types of heavy chains. One of these domains will show considerable sequence variation (V_H) whereas the others are constant (C_H) for the same isotype. The tertiary structure generated by the combina-

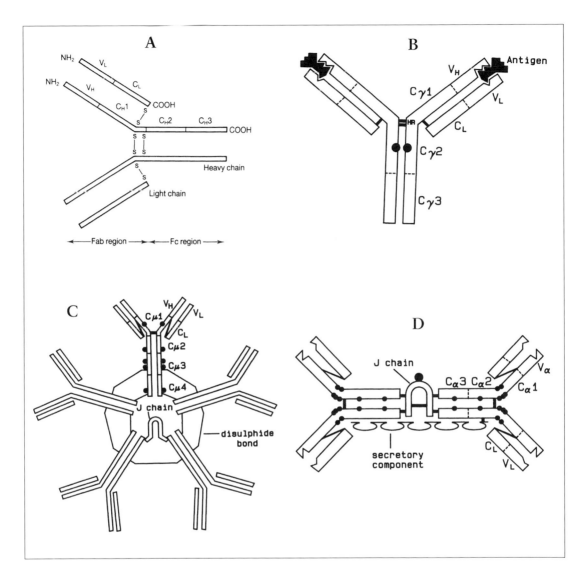

Figure 1

(A) Simplified diagram of basic immunoglobulin molecule showing 4 chain structure of 2 heavy and 2 light chains with their variable (V) and constant (C) regions held together by disulphide bonds (S–S). (B) Simplified structure of IgG showing the position of the paratope with a complementary epitope of an antigen molecule fitting into the paratope. The carbohydrate is shown by the black circles and HR indicates the hinge region. (C) Simplified structure of IgM showing its pentameric form with the subunits joined by disulphide bonds and the J chain. The carbohydrate is shown in the top monomer as black circles. (D) Secretory IgA dimer joined by the J chain and showing the secretory component. The black circles represent carbohydrate components.

tion of the V_L and V_H domains determines the shape of the antigen-combining site or paratope. Since the two light and two heavy-chains are identical, each antibody unit will have two identical paratopes, situated at the amino-terminal end of the molecule, that recognize the antigen. The carboxyl end of the antibody will be the same for all members of the same class or subclass and is involved in the biological activities of the molecule.

hinge region

The area of the heavy-chains between the C_H1 and C_H2 domains contains a varying number of interchain disulphide bonds and is known as the hinge region. A number of enzymes cleave immunoglobulins at distinct points to generate different peptide fragments. These have been used to study the structure and function of immunoglobulins and generate useful reagents. The sites of cleavage of pepsin are to the carboxyl side of the hinge. This enzyme generates a single F(ab')$_2$ fragment, containing two paratopes joined at the hinge, and a number of small peptides from the Fc portion. Papain cleaves the molecule in the hinge region to generate two identical Fab fragments, each containing a paratope, and a single Fc fragment.

enzyme cleavage

IgG

IgG is the major immunoglobulin of serum making up 75% of the total and having a molecular weight of 150 000 Da in humans. The molecule is composed of a single basic unit with γ heavy-chains (Fig. 1B). Four subclasses are found in man – IgG$_1$, IgG$_2$, IgG$_3$ and IgG$_4$ – that differ in their relative concentrations, amino acid composition, number and position of interchain disulphide bonds and biological function. IgG is the major antibody of the secondary immune response and is found in both the serum and tissue fluids.

IgG subclasses

IgA

In humans most of the serum IgA occurs as a monomer, but in many other mammals it is mostly found as a dimer. The dimer is held together by a J chain which is produced by the antibody-producing plasma cells. IgA is the predominant antibody class in seromucous secretions such as saliva, tears, colostrum and respiratory, gastrointestinal and genitourinary secretions. This secretory IgA (sIgA) is always in the dimeric form and is composed of two basic four-chain units (two light-chains and two α heavy-chains), a J chain and the secretory component (Fig. 1C). The se-

J chain

secretory IgA

cretory component is part of the molecule that transports the dimer produced by a submucosal plasma cell to the mucosal surface. It not only fa-
cilitates passage through the epithelial cells but protects the secreted molecule from proteolytic digestion. There are two subclasses of IgA – IgA_1
and IgA_2.

**secretory
component**

IgM

IgM is a pentamer of the basic unit with its heavy-chains that is composed
of five domains (Fig. 1C). The five basic units are held together by disulphide bonds between their $C\mu3$ domains, and the complete pentamer also contains a single J chain. Because of its large size this isotype is mainly confined to the intravascular pool and is the antibody type produced
during the primary immune response.

IgD

Many circulating B-cells have IgD present on their surface, but it accounts for less than 1% of the circulating antibody. It is composed of the
basic unit with δ heavy-chains. The protein is very susceptible to proteolytic attack and therefore has a very short half-life.

IgE

The IgE heavy-chain (ϵ) has five domains and is present in extremely low
levels in the serum. However, it is found on the surface of mast cells and
basophils which possess a receptor specific for the Fc part of this molecule. Interaction of this antibody with antigen leads to histamine release
from the mast cells and basophils in allergic reactions (Chapter A9).

Antigen binding

Despite the different characteristics of the various isotypes, as shown in
Table 1, all antibody molecules are composed of the same basic unit
structure with the Fab portion containing the antigen-recognizing
paratope and the Fc region carrying out the activities that protect the
host, i.e. effector functions. The diversity seen in the Fc region between
the various heavy-chains is responsible for the different biological activ-

**Fab portion
Fc region**

ities of the antibody isotypes. However, the amino acid sequences found within the variable domains, i.e. parts responsible for binding antigen, of different antibody molecules exhibit considerable diversity.

hypervariable regions

framework residues

The variability in amino acid sequence in the V domains of light and heavy-chains is not spread evenly over their entire length but is restricted to short segments. These segments show considerable variation and are termed hypervariable regions. Hypervariable regions contain the residues that make direct contact with the antigen and are sometimes referred to as complementarity determining regions (CDRs). Although the remaining framework residues do not come into direct contact with the antigen, they are essential for the formation of the correct tertiary structure of the V domain and maintenance of the integrity of the binding site. In both light and heavy-chains there are three CDRs which, in combination, form the paratope.

Antigen and antibody are held together by individually weak noncovalent interactions. When large numbers of these interactions occur involving hydrogen bonds' electrostatic van der Waals and hydrophobic interactions, considerable binding energy develops. These attractive forces are only active over extremely short distances, and therefore the epitope and paratope must have close fitting (complementary) structures to enable them to combine. If the electron clouds overlap or residues of similar charge are brought together, then repulsive forces will come into play. The balance of attraction and repulsion determines the strength of the interaction between an antibody and a particular antigen, i.e. the affinity of the antibody for the antigen.

affinity

Generation of antibody diversity

Over the last few decades progress in molecular genetics has led to substantial advances in the understanding of how antibody diversity is generated.

When introduced into the body an antigen selects from the available antibodies only those that can combine with its epitopes. It therefore follows that an individual must have an extremely large number of different antibodies to cope with the vast array of different antigens present in the environment. It has been estimated that more than 10^{11} different combining sites can be produced. There are not enough genes in a cell for each antibody molecule to have its own unique set of genes. In addition, as has been noted above, half of each light and a quarter of each heavy-chain are variable, but the rest is constant for a particular isotype. The genes for the light and heavy-chains are composed of coding exons separated by noncoding (silent) introns. A relatively small number of different germ line genes are present with the variable domain coded for by separate gene segments. Additional diversity is produced by somatic mutation and by introducing variable recombinations when the complete antibody variable exon is being assembled. Each constant domain is coded for by a different exon.

somatic mutation

Light-chain genes

Light-chains are composed of two domains, C_L and V_L. The structure of the constant region will determine if the light-chain will be Kappa (κ) or Lambda (λ) and the primary amino acid sequence of the variable domain determines its antigen specificity.

Kappa and Lambda light chains

The genes for the K chain are on chromosome 2 in humans. In cells not producing antibodies the gene segments that form the complete light-chain are separate. Even in a fully differentiated B-lymphocyte the VK and CK gene segments are not joined together. The V and C gene segments are separated by a small section of DNA known as the J gene segment.

In humans, there are about 100 Vκ and 5 Jκ gene segments associated with a single Cκ gene segment. As the B-cell develops, rearrangement of the DNA takes place to bring a V and J gene segment together. If this V-J joining is successful in producing a variable exon that can give rise to a functional product, then this is the structure produced in the mature B-cell. The rearranged DNA will then be transcribed into a large primary transcript known as heterogeneous nuclear messenger RNA (mRNA). Mature mRNA will be formed after splicing out the noncoding regions, i.e. introns, and any extra nonrelevant gene segments between the variable and constant exons. Translation of this mRNA will generate a κ light-chain where the V domain is formed from the V and J gene segments. Two CDRs will have come from the V gene segment and a third will be generated at the site of V-J joining. Therefore, the combination of different V and J segments will generate different antigen-combining sites. As a result the number of possible κ light-chains will be at least 500 (100×5). The same V gene segment associating with different J gene segments will also give two different paratopes sharing CDRs.

antigen combining sites

A similar mechanism for generating diversity applies to the λ light-chains. In the germ line configuration there are more than 100 V gene segments and there are 6 functional J gene segments each associated with its own C gene segment. As with κ the first event is V-J joining to give a variable exon. After transcription and splicing this gives rise to mRNA that can be translated into a functional λ light-chain.

Heavy-chain genes

The heavy-chain V domain is generated by the same mechanisms as outlined for the light-chain. In addition to the V and J gene segments there are D gene segments. In humans there are 12 germ line D gene segments together with 100–200 V_H gene segments and 6 functional J_H gene segments. The rearrangements take place in a defined order: a D gene segment joins with a J gene segment and then a V gene segment is joined. Again, two CDRs are coded for in the V_H segment and the site of the third is generated by the combination of V, D and J (Fig. 2).

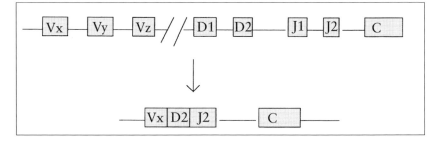

Figure 2 Schematic view of an antigen receptor gene locus (immunoglobulin or TCR)
Recombination of a particular V-D-J gene segment to form a rearranged variable gene region. The variable region (V) is separated from the constant region (C) by an intron that is removed by RNA splicing (light-chain genes of immunoglobulin lack the D segments).

allelic exclusion

Once a functional V_H exon has been constructed from the V, D and J gene segments on one chromosome, rearrangements of the gene segments on the other chromosome are inhibited. This is known as allelic exclusion. Allelic exclusion also acts on light-chain genes which are also restricted to the production of only one isotype per cell, i.e. light-chain isotype exclusion. This ensures that one particular cell, and its progeny, will produce antibody with a single specificity.

Thus the mature B-cell has a rearranged heavy-chain with a complete V_H exon, composed of V, D and J gene segments, upstream of the C_H gene segments. The light-chain will be produced from either a successfully rearranged κ or λ gene.

Additional diversity

The random joining together of any V with any D and any J gene segments gives a vast number of possible combinations. However, in addition to this, the exact place where these recombinations occur can vary. In certain cases imprecise joining will result in the formation of a modified codon and the subsequent insertion of a different amino acid.

inaccuracies

Table 2 lists the various mechanisms leading to generation of antibody diversity. Multiple germ line variable gene segments combine with J and D gene segments. There are inaccuracies in these recombination events that generate the part of the protein that contains the third CDR. Somatic point mutations occur, introducing additional variation in specificity. Finally, since any light-chain can associate with any heavy-chain, diversity is increased enormously.

additional diversity

Table 2 Generation of antibody diversity

1. Multiple germ line V gene segments
2. V-J and V-D-J recombinations
3. Junctional diversity (imprecise joining and N-region additions)
4. Somatic mutation
5. Assorted heavy- and light- chain combinations

During the production of the V gene segment all of these mechanisms can occur.

Heavy-chain constant region genes

A particular plasma cell and its progeny will produce different classes of antibodies as an immune response develops. However, the same variable exon generated by V-D-J joining will be used. All that is altered, or switched, is the heavy-chain constant region. The gene segments that code for the different types of heavy chains are arranged downstream from the J gene segments. Various switch sequences control the recombination processes that mediate class switch.

class switch

The first transcript to be produced as a B-cell develops, after V-D-J joining, contains the exon for V_H and the exons for the constant regions domains of μ and δ. This product is differentially spliced to give a μ mRNA and a δ mRNA both containing the same V_H exon. Therefore, the first heavy-chains to be produced will be μ and δ. These combine with the light-chains to give IgM and IgD molecules that are inserted into the membrane. When the B-cell is stimulated by antigen, the cell will first secrete IgM in a pentameric form. As the immune response develops, the class of antibody being produced changes. There are further DNA rearrangements resulting in the bringing together of a different constant region gene segment to the original V_H exon and the elimination of intervening DNA with its μ and δ heavy-chain gene segments. Thus the progeny of a single B-cell will produce different immunoglobulin isotypes as the response to a particular antigen develops, but each will have the same paratope (see also Chapter A2).

T-cell receptor

CD nomenclature

The complex on T-lymphocytes that is involved in antigen recognition is composed of a number of glycoproteins. Some of these molecules have been systematically named by CD (cluster of differentiation) nomenclature using antibodies produced by immunization of an appropriate species (e.g. sheep or goat) with T-cells carrying the glycoprotein.

The T-cell antigen receptor (TCR), also known as Ti, is a heterodimer composed of an α and a β, or a γ and a δ chain. The majority of T-cells (approx. 95%) use the αβ heterodimer in antigen recognition. The role of cells that possess the γδ molecules is unknown, but they may be involved in the immune response to particular types of antigens at specific anatomical sites. The two glycoprotein chains that form the T-cell receptor are linked together by disulphide bonds. These molecules are structurally similar to immunoglobulin, having a variable and a constant region. Within these regions, domains are present that fold into a secondary structure with many of the characteristics of immunoglobulin variable and constant domains.

The V region forms a domain that contains the antigen-binding site of the T-cell receptor. The C region contains four domains. The most amino-terminal portion forms an immunoglobulin constant-like domain with an intrachain disulphide bond. There is a short hinge or connecting peptide, a transmembrane portion with many hydrophobic amino acids and a short cytoplasmic tail. The transmembrane portion contains positively charged amino acid residues which appear to be involved with the interaction of the T-cell receptor with other membrane components.

The T-cell receptor is the molecule that is responsible for the recognition of specific major histocompatibility complex (MHC)/antigen complexes and will be different for every T-cell. Therefore, as for antibody, there are mechanisms for the generation of diversity. In humans, the α genes are on chromosome 14 and are arranged in a way similar to the antibody light-chain genes. There are about 100 Vα segments, around 100 Jα segments and a single Cα gene segment. On chromosome 7 the β variable gene segments are orientated in a manner similar to that found for the antibody heavy-chain gene. There are between 75 and 100 Vβ, 2

Dβ and about 14 Jβ gene segments upstream of 2 Cβ gene segments. The γ chain locus, also on chromosome 13, is similar to the γ light-chain locus with 2 functional C segments, each associated with 2–3 J segments, and 8 known V segments. The δ chain locus is found between Vα and Jα. There are 4 V, 3 J, 2 D and a single C gene segment.

Genetic rearrangement of these multiple germ line gene segments, similar to that seen in B-cells, is necessary before a functional T-cell receptor can be produced. The β chain locus rearranges prior to the α locus, with the joining of Dβ and Jβ as the first step. This is followed by the formation of a complete V exon (V-D-J gene segments joined together) and allelic exclusion occurs if the V exon formed is functional. Production of a β gene product stimulates rearrangements at the α locus where the V exon is formed by the joining of a Vα and a J. gene segment. The primary nuclear transcript of the T-cell receptor genes contains the V and C exons separated by an intron. As with immunoglobulin genes, this RNA is processed to give mRNA that is then translated into the final product. Imprecise joining and N-region additions (discussed above for immunoglobulins) add to the diversity of structures that can be generated. In addition, more than one Dβ and Dδ gene segment can be used.

There are many fewer V gene segments for the T-cell receptor compared with those present in the immunoglobulin loci. Since the first two CDRs are present within the V gene segment, this suggests that there will be less diversity in these areas of the T-cell receptor compared with immunoglobulin. However, there is great potential to develop variation in the amino acid sequence of the third CDR because of the large contribution to diversity generation by imprecise joining, N-region additions and the use of multiple D gene segments in T-cells. This imbalance in diversity between CDR1/CDR2 and CDR3 may be important in T-cell recognition. The T-cell binds antigen fragments associated with MHC molecules (cf. p. 17), its receptor interacting with both the antigen fragment and MHC molecule. It is thought that the CDR1/CDR2 portion, which exhibits less diversity, might interact with the MHC molecule, and the CDR3 with the antigen fragment.

imprecise joining

N-region additions

multiple D gene segements

Other molecules associated with the T-cell receptor

The T-cell receptor heterodimer gives specificity for antigen recognition to the T-cell, but other cell membrane molecules are needed for T-cells to function. The CD3 complex (T3 in humans) is present on all T-cells and has a constant structure. It is composed of four noncovalently associated polypeptide chains, γ, δ, ε and z, and may also transiently associ-

CD3 complex

ate with another peptide termed *eta* (η). The constituent molecules have a negative charge in their transmembrane portion. These seem to be important in the association of the complex with the T-cell receptor which has positively charged residues in the corresponding region. The CD3 complex is involved in signal transduction. and residues present in the cytoplasmic domain are susceptible to phosphorylation which is a commonly used activation signal.

CD4
CD8

CD4 and CD8 (T4 and T8 in humans; L3T4 and Ly2 in mouse) are mutually exclusive molecules (Fig. 3). They are present on T-cells that are restricted in their recognition of antigen by MHC class II and class I molecules respectively. CD4 is a monomeric transmembrane glycoprotein that folds into four extracellular immunoglobulin-like domains. CD8 is a disulphide-linked dimer. Each chain has an N-terminal immunoglobulin-like domain, a non-immunoglobulin-like domain, a transmembrane portion and a cytoplasmic tail. Due to their almost exclusive correlation with a specific MHC class it is thought that these molecules bind to nonpolymorphic determinants on the MHC molecules. This interaction could stabilize the binding of the T-cell receptor to the

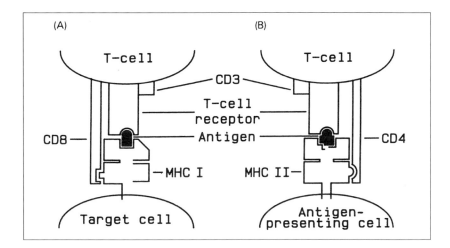

Figure 3 Interaction between MHC class I and class II molecules with the T-cell receptor and associated CD4 or CD8 molecules

(A) The CD8 T-cell receptor binds to both antigen and the MHC class I molecule with resulting lysis of the target cell (e.g. virus-infected). The CD3 molecule is involved in signal transduction to activate the T-cell to produce lytic materials. (B) The CD4 T-cell receptor binds to the MHC class II molecule on an antigen-presenting cell (e.g. macrophage) in a similar way as the class I receptor with the CD3 molecule activating the T-cell so that it leads to induction of antibody- and cell-mediated immunity. Modified from Weir DM and Stewart J (1997) Immunology, 8th edn., Churchill Livingstone, Edinburgh, with permission.

MHC/antigen complex, or it may have a coreceptor function. In the former case the CD4 or CD8 molecule could interact with the same MHC molecule as the TCR or with a different one, and this interaction does not generate a stimulatory signal, i.e. it solely stabilizes the specific interaction (TCR with antigen/MHC). In the latter case the T-cell receptor and CD4 or CD8 bind to the same MHC molecule but at different sites, and the joint signal that is generated leads to the stimulation of the T-cell. T-cells that have an $\alpha\beta$ receptor possess CD4 or CD8, whereas only a few $\gamma\delta$ T-cells have been shown to be CD8$^+$, and none appear to have the CD4 molecule (see also Chapter A3).

coreceptor function

Major histocompatibility complex

The major histocompatibility complex (MHC) is part of the genome that codes for molecules that are important in immune recognition, including interactions between lymphoid cells and other cell types. It is also involved in the rejection of allografts. The major histocompatibility complex of a number of species has been studied, but most is known about mouse and humans.

The gene complex contains a large number of individual genes that can be grouped into three classes on the basis of the structure and function of their products. The products of the genes are sometimes referred to as MHC antigens because they were first defined by serological analysis, i.e. using antibodies.

MHC class I and class II molecules are involved in immune recognition by presenting antigen fragments to T-lymphocytes. MHC class I molecules bind peptides produced from endogenously produced proteins, e.g. viral protein, and present them to CD8$^+$ T-cells. Exogenous antigens, i.e. foreign material taken into a cell by endocytosis, are processed within cells, and the resultant peptides presented by MHC class II molecules to CD4$^+$ T-cells. Other genes that play a role in generating the antigen fragments have recently been mapped to the MHC.

class I and class II MHC molecules

The MHC of humans is known as human leucocyte group A (HLA), and in mice it is referred to as histocompatibility-2 (H-2). There are other histocompatibility loci (e.g. H-1, H-3, H-4 etc.) that mediate graft rejection, but the reactions they stimulate are much weaker. These so-called minor histocompatibility antigens are not involved in immunological recognition of pathogenic organisms.

**HLA in humans
H-2 in mice**

MHC antigen structure and distribution

The MHC class I molecule is a dimer composed of a glycosylated trans-membrane peptide of molecular weight 45 000, coded for within the MHC, noncovalently linked to a 12-kDa peptide, β2-microglobulin (Fig. 4A). The globular protein formed by these two peptides is present on the surface of virtually all nucleated cells in humans. β2-microglobulin is required for the processing and expression of MHC-encoded molecules on the cell membrane. The complete molecule has four extracellular domains, three formed by the MHC-encoded α or heavy-chain and one by β2-microglobulin. In addition, the heavy-chain has a transmembrane portion and a cytoplasmic tail of about 30 amino acids. The extracellular portion has an immunoglobulin-like region composed of the α3 domain and β_2-microglobulin and a peptide-binding region formed by the α_1, and α_2 domains. The polypeptide backbones of the α_1 and α_2

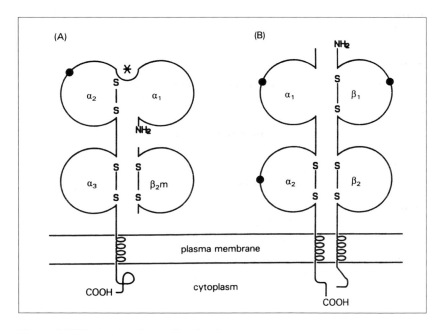

Figure 4 MHC class I and class II molecules

(A) The class I molecule consists of three globular domains, α_1, α_2 and α_3, held together by disulphide and noncovalent bonds. β_2 microglobulin (β2M) is noncovalently attached to the α_3 domain. The antigen binding cleft is indicated by *. (B) The class II molecule is made up of two noncovalently associated peptides, α and β, each with two domains, a transmembrane portion and a cytoplasmic tail. Carbohydrate is shown by black circles. The α_1 and α_2 domains fold to make an antigen cleft (see text). Modified from Weir DM and Stewart J (1997) Immunology, Churchill Livingstone, Edinburgh, with permission.

domains fold in such a way that they form a platform of a β-pleated sheet supporting a peptide-binding cleft. The sides of this cleft are formed by two α-helices, one from α_1 and one from α_2. It is within this cleft that antigen fragments are held and presented to T-cells.

The MHC class II molecules consist of two polypeptide chains (α 34-kDa and β 28-kDa) held together by noncovalent interactions (Fig. 4B). They have a much more limited cellular distribution, being limited to the surface of certain cells of the immune system. In humans, they are normally found on B-lymphocytes, macrophages, monocytes and activated T-lymphocytes. Each polypeptide chain has two extracellular domains, a transmembrane portion and a cytoplasmic tail.

Gene organization

The genes that code for the HLA antigens are found on the short arm of chromosome 6. They are arranged over a region of between 2000 and 4000 kbp containing enough DNA for over 200 genes. The MHC genes are contained within regions known as A, B, C and D. An MHC class I gene that codes for the heavy-chain is present in the A, B and C regions, whereas β2-microglobulin is coded for elsewhere in the genome. The genes that code for class II molecules are found within the D region. There are three class II molecules, DP, DQ and DR. The class III genes that code for a number of complement components and other molecules are grouped together in a region between D and B.

HLA antigens

The H-2 complex on chromosome 17 contains the same types of genes, but they are arranged slightly differently. The class I genes are present in the K and D regions that are at either extremity of the locus. The I region contains the genes that code for the two class II molecules A and E (sometimes referred to as I-A and I-E). MHC class II molecules are sometimes known as Ia (immune associated) antigens because they are coded for by the H-2 I region. There is also a region in the mouse coding for class III molecules known as the S region.

H-2 complex

I region

MHC polymorphism

There are a number of different MHC class I and class II molecules, with those of each class having a similar basic structure. Fine structural differences can be detected in the α_1 and α_2 domains of class I molecules and in α_1 and β_1 domains of class II molecules. The variations found are due to differences in the amino acid sequence and can be detected serologically. The variable residues will give rise to different three-dimensional shapes on the MHC molecules. Since most of the residues involved form part of the peptide-binding cleft, this will influence the way antigen fragments can bind to the MHC molecule, i.e. different MHC molecules will bind different peptides.

polymorphism

haplotype

codominance

These differences are found not only between the different MHC class I and class II molecules of an individual but also between the same molecules in different individuals. Therefore many different forms of these molecules can be identified in a population – they are highly polymorphic. Thus it is unlikely that two individuals will have exactly the same MHC antigens. The MHC molecules of a particular individual, their haplotype, can be given a designation using tissue-typing reagents. So on each chromosome an individual will have the genes that code for an A, B, C, DP, DQ and DR molecule. The MHC genes are codominant; thus the products of both alleles are expressed on the cell surface. Consequently, all the nucleated cells in the body will express multiple copies of two HLA-A, two HLA-B and two HLA-C molecules. On certain cells there will also be HLA-DP, -DQ and -DR molecules that were inherited from both parents. The polymorphism maps mainly to the α_1 and α_2 domains of MHC class I molecules and to the α_1 and β_1 domains of MHC class II. The rest of the molecules are conserved. Since CD4 and CD8 are monomorphic, it is likely that they bind to conserved regions. Experimental evidence suggests that CD8 binds to a site on the α_3 domain of MHC class I molecules and CD4 to a site in the α_2 or β_2 domains of MHC class II molecules.

CD4 and CD8 restriction

MHC antigens are essential for immune recognition by T-lymphocytes, which are only able to bind to antigens when they are associated with these molecules. The different classes of MHC antigens are involved in the restriction of different T-cell types or subsets. T-lymphocytes that have CD4 molecules on their surface recognize antigen in association with MHC class II molecules, whereas those that have CD8 molecules are restricted by MHC class I molecules.

Functional aspects

Initially naive CD4 T-cells when activated by the antigen-MHC class II complex secrete a broad range of cytokines including interleukin (IL)-2,3,4,5,10 and interferon (IFN)γ. These cells then differentiate, on contact with the antigen-MHC complex, into either Th1, (inflammatory T-cells), which secrete mainly IL-2, IFNγ and tumor necrosis factor (TNF), or Th2 (helper T-cells), which secrete mainly IL-4,5,6 and 10. The

Th1 cytokines are potent activators of macrophages, increasing their ability to kill phagocytosed microorganisms and to recruit macrophages, lymphocytes and neutrophils to the site of activation. Activated macrophages also express increased levels of receptors for the Fc component of immunoglobulins, thus enhancing their ability to phagocytose immune complexes and antibody-coated pathogens. In contrast, the Th2 cytokines activate B-cells that differentiate into antibody-secreting cells. Cytokines from both Th1 and Th2 subsets of T-cells regulate the isotype switching of B-cells from the initial IgM to the other isotypes.

cytokines

Antigen-MHC class I complexes serve a different function and present their antigen to the CD8 cytolytic T-cells that are activated to produce a group of effector molecules, perforin and granzymes, in their secretory granules. This enables the activated T-cell, on recognizing its target, to release the effector molecules on the surface of the target cell. Perforin that shows homology with the C9 complement component induces pores in the target-cell membrane, thus allowing the granzymes into the cytoplasm and activating the process of apoptosis (programmed cell death) in the target cell. Thus it can be seen that there are two receptors on T-cells that determine antigen-MHC recognition, the variable $\alpha\beta$TCR and the invariant CD4 or CD8 molecules, CD4 binding to the β_2 domain of the class 2 MHC and CD8 to the α_3 domain of the class I MHC molecule (see also Chapter A3).

activated T-cells

effector molecules

In some disease situations an imbalance may occur in the expression of the Th1 or Th2 subsets perhaps brought about by the type of antigen encountered, its dose, the form or route in which it is presented or in some instances a genetic predisposition of the individual. For example, it is suggested that autoimmunity may be due to excessive activity of the Th1 cells, their cytokines inducing an inflammatory response. Restoration of the balance between the Th1 and Th2 cells could lead to abolition or prevention of tissue destruction. An example of this has been shown in animal experiments in which colitis (induced by haptenated colonic proteins) can be prevented by prior feeding of the mice with the antigen, thus inducing oral tolerance. This results in production of Th1-like cells that produce high amounts of TGFβ (transforming growth factor β), a potent inhibitor of the Th1 response. The possible application of such procedures to human disease is indicated by the finding that T-cells extracted from Crohn's disease tissues are skewed towards the Th1 type.

autoimmunity

Development and maturation of T- and B-cells

Henk-Jan Schuurman and Valerie F.J. Quesniaux

Introduction: acquisition of specificity

The immune system has unique properties which distinguish it from other homeostatic systems in the body. First, it shows an extreme specificity and discrimination in recognition of "self" antigens and "nonself" antigens of potentially pathogenic microorganisms or substances in the external environment. Second, it carries "memory", resulting in a more rapid and avid response to antigens upon secondary contact. Third, it responds to antigen in multiple ways, resulting in a variety of potential mechanisms to inactivate or destruct its targets. Related to this, there is a finely tuned regulatory network of cells and their products that maintain homeostasis in the system or dampen reactions when imbalances arise. Lymphocytes have a central function; for instance, specificity is a characteristic of these cells. This chapter describes their development and maturation, up to the stage at which the cells are able to exert their function in host defence. The focus is on the acquisition of specificity, because this is the major event during development and maturation. Memory is a typical characteristic of the competent immune system, and is only touched upon in describing affinity maturation of matured B-cells. Most information described in this chapter is based on studies in mice: T- and B-lymphocyte maturation in other species relevant for the discipline of immunopharmacology (rat, humans) follows similar principles.

specificity

memory

many pathways

T- and B-lymphocytes: common origin from hematopoietic stem cells

T-lymphocytes gained their name because they develop in the microenvironment of the thymus, an organ located in the mediastinum anterior to the heart; the molecular basis of antigen recognition by these cells is the T-cell receptor complex described in Chapter A1. B-lymphocytes

T- and B-cell origin

**pluripotent
stem cell**

**adhesion factors
and stromal cells**

gained their name because they develop in avian species in the microenvironment of the bursa of Fabricius, an organ located in the intestine near the cloaca, just underneath the epithelium; this organ does not exist in mammalian species, and in these species the bone marrow functions as the bursa equivalent. The molecular basis of antigen recognition of B-lymphocytes is the immunoglobulin molecule described in Chapters A1 and C2. The major B and T types of lymphocytes are divided into subsets with different functions, e.g. T-helper and T-cytotoxic lymphocytes, which are further described in Chapter A3.

The development of lymphocytes starts with the pluripotent hematopoietic stem cell [1, 2]. In embryogenesis these cells are found first in the yolk sac, thereafter in fetal liver and finally in the bone marrow. In adults, hematopoietic stem cells occur almost uniquely in the bone marrow; only a very small subset of hematopoietic cells in the peripheral circulation have stem-cell potential. In rodents, extramedullary hematopoietic activity can also be observed in the red pulp of the spleen. Hematopoietic stem cells are self-renewing and produce a continuous supply of hematopoietic mature cells for the whole life span. The progeny of the pluripotent hematopoietic stem cell comprise cells committed to different lineages in the hematopoietic system (Fig. 1): a first differentiation involves the myeloid and lymphoid progenitor cell. The myeloid progenitor subsequently gives rise to precursors of erythrocytes, thrombocytes, granulocytes and monocytes. The existence of a commmon lymphoid progenitor cell is still controversial, but there is evidence for the presence of progenitor cells that are committed to the T- or B-cell lineage. A cell surface marker that is widely used to identify (and enrich) hematopoietic stem and progenitor cells is the CD34 molecule, a molecule with a mucin-like structure and a possible ligand function for lectin-like adhesion molecules. The differentiation of pluripotent stem cells into committed progenitors of T- or B-cell lineage is poorly understood. The process seems to involve tight interactions between stem cells and the bone marrow microenvironment (stromal cells), and to be under the control of cytokines. VLA-4 is an example of a cell adhesion molecule of the integrin series for which a pivotal role in differentiation of stem cells into lineage-specific progenitors (lymphoid, myeloid) has been demonstrated. Another example is hyaluronic acid on stromal cells, which binds the CD44 molecule on lymphoid progenitor cells. Major cytokines promoting the differentiation of pluripotent stem cells into stem cells of the T- and B-lymphocyte lineage are stem-cell factor (SCF, the c-kit ligand) and interleukin 7 (IL-7). The adhesion of lymphoid progenitor cells to the stroma probably promotes the binding of SCF from the stromal cells to the c-kit receptor on the progenitor cell. In B-lymphocyte matu-

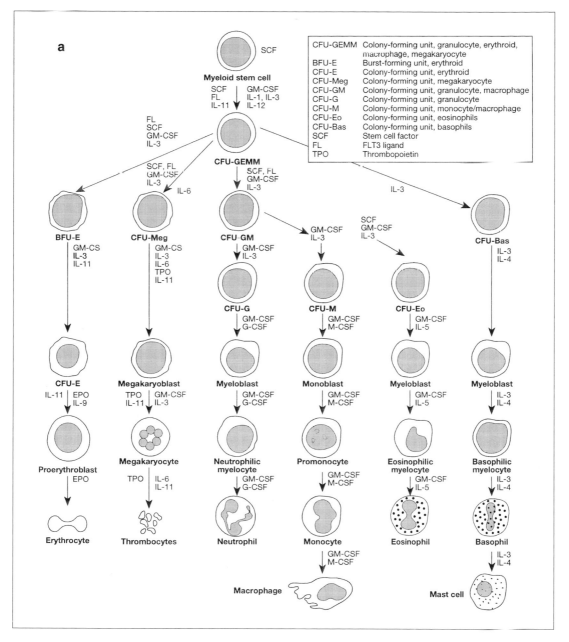

Figure 1 (continued on next page)

(a) Schematic representation of the differentiation of myeloid cell lineages and the effect of certain cytokines on the development of hematopoietic cells in distinct lineages.

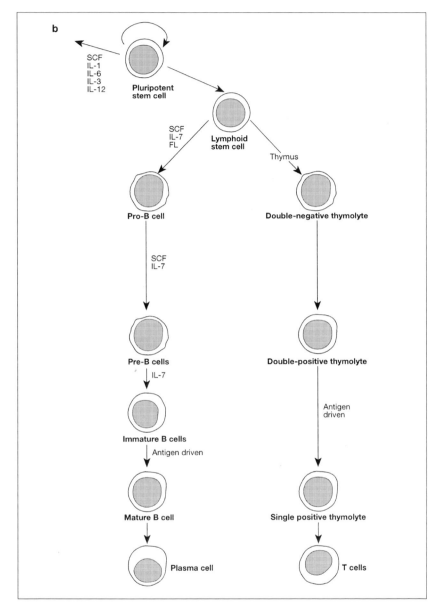

Figure 1 (continued)

(b) Schematic representation of the differentiation of and lymphoid cell lineages and the effect of certain cytokines on the development of hematopoietic cells in distinct lineages.

ration, late pro-B-cells (decribed in more detail below, see Fig. 3) would then respond to IL-7 for their growth and maturation. Finally, lineage-specific transcription factors promote the development of various cell lineages from hematopoietic stem cells [3]. One of these is the Ikaros gene, which encodes a family of zinc-finger DNA binding proteins, that is crucial for early development into the T- or B-lymphoid stem cell.

Specificity: rearrangement of genes encoding antigen receptors

A major event in the differentiation of lineage-specific stem cells into mature T- or B-lymphocytes is the synthesis and surface expression of antigen receptors. This involves the generation of all potential specificities required for a functionally active immune system, namely for T-cells the α and β chain of the T-cell receptor complex, and for B-lymphocytes the light and heavy-chains of the immunoglobulin molecule. The germline genome comprises a complex set of gene segments, called V (variable), D (diversity), J (joining) and C (constant) gene segments. A particular combination of one V, D, J and C gene segment has to be generated before transcription and translation into a chain of the antigen receptor is possible. This is achieved by gene rearrangement: one combination is prepared by excision of intervening genes. As soon as a translocation on one of the two chromosomes encoding a receptor chain is obtained that is in-frame (productive rearrangement), the potential gene rearrangement of the other chromosome is blocked, so that the cell only encodes the product of one single V-D-J-C gene segment leading to a given receptor specificity. Gene rearrangement is an error-prone process, however, and can produce nonproductive translocations. Thus, most B-lymphocytes have rearranged the D-J gene segments of the heavy-chain of the immunoglobulin molecule on both chromosomes, which is the first step in B-lymphopoiesis.

V-D-J-C gene segments

The process of gene rearrangement is unique to T- or B-lymphocytes, i.e. the molecular basis of the definition of a B-cell is the presence of rearranged genes encoding immunoglobulin chains, and that of a T-cell is the presence of rearranged genes encoding the T-cell receptor α and β chains. Classical T-cells use the α and β chains in the T-cell receptor complex. A small subset of T-cells use two other chains instead, the γ and δ chains. This subset is the so-called γ/δ T-cell population. Because it expresses a smaller repertoire of antigen-recognition specificities, it is considered a more "primitive" (less well developed) T-cell population than α/β T-lymphocytes. The γ/δ T-cell population is particularly present during embryonic life. In adults, it apparently has a special function, as a "sentinel" in initial defence at secretory surfaces.

T-/B-cell receptor chains

factors influencing rearrangement

The process of gene rearrangement is essentially random, ocurring under the influence of recombination activation proteins, RAG-1 and RAG-2. These molecules are upregulated in cells during the rearrangement phase, bind to recombination signal sequences in the DNA and so promote cutting (double-stranded DNA breaks), hairpin formation and splicing out of intervening gene segments. Specific DNA-dependent protein kinases are involved in opening the coding sequences. In addition to rearrangement of gene segments, diversity is further increased by N-region addition of non-germline-encoded nucleotides to V-(D)-J junctions, which is a random process under the influence of the enzyme terminal deoxynucleotidyl transferase (TdT). This nuclear enzyme is present in lymphocytes during the immature phase of development. It seems plausible that cytokines in the environment, such as IL-7, play a role in initiating gene rearrangement by upregulation of the DNA binding proteins and kinases involved. Gene rearrangement occurs in a sequential manner for the different receptor chains, and different stages of development can be distinguished within the rearrangement phase. This is described below separately for T- and B-lymphocytes.

Selection of the antigen-recognition repertoire

selection: positive and negative

Essentially, the specificity of the immune system is shaped after receptor gene rearrangement in the contributing T- and B-cells: the progeny of each distinct cell with a given specificity is considered to be a distinct clone, together constituting the whole repertoire of antigen-recognition specificities. The only way to change specificity within a given clone is by somatic mutation, a process which occurs later in B-cell maturation. However, not all potential rearrangements prove to be useful: the required repertoire must be selected out of the total potential repertoire. Unwanted (potentially deleterious, e.g. self-reactive) specificities must be deleted and those needed for proper functioning allowed to expand. This selection occurs according to various processes that are essentially similar for B- and T-lymphocytes, although the requirements for the selection of specificities apparently differ. When the lymphocyte expressing the relevant receptor on its surface is exposed to antigen, should the cell exhibit an unwanted specificity, e.g. an autoreactive lymphocyte with anti-"self" receptor specificity, the cell is activated to initiate cell death by apoptosis (programmed cell death). Should the cell exhibit a desired specificity, it is activated to expand. The first process is called negative selection, the second one positive selection. Apart from environmental factors, such as the nature of the antigen and the antigen-presenting cell, intrinsic characteristics of the lymphocyte with a particular maturation phase determine the outcome of activation, either cell death or expansion. For example, immature T-cells undergoing negative selection exhibit an intrinsic purine/pyrimidine metabolism, such that cell activation results in cell death by accumulation of toxic nucleotide triphosphatases. Immature cells undergoing selection also express receptors (Fas/Apo-1) which, upon activation, induce apoptosis in the cell. The hallmark of apoptosis is the endonuclease-induced fragmentation of chromosomes into about 200-bp fragments.

T-lymphocyte maturation in the thymus

The thymus plays a pivotal role in shaping the T-cell repertoire, as exemplified by the absence of a functionally active T-lymphocyte system in individuals with a congenital absence of the thymus (humans with DiGeorge syndrome, rats and mice with the *rnu* or *nu* mutation). Committed hematopoietic progenitors require the thymic microenvironment for differentiation, gene rearrangement and the subsequent selection processes (Fig. 2) [4–7]. The thymus has a unique microenvironment of reticular epithelium which is not observed in other lymphoid organs. Other cell populations contributing to T-cell development are dendritic cells and cells of the monocyte-macrophage cell lineage of bone marrow origin which play a main role in antigen presentation and are mainly found in the medulla of the thymic lobes.

thymus microenvironment

Lymphocytes

Four main T-lymphocyte subsets, corresponding to various stages of development, are differentiated based on their expression of CD3, CD4, CD8 and CD25 antigens. As outlined in other chapters, CD4 and CD8 antigens are closely linked to the antigen-receptor complex and are involved in antigen recognition in association with major histocompatibility complex (MHC) class I or class II molecules on antigen-presenting cells. CD4 expression in mature T-lymphocytes is linked to helper cell activity and recognition of antigen by MHC class II molecules, and CD8 expression is linked to cytotoxic cell activity and recognition of antigen by MHC class I molecules (see Chapter A.1). The expression of CD25 (IL-2 receptor α chain) on mature T-lymphocytes is associated with a

four main subsets

29

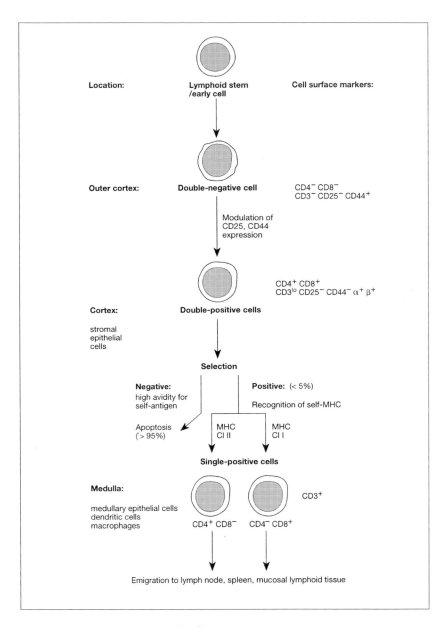

Figure 2 T-cell development in the thymus

Various stages in development can be followed by the expression of cell surface markers and T-cell receptor α and β chains. The process starts after entry of the lymphoid progenitor cell from the bone marrow. "Double-negative" cells in the outer cortex differentiate into "double-positive" (CD4⁺CD8⁺) cells. After positive selection a small percentage of these cells differentiate into mature "single-positive" cells expressing either CD4 or CD8. These cells emigrate from the thymus to peripheral lymphoid organs.

state of activation; together with antigen- or mitogen-induced IL-2 receptor β and γ chains, it confers responsiveness to the T-cell growth factor IL-2.

In the thymus, hematopoietic progenitors which form a small subset in the outer cortex show a low expression of CD4 and are negative for CD8 and CD25. These cells develop into so-called double-negative cells, being CD4$^-$CD8$^-$ and CD3$^-$CD25$^-$. Upon expression of CD25, and presumably under the influence of cytokines (stem-cell factor, IL7?), cells start to rearrange the genes encoding the antigen-receptor complex, first those encoding the β chain (Vβ-D-Jβ) and subsequently the α chain (Vα–Jα). If this rearrangement is successfully completed (e.g. a productive rearrangement from either one of the two chromosomes), the cells develop into the so-called double-positive CD4$^+$CD8$^+$ stage, which is the major lymphocyte subset in the cortex. At this stage, selection of relevant populations (clones) occurs, with first positive and subsequently negative selection. Upon completion of this process, cells develop into so-called single-positive cells, either CD4$^+$CD8$^-$ or CD4$^-$CD8$^+$ cells, which form the major populations of lymphocytes in the medullary areas of thymic lobules. The transmembrane tyrosine phosphatase CD45 isoforms have been implicated in the transition from CD4$^-$CD8$^-$ to CD4$^+$CD8$^+$ thymocytes and the further transition into single-positive cells, since these transitions do not occur in mice in which the CD45 gene has been "knocked out". These mice show accumulation of CD25$^+$CD44$^-$ double-negative cells, which in the absence of CD44 expression are unable to attach to the stroma via the adhesion between CD44 and hyaluronic acid mentioned above. CD4$^+$CD8$^-$ or CD4$^-$CD8$^+$ cells are the main populations emigrating from the thymus into the periphery (e.g. lymph nodes, spleen, mucosal lymphoid tissue). While still considered immature upon migration from the thymus, the cells become fully mature and immunocompetent shortly after arrival in the peripheral immune system. This has been demonstrated in rats using the RT.6 marker, which is a marker for immature cells present on these so-called recent thymic emigrants [8].

sequential expression of markers and gene rearrangement

role of CD45

Selection

Selection is crucial in intrathymic T-cell development. It requires recognition of antigen and MHC molecules by the receptor complex on the developing lymphocyte. Initially, this is an "immature" type of receptor comprising only the β chain with an α-like chain and the CD3 molecule. After rearrangement of the α chain, the receptor complex is similar to

positive selection

that found on mature lymphocytes. Positive selection involves the recognition of MHC antigens: in the case of MHC class I linked to CD8, the double-positive cell expands into a $CD4^-CD8^+$ cell population (cytotoxic subset), and in the case of MHC class II linked to CD4, the double-positive cell expands into a $CD4^+CD8^-$ population (helper subset). Epithelial cells represent the major stromal cell population involved in positive selection, which most probably occurs in the thymic cortex. MHC molecules on this cell population are not "empty" but contain peptides of thymic origin required not only for stabilization of MHC molecules but also for recognition by the T-cell receptor. The exact nature of this self-peptide recognition in positive selection remains to be determined. If not positively selected, the cells die in the thymus cortex, presumably

negative selection

by apoptosis. Negative selection involves the high avidity recognition of self-antigens, e.g. self-peptides presented by MHC molecules. Should recognition occur with sufficient avidity, the cells are deleted by induction of apoptosis. It has not been completely established which cells in the thymus microenvironment mediate negative selection: originally this property was ascribed to a unique population of dendritic cells in the medulla, but a number of studies suggest that epithelial cells themselves are also able to induce negative selection. This means that positive and negative selection do not necessarily have to be performed in strict order; for example, cells can be negatively selected without being first positively selected.

Consequences of selection

total repertoire

The selection process of immature T-lymphocytes has two relevant consequences for the immunocompetent T-cell population. First, it is much reduced in its repertoire. The number of V and J gene segments in the human genome for the α chain is more than 60 and 61, respectively; for the β chain the number of V, D and J gene segments is more than 106, 2 and 13, respectively. Combined with the potential N-region addition of non-germline-encoded nucleotides, the total possible repertoire of the T-cell population is estimated at about 10^{12}. The actual T-cell repertoire

actual repertoire

is about 10^6-10^7; this large difference from the total repertoire is ascribed either to a failure to perform all potential rearrangements, or to the high power of intrathymic selection. Arguments for the latter also come from thymocyte kinetics, i.e. only a very small fraction of cells entering the thymus and generated during development actually emigrate as mature lymphocytes. Second, in outbred populations, the repertoire generated is unique for each individual, as it is biased to recognition of self-MHC antigens, and various class I and II loci manifest considerable polymorphism.

B-cell development in the bone marrow

The main site of B-cell development in mammals is the bone marrow (Fig. 3) [1]. There are claims that in some species the Peyer's patches along the intestine are not only a major site for mucosal immune responses but also contribute to B-cell development [9]. Different stages in B-cell maturation have been identified [10].

First, hematopoietic stem cells or lymphoid progenitors develop into pro-B-cells and rearrange gene segments encoding the V, D and J part of the immunoglobulin heavy-chain. During this phase the cell expresses recombination activation proteins (RAG-1 and -2 proteins) and TdT, which all promote rearrangement processes. In the case of a productive rearrangement, the cell develops into a (large-sized) pre-B-cell which is negative for RAG proteins and TdT. The first gene segment adjacent to the VDJ recombinant that encodes the constant part of the heavy-chain is the μ-chain segment: in this phase of maturation the cell is able to synthesize heavy-chains of the immunoglobulin M molecule, which are present in the cytoplasm as monomeric proteins.

first: to μ-chain

Upon reexpression of RAG and TdT, the cell starts to rearrange the V and J gene segments encoding the light-chain of immunoglobulins. The light-chain in immunoglobulin molecules is exceptional among antigen-receptor chains, because two gene complexes encode this chain, either the κ or the λ chain. However, each individual B-cell synthesizes only one light-chain isotype: first the κ gene complex rearranges, and if this has resulted in a productive rearrangement, subsequent rearrangement of the λ genome is blocked. After rearrangement of the light-chain, the cell ends as a so-called (small-sized) immature B-cell with surface expression of IgM.

then: to IgM

In a subsequent phase, the mature B-cell starts to express IgD on the cell membrane, i.e. the same VDJ transcript is combined with either the Cμ or Cδ gene segment. The simultaneous expression of surface IgM and IgD is possible by alternative RNA processing and termination of transcription. B-lymphocytes showing surface expression of both IgM and IgD are mature B-cells capable of responding to antigen stimulation. They form the major resting B-cell population found in the blood circulation and peripheral lymphoid organs.

then: to IgM/IgD

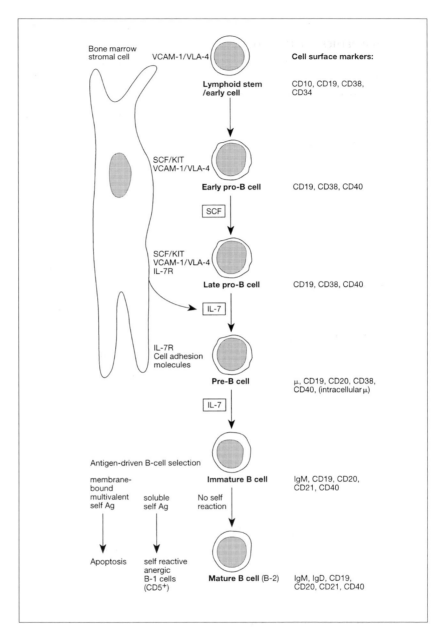

Figure 3 Stages of B-cell development

Early B-cell development occurs in the bone marrow in close contact with stromal cells through adhesion molecules or interactions between cytokines and their receptors. Prominent in B-cell development are stem-cell factor (SCF) and IL-7. Various cell surface molecules are expressed during development and can be used as markers. MHC class II and CD45R are expressed at all stages. CD45, CD19 and CD21 exhibit signalling functions. CD40 is involved both in B-T-cell interaction and signalling; it acts as a receptor for CD40 ligand, which is expressed on T-cells.

During B-cell development changes occur in cell surface markers. One of the earliest markers of developing B-cells is the tyrosine phosphatase CD45R (B220 in mice), which has an as yet unknown function in B-cell development. The expression of CD34 (hematopoietic cell marker) is lost at the (large-sized) pre-B-cell stage. Pre-B-cells (small-sized) in the bone marrow express CD25. The coreceptor CD19, a molecule tightly connected to the B-cell antigen-receptor complex with transmembrane signalling function, as well as MHC class II and CD40 are expressed already at the pro-B-cell stage. Interactions between CD40 and CD40 ligand are essential for the induction of B-lymphocyte mediated co-stimulation in T-cell activation.

B-cell markers

Selection

Since the generation of the antibody repertoire is a random process, it also includes specificities for self-components. The restriction and demands for selection between self and nonself are considered less stringent for B-lymphocytes than for the T-cell population. A main difference is that B-cells and their antibody products recognize antigen as such (nominal antigen), unlike T-cells, which recognize antigen after processing to peptides and linking with an MHC molecule. So there is no apparent need for positive selection.

B-1 B-cells

Self-reactive B-cells are allowed to exist in the body, and their antibody products are assumed to play a regulatory function in immune reactivity. This has been best demonstrated for a particular subset of murine B-cells, the so-called B-1 (formerly "Ly-1" or "CD5$^+$") B-cell population, which differs from conventional (B-2) B-lymphocytes and comprises two populations, the B-1a and B-1b-cells [11]. Conventional B (B-2) cells form the bulk of circulating B-lymphocytes and are replenished throughout life from progenitor cells. B-1a cells arise early in embryogenesis, and originate from a fetal liver bipotential precursor which has the potential to generate either B-cells or macrophages; these cells constitute a few percent of the total B-cells and maintain their numbers by self-replenishment. B-1b-cells share many properties with B-1a cells, but in adults can also develop from bone marrow progenitors. B-1 cells are most frequent in early embryonic and postnatal life. They preferentially use certain heavy and light-chain variable genes, encoding antibodies reactive with multi-

B1a and B1b subsets

ple antigens (polyreactive antibodies). Their specificities include those with low affinity for self-antigens; based on these specificities, a role of these cells in immunoregulation has been speculated. B-1 cells constitutively express the IL-12 receptor β1 subunit and bind IL-12, whereas B-2 cells express IL-12 receptor only after appropriate stimulation.

Negative selection

Selection in the "classical" B-cell population, similar to that of immature T-cells, has only been documented in recent years. Immature B-cells in the bone marrow can be eliminated when they encounter multivalent membrane-bound antigens. This elimination is associated with down-regulation of membrane-bound IgM, an arrest of further maturation and apoptosis. It appears that cells can escape this negative selection by changing their specificity, e.g. by hypermutation or rearrangement of light-chain genes [10, 12, 13].

Competitive selection

the lymphoid follicle

A second process of B-lymphocyte selection occurs at the stage when the cells are mature, in secondary follicles of lymphoid tissue (so-called germinal centres) [14]. The microenvironment at this location is provided by follicular dendritic cells, which, unlike the dendritic cells mentioned above do not originate from the bone marrow but develop from mesenchymal fibroblasts. Follicular dendritic cells trap antigen on their surface, presumably in the form of immune complexes, and present it to differentiating mature B-cells (so-called centroblasts and centrocytes). At this stage of differentiation B-cells are particularly prone to somatic hypermutation of genes encoding the variable parts of the immunoglobulin molecules. Under the influence of T-cells and of T-cell factors such as IL-2, rearrangements also take place in the gene segments encoding the

to: IgG, IgA, IgE

constant part of the immunoglobulin heavy-chain, resulting in a loss of IgM- or IgD-synthesizing capacity and initiation of the synthesis of IgG, IgA or IgE.

to: plasma cell differentiation

These two processes of the T-cell dependent B-cell antibody response, namely immunoglobulin class-switch and affinity maturation by somatic mutation, are unique to germinal centres and precede the final differentiation of B-cells into plasma cells. In binding to the antigen on follicular dendritic cells, some competition emerges between B-cell populations, in that populations with a high affinity for exogenous antigens survive and those with low affinity (including self-reactive B-cells) are deemed to die by apoptosis. In this way, negative selection of self-reactive B-cells particularly applies to those B-cell populations that are intended to make antibodies in a T-cell-dependent manner. It does not include the B-lymphocytes involved in T-cell independent IgM-class autoantibody synthesis, as these B-cells are not subjected to follicular maturation.

Mature T- and B-cells: tolerance

The process of development and maturation of T- and B-cells includes, to some extent, the discrimination between self and nonself. The elimination of self-reactive cells by negative selection early after cells have expressed their antigen receptors is described as deletional tolerance and essentially avoids strong reactions to self-components [15]. The T-cell repertoire shaped by intrathymic maturation is considered to be rather stable, so that new specificities normally do not emerge in mature populations. Somatic mutation in the B-cell population essentially allows the generation of autoreactive cells. Because the competitive selection in germinal centres mainly involves antigens from exogenous sources in locally trapped immune complexes, it is unlikeley that new autoreactive populations will emerge.

tolerance and stability of repertoire

However, to delete for all potential autoantigens in the body would be essentially impossible, first because all autoantigens have to be presented to developing lymphocytes, and secondly because this could form exessively large "holes" in the repertoire. It is therefore assumed that the stringent mechanism of deletional tolerance only holds for those antigens that are directly exposed to (T) cells of the immune system; otherwise regulatory mechanisms exist in the mature immune system that prevent damage by autoreactive effector cells or their products. This includes the induction of anergy after inappropriate cell stimulation (e.g. for T-cells the absence of costimulatory signals in antigen stimulation), or the presence of immunoregulatory circuits by which potentially autoreactive cells are suppressed. The idiotype-anti-idiotype network comprising antibodies with a specificity for the variable part of other antibodies is often quoted as an example of such a network; otherwise T-cells with suppressor function also play a role in this respect. As these mechanisms of tolerance in the strictest sence do not form part of the development and maturation process of T- and B-lymphocytes, they are not discussed further in this chapter.

deletional tolerance and anergy

antibody network

T- and B-cell development and maturation: relevance for immunopharmacology

sharing cytokines and adhesion factors

The discipline of immunopharmacology is mainly focussed on mechanisms of and intervention in the process of a competent immune system. The way in which lymphocytes develop and mature is secondary in this respect. However, cell biological processes during lymphocyte development are in many ways similar to reactions of mature cells upon antigenic stimulation. This not only applies to the basic response of cell proliferation, but also to the involvement of growth factors and intracellular signalling pathways. For instance, besides IL-7, cytokines with a role during intrathymic T-cell development include IL-2, -4, -6 and -10, as well as interferon-γ and tumor necrosis factor α (TNFα). Also, with regard to adhesion molecules, interference with the integrin-mediated adhesion of VLA-4 (binding to VCAM-1, see Fig. 3) not only blocks immune responses (e.g. transplant rejection), but also blocks early events in hematopoiesis in the bone marrow.

immunomodulatory drugs

Some currently used immunomodulatory drugs (see Chapter C8) serve to illustrate this principle. Antiproliferative drugs used in the treatment of cancer suffer from the significant side effect of bone marrow depletion. The macrolide rapamycin is an immunosuppressive drug that blocks growth factor-induced cell proliferation. Although rodent studies have indicated that its effect on bone marrow hematopoietic activity at pharmacological doses is negligible, it induces almost complete atrophy of the thymus at these dosages and hence blocks T-cell differentiation. The immunosuppressives cyclosporin A and FK-506 have a more restricted mechanism of action, i.e. inhibition of calcineurin activity with subsequent blockade of intracellular signal transduction leading to synthesis of cytokines, most notably IL-2. These drugs have a peculiar activity on T-cell development, as they appear to block apoptosis during negative selection of T-cells. It is not known whether this bears any relevance for generation of autoreactivity in humans. However, under special conditions, namely total bone marrow depletion by irradiation and/or antiproliferative drugs followed by autologous bone marrow transplantation, which is a procedure in cancer treatment, a short course of cyclosporine treatment results in autoreactive cells [16] (see Chapter C8).

making a new repertoire

Thymic "re-education" is nowadays under consideration as an alternative therapeutic approach to autoimmune diseases such as severe rheumatoid arthritis in which the causative agent is not known. Immunoablation would eradicate the pathogenic T-lymphocytes, followed by reintroduction of tolerance (or restoration of T-T-cell control) by transplantation of hematopoietic stem cells which have to undergo re-education leading to an altered repertoire in view of the antigens present.

In conclusion, it is of utmost importance to understand mechanistic similarities between the developing immune system and the responses of the competent immune system when immunopharmacological events require interpretation. In addition, it is likely that immunopharmacology will add to our understanding of lymphocyte development, through the effects of specific pharmacological intervention in the biological pathways for T- and B-cell development and maturation.

T-cell-mediated immunity

Sergey G. Apasov and Michail V. Sitkovsky

Introduction

T-lymphocyte-mediated immunity includes the primary immune response, effector functions and immunological memory (Fig. 1). The primary immune response begins in peripheral lymphoid organs when naive
T-lymphocytes are stimulated by "professional" antigen-presenting cells
(APCs). This step requires cell-cell contact, antigen recognition and costimulatory signals. The primary immune response results in activation
and differentiation of *naive* T-cells into *effector* cells and in generation
of *memory* T-lymphocytes. Effector T-cells are able either to destroy infected cells directly or to produce soluble factors – lymphokines. Various lymphokines can regulate the immune response by serving as growth
factors for different cells of the immune system. Effector cells also make
cell-cell contact and recognize antigen on the surface of any antigen-bearing cells, but may not need costimulatory signals to execute their functions. Effector cells are short-lived and disappear shortly after clearance
of antigen. Memory T-lymphocytes develop after the primary immune response and persist in the host for an extended period. Reexposure of
memory T-cell to the same or similar (cross-reactive) antigen causes a
rapid effector response which is early enough to block widespread
pathogen expansion, so that disease can be prevented.

Activated T-cells of the immune system function either as cytotoxic
or helper effector lymphocytes and can be further subdivided into functionally distinct subpopulations.

**primary immune
response**

Th1 and Th2 subpopulations of effector T-cells

The definitions of two major subpopulations among T helper effector cells
are based on the different patterns of secreted cytokines which result in
distinct functional contributions to immunological processes. T helper 1

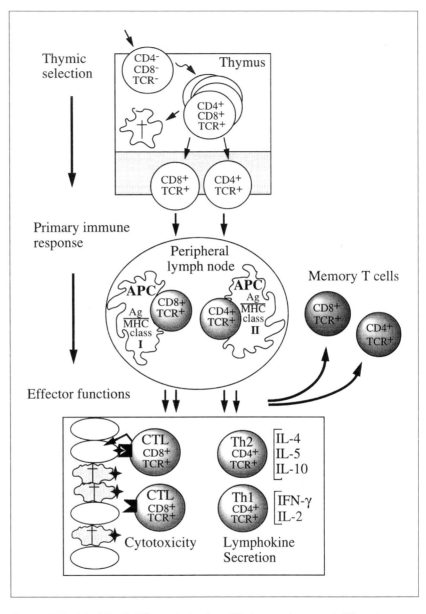

Figure 1 Model of T-cell differentiation into T helper and cytotoxic T-lymphocytes (CTLs)

Once they complete thymic development, naive T-cells mediate the primary immune response and generate effector cytotoxic and helper T-cells as well as long-lived memory T-cells. Effector CTLs destroy infected cells, whereas T helper (Th) cells produce lymphokines. Th1-type helpers stimulate cellular immune response; Th2 effectors help to develop humoral immunity. TCR, T-cell receptor; APC, antigen-presenting cell; MHC, major histocompatibility complex; IL-2, -4, -5, -10, interleukin- 2, -4, -5, -10; IFNγ, interferon-γ.

cells (Th1) produce lymphokines such as interleukin-2 (IL-2), interferon γ (IFNγ), and lymphotoxin that promote cell-mediated cytotoxicity and the inflammatory response. T helper 2 (Th2) cells are responsible for the secretion of lymphokines that are stimulatory for allergic reactions and antibody production, including IL-4, IL-5, IL-6, IL-9, IL-10 and IL-13. Patterns of secreted lymphokines overlap somewhat between Th1 and Th2 types. IL-3, granulocyte-macrophage colony-stimulating factor (GM-CSF), tumor necrosis factor α (TNFα) and some chemokines are produced by both types of helper T-cells. There is also a transient subset of T helper cells with broad lymphokine-producing ability which is known as the Th0 type. Th1 and Th2 cell subsets develop upon antigenic activation of the common naive $CD4^+$ T-cell precursors that produce mainly IL-2. Restimulation of these activated T-cells in the presence of transforming growth factor β (TGFβ) or IL-4 results in subsequent development of Th1 or Th2 phenotypes, respectively. It is therefore believed that different pathogens may trigger the differentiation of naive T-cells into Th1-or Th2-type immune responses depending on the ability of the particular antigen to stimulate specific cytokine production. The secretion of IFNγ, IL-12 and TGFβ promotes development of Th1-type effector cells, whereas IL-4 stimulates differentiation of Th2 cells. Development of Th1 and Th2 subsets are mutually inhibitory. Thus, production of IFNγ while promoting the Th1-type effector T-cells is inhibitory for development of the Th2 type, and the opposite effect is seen with IL-10. The choice of a Th1 versus a Th2 immune response is dependent on the nature of the particular pathogen and the microenvironment of activated T helper cells. For example, Th1 immune responses were found to predominate against protozoans such as *Leishmania* and *Trypanosoma* and in autoimmune diseases, whereas Th2 cells appeared exclusively in immune reactions against different helminths or in different allergic reactions.

It should be mentioned that other cells of the immune system also produce cytokines that contribute to the development of the immune response. Most studied cells are phagocytic macrophages producing inflammatory cytokines, such as IL-1, IL-6, IL-8, IL-12 and TNFα. While IL-1 was long time considered as the major inflammatory cytokine, recent studies emphasize the important role of IL-12 to turn on Th1 versus Th2 pathway (see Chapter A4).

Th1 and Th2: different patterns of secreted cytokines

cytokines from macrophages

CD8$^+$ Cytotoxic T-lymphocytes

Differentiation of naive CD8$^+$ T-cells into cytotoxic effectors requires T-cell receptor (TCR) costimulatory molecule signalling and is known to

enhancement of cytotoxic effects

be enhanced by soluble cytokines including IL-1, IL-2, IL-4, IL-12 and IFNγ. It has also been found that CD8⁺ cytotoxic cells are capable of producing lymphokines in a pattern similar to that of T helper cells. It was therefore proposed that cytotoxic T-lymphocytes be divided into Tc1 and Tc2 phenotypes according to IL-2/IFNγ and IL-4 secretion, respectively, in a manner similar to the Th1 and Th2 classification. Despite the fact that cytotoxic lymphocytes (CTLs) can produce cytokines, they are not able to provide cognate help for B-cell antibody production.

functions

The major functional activity of effector cytotoxic T-cells is elimination of any other cell bearing a "foreign" antigen on the surface. The main features of CTL activities are their specificity and efficiency. The basis of immunologic efficiency of CTLs is the ability of a single T-cell to kill more than one individual specific "target" cell. The immunologic specificity of CTLs is reflected in their ability to spare surrounding "innocent" *bystander* cells.

Mechanisms of cytotoxicity by CTLs

secretory granule exocytosis

There are two major mechanisms of cytotoxicity that are currently characterized among CD8⁺ CTLs. Secretory granule exocytosis was the mechanism discovered first. The CTL granules are small internal vesicles structurally similar to lysosomes that contain the cytolysin/perforin proteins as well as granzyme proteases. Activated CTLs are able to form conjugates with potential target cells and, upon TCR stimulation, to secrete the contents of the cytolytic granules into the extracellular synapse-like junctional cleft formed between the CTL and the target cell. Perforin/cytolysin forms pores in the plasma membrane of target cells, thereby permeabilizing them for ions and large proteins such as granzymes that diffuse into the target-cell cytoplasm. This process is dependent on Ca^{2+}, induces apoptotic (genetically programmed cell death) changes in the target including DNA fragmentation and results in the complete destruction of the target cell.

triggering of programmed cell death

Another mechanism was described more recently; this involves triggering of programmed cell death by surface Fas receptor (APO-1, CD95). Activated CTLs upregulate surface expression of Fas ligands that cross-link Fas molecules on target-cells during target-CTL conjugate formation. Cross-linking of Fas molecules induces apoptosis and cell death within hours and does not require the presence of Ca^{2+}, or the synthesis of RNA or protein. This mechanism, however, is not restricted to CTL function, but appears to be more general in regulation of the immune response. T-lymphocytes express both Fas and Fas ligand on their surface, and loss of function of either of these molecules, due to naturally occurring genetic mutations, results in lymphoproliferative disorders and development of autoimmune disease.

Ts cells

Under certain conditions, T-lymphocytes are capable of inhibiting immune responses in an antigen-specific manner, and the existence of specific T suppressor (Ts) cells has been proposed. Despite many reports of antigen-specific suppressor factors, the molecular mechanisms of suppression are still unknown, and no specific surface markers for suppressor cells have been found to establish a class of specialized T suppressor cells. Alternatively, a wide range of immune response downregulating mechanisms have been described recently. Among these are inhibitory coreceptors such as CTLA-4, killer inhibitory receptors (KIR), inhibitory cytokines and induction of apoptosis – a self-destructive intracellular process in overactivated T-cells. Clearance of "foreign" antigen will eventually stop activation and clonal expansion of mature T-lymphocytes.

no Ts specific surface markers

Molecular mechanisms of T-cell-mediated immunity

Central to the study of antigen-specific T-lymphocyte differentiation and effector functions are the surface receptors which are involved in cell-cell contact, antigen recognition and signalling. Thus, *integrins* mediate adhesion between cells; *TCR complex* is responsible for antigen-dependent recognition, binding and signalling; *costimulatory* receptors such as CD28 and CTLA-4 regulate TCR-triggered activation of T-lymphocytes (Fig. 2).

surface receptors

The common feature of T-cells is that their activation and functions are critically dependent on the recognition of antigenic peptides on the surface of APCs by the TCR complex on the surface of T-cells.

Recognition of intracellular infection by T-cells is possible because peptide fragments, for example, of viral proteins are displayed (become visible) on the surface of infected cells or phagocytic cells due to the functioning of a well-coordinated intracellular system of antigen processing

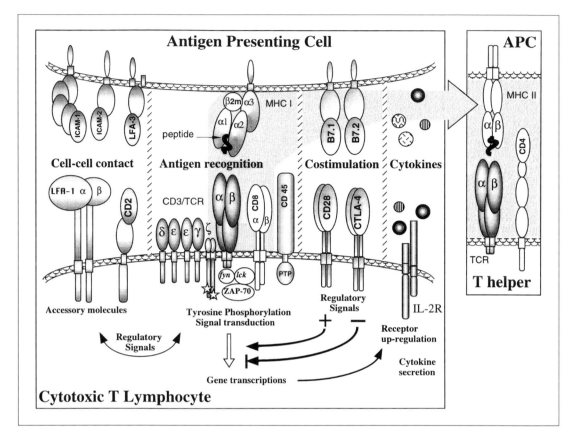

Figure 2 Molecular requirements for T-cell activation

T-lymphocyte differentiation and effector functions depend on surface receptors which provide cell-cell contact, antigen recognition and signalling. TCR complex is responsible for antigen-dependent recognition, binding and signalling; integrins mediate adhesion between cells; costimulatory receptors regulate TCR-triggered activation of T-lymphocytes. Insert: Th cell differs from cytotoxic T-cell in antigen recognition. T helpers recognize the complex of an antigenic peptide which MHC class II molecules by using TCR and CD4 molecules as coreceptors. See text for explanation.

MHC

by APCs. The main participants of this system are glycoproteins encoded by genes of the major histocompatibility complex (MHC). Two different classes of MHC are involved in the presentation of peptide antigens for two major subpopulations of T-lymphocytes. MHC class I molecules present cytoplasmic antigens that can be recognized by CD8[+] CTLs, whereas MHC class II/peptide complexes present antigens for CD4[+] T helper cells. Antigenic peptides trapped in a special groove of MHC molecules form a structure that is recognized by the TCR complex, whereas CD8 and CD4 – serving as coreceptors – are able to bind directly to MHC molecules.

Presentation of antigen by MHC class I and II molecules

An important advance in our understanding of antigen presentation came with the realization that different strategies are used by the immune system to recognize pathogens residing in the cytosol as compared with other pathogens that are localized in vesicular compartments of cells. MHC class I molecules bind to the antigenic peptide generated in the cytoplasm by a multimolecular complex of proteases called proteosomes and transported to the endoplasmic reticulum by transporters associated with antigen processing (TAP-1 and TAP-2). The newly formed MHC class I/peptide complexes in the endoplasmic reticulum are subsequently transported through the Golgi to the cell surface.

MHC class I

In contrast, MHC class II molecules bind peptides that are generated in lysosomes from pathogens that reside in intracellular vesicles or from extracellular proteins that are internalized by endocytosis. An additional nonpolymorphic invariant chain plays an important role in the formation and expression of MHC class II/peptide complexes. The invariant chain binds to the MHC class II binding site, stabilizing the MHC molecules that are transported from the Golgi to endosomes and lysosomes, where the invariant chain is degraded and replaced with peptides. Peptides loaded into MHC class II molecules, therefore, are generated from proteins in endosomal compartments by vesicular acid proteases at acidic pH.

MHC class II

MHC class I molecules are expressed, in varying degrees, on almost all cells, and the level of expression of MHC class I may determine the ability of CTLs to recognize and to kill these cells. MHC class II molecules are almost exclusively expressed on antigen-presenting cells, such as macrophages, B-lymphocytes and dendritic cells. Macrophages are phagocytic cells providing the first line of host defense against infection. B-cells are efficient in presenting soluble antigens because they can use their surface immunoglobulins to capture antigenic protein followed by endocytosis, internalization and presentation of peptide fragments in MHC class II/peptide complexes. Most important, APCs are dendritic cells specializing in antigen presentation. Dendritic cells in lymphoid, connective tissues and epithelia (e.g. Langerhans' cells in skin) are the most efficient "professional" antigen presenters and T-cell stimulators by virtue of high levels of expression of MHC class I and II and costimulatory molecules.

expression of MHC class I and II

Superantigens

description of superantigens

An unusual class of antigens known as "superantigens" stimulate the immune system without processing by APC. Superantigens are products of many viral, bacterial and mycoplasmal pathogens which bind directly to the MHC class II molecules outside of the antigen-binding groove. Superantigens stimulate a large proportion of T-lymphocytes, bypassing the TCR antigen-recognition site and binding to variable regions of TCR β chains. This results in activation of T-cells, massive proliferation, large-scale production of cytokines and eventual cell death, thereby explaining the pathogenesis (systemic toxicity and immunosuppression) of diseases involving such molecules.

Recognition of antigen by TCR and the TCR complex on T-cells

structure of the TCR

The understanding of the structure of the TCR eluded researchers for a long time. Only with the development of clonotypic monoclonal antibodies (mAbs) and creative use of recombinant DNA techniques did it become possible to describe the complexity of the TCR multimolecular complex. One explanation for the difficulties encountered in obtaining mAbs to TCR is the relatively small number (only several tens of thousands) of TCR molecules on the surface of T-cells.

diversity of TCR molecules

The TCR consists of two polypeptide chains, which are linked by a disulfide bond into an immunoglobulin-like three-dimensional structure. TCR molecules have a variable region, a constant region and a short hinge region. The diversity of TCR molecules recognizing peptide/MHC complexes is created during rearrangement of TCR genes and is most evident in the complementarity-determining regions (CDRs) of the antigen-binding site of TCR α and β chains. TCR α and β chains are associated with the CD3 complex which consists of six transmembrane proteins including two ε, δ, γ and two ζ chains. The formation of the complete TCR-CD3 complex is critical for the surface expression of the α, β chains of TCR as well for signal transduction. Proteins of the CD3 complex have homology with the immunoglobulin superfamily, and their cytoplasmic portions contain specialized sequences called immunoreceptor tyrosine-based activation motifs (ITAMs). These motifs are important in recruit-

immunoreceptor tyrosine-based activation motify

ment of intracellular tyrosine protein kinases and transduction of intracellular signalling.

TCR signalling

The engagement of the TCR complex in recognition of peptide/MHC
molecules results in aggregation of TCR molecules and coreceptors, and
induction of a series of biochemical events resulting in signal transduction. Activation of the intracellular protein tyrosine kinase (PTK) *lck* is
one of the earliest events of this pathway. p56 *lck* together with *fyn* PTK
induces tyrosine phosphorylation of the CD3 complex, most importantly of CD3 γ chains, which in turn leads to the recruitment of
ZAP-70/p72 *syk* PTK and tyrosine phosphorylation of phospholipase
C-γ, phosphatidyl inositol-3 kinase and several other intracellular substrates. TCR-mediated signal transduction, together with other signals,
results in the activation, proliferation and differentiation of T-cells as discussed above. TCR engagement alone may trigger effector T-cells to realize their functions but is not sufficient for induction of the primary response and differentiation of naive T-cells into activated effector T-cells.

**TCR-mediated
signal
transduction**

Costimulatory molecules

T-lymphocytes must receive two signals in order to develop a productive
immune response. TCR/MHC I/peptide interactions generate signal one
while costimulatory molecules produce signal two. Failure to receive the
costimulatory signal may result in long-lasting antigen-specific unresponsiveness of T-cells, termed anergy. The primary source of costimulatory signals is interaction of CD28 molecules on naive T-cells with the
proteins of the B7 family, B7.1(CD80) and B7.2(CD86) on the surface
of "professional" APCs (Fig. 2). Following the TCR-mediated signal,
binding of CD28 to B7 induces upregulation of the IL-2 receptor, lymphokine production and upregulation of other accessory molecules such
as CD40 ligand and CTLA-4 receptor. CD40 ligand binds to CD40 receptor on APCs, and this interaction transduces an activating signal to
the T-cells and induces upregulation of B7 molecules on APCs. CD40 lig-
and expression thus prolongs costimulatory activity and may be especially important in T- and B-cell interaction.

**Mechanism of
costimulatory
signaling**

The requirement for costimulatory signals may reflect the mechanism of protection from an antiself immune response. Indeed, the absence of a costimulatory signal will prevent a self-reactive immune response, for example due to cross-reaction of TCR to "self" peptide in the MHC complex.

CTLA-4

Transiently expressed CTLA-4 molecules also bind to B7 but provide signalling that is inhibitory and helps to stop the immune response and inflammation. CTLA-4 thus functions as a negative regulator of T-cell activation. Cross-linking of CTLA-4 inhibits cell cycle progression without inducing apoptotic death, thus saving potentially useful antigen-specific effector T-cells.

There are a number of other accessory molecules on the T-cell surface (Fig. 2) that function as adhesion molecules or as signalling receptors or both. Most interesting are CD2 and CD45 molecules, which may induce stimulatory or inhibitory signals under different circumstances, and integrins, which are discussed in the next section.

TCR dependent cell-cell contacts in interactions of T-cells with antigen-presenting cells

the adhesion molecules LFA-1

The interactions between T-cells and surrounding cells are mediated by adhesion molecules, including integrins. Some of the integrins, such as LFA-1, mediate direct cell-cell adhesion of T-cells with antigen-presenting cells. LFA-1 molecules recognize integral membrane proteins of the immunoglobulin superfamily, ICAM-1, -2 and -3 on the surface of APCs. Integrins have low adhesion activity on naive and resting T-cells; however, the functional activity of integrin receptors rapidly increases upon cellular activation. Modulation of integrin activity is important for T-cell functions. Naive T-cells must form transient and weak conjugates with every surrounding cell, enabling them to screen for the presence of rare infected cells and easily disengaging if no antigen is detected; however, if the antigen is present, the antigen/TCR interactions trigger conformational changes in adhesion molecule LFA-1. The activated LFA-1 mediates stronger and long-lasting conjugates, thereby providing sufficient time for early biochemical changes that are required to initiate the ensuing T-cell response. Costimulatory signals and cytokines may also increase integrin receptor affinity and regulate cell-cell interactions.

Immunological studies in recent years have focused on identification of different surface receptors, as well as molecular structure analysis and biochemical study of receptor-mediated signal transduction. Structure and function of immunoreceptors are the keys in understanding the mechanisms of immune reactions and in developing a clinical approach and strategy in an attempt to manipulate immune functions.

Cytokines

Klaus Resch

Introduction

For each immune response several cells have to cooperate. Within the lymphoid organs, such as lymph nodes, spleen or Peyer's plaques, the cells of the immune system do not form fixed anatomical structures but interact in a dynamic fashion, some cells, especially T-lymphocytes leaving the lymphoid organ to circulate through the body before returning. As a consequence, the communication between the cells – lymphocytes, monocytic cells and granulocytes – depends on secreted diffusible mediators, the most important of which are the cytokines.

communication between cells

An unambiguous definition for these molecules does not exist, with the exception that they are all proteins. The majority of cytokines are not synthesized exclusively by the cells of the immune system but by many other cells, and cytokines, too, may have effects on many cells. Therefore they cannot be clearly distinguished from general growth factors (or hormones), most of which also affect cells of the immune system, although their primary function – e.g. that of the nerve growth factor (NGF) – involves other organs. For practical purposes cytokines can be defined as protein mediators which are (1) primarily synthesized by cells of the immune system, (2) predominantly regulate differentiation and activation of these cells and (3) are partially responsible for the effector functions of these cells, including inflammation.

definition of cytokines

All cytokines exert their biological functions by binding to high-affinity plasma membrane receptors. The structures of the known cytokines as well as of most of their respective receptors have been elucidated by molecular cloning [1–4].

Principles of Immunopharmacology, ed. by F. P. Nijkamp and M. J. Parnham
©1999 Birkhäuser Verlag Basel/Switzerland

Differentiation factors

The mature cells of the immune system have a finite life span. Their physiological half-life ranges from several hours (neutrophilic granulocytes) to months (monocytes and most lymphocytes); some lymphocytes survive longer, memory Th lymphocytes for many years. Therefore the cells must be continuously renewed from a stem-cell pool, which in adult humans is located in the bone marrow. How the pool (reservoir) of stem cells is kept constant by self-renewal is not clear. Besides a direct influence of the stromal microenvironment, the cytokines interleukin(IL)-1 and IL-6 (see below) appear to be involved. The hematopoietic stem cells, of which low numbers are also present in blood – carrying the surface marker CD34 – give rise to lymphocytic or myelomonocytic cells, as well as platelets and erythrocytes (Fig. 1) (see also Chapter A2).

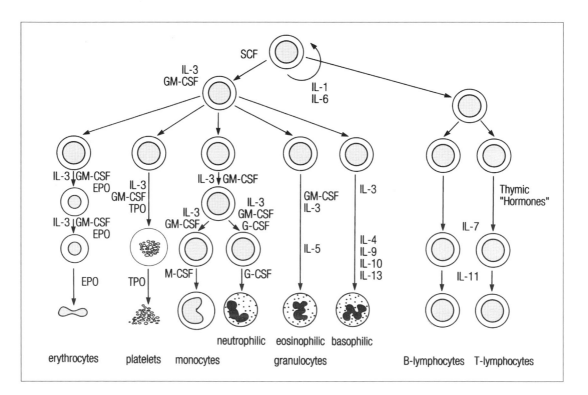

Figure 1 Cytokines involved in the differentiation of cells of the immune system
CSF, colony-stimulating factor; EPO, erythropoietin; G, granulocyte; IL, interleukin; M; macrophage; SCF, stem-cell factor; TPO, thrombopoietin.

The major differentiation factors of the myelomonocytic cell lineage are known best. Several of them are named according to the observation which led to their discovery, to stimulate outgrowth of colonies from bone marrow cell cultures, i.e. colony-stimulating factors (CSFs). Some of these factors – e.g. stem-cell factor (SCF), multi-CSF (synonymous with IL-3) – regulate early differentiation steps. Others, such as granulocyte/monocyte (GM) CSF control intermediate steps or selectively induce end differentiation into mature (neutrophilic) granulocytes (G-CSF) or monocytes (M-CSF). Similarly erythropoietin, synthesized in the kidney, promotes generation of erythrocytes, and thrombopoietin, which is synthesized in the liver and spleen, promotes formation of platelets. Table 1 summarizes their predominant physiological properties. As gene technology has facilitated the production of sufficient amounts, CSFs are now exploited as drugs (Table 2) [5].

differentiation factors of the myelomonocytic cell lineage

Thus erythropoietin has become established as the drug of choice for the treatment of severe anemias during terminal renal disease or due to cytostatic therapy [6]. Although discovered only recently, thrombopoietin has been applied successfully in clinical trials for the treatment of thrombocytopenias [7]. Filgrastim (human recombinant G-CSF with an additional methionine, generated from bacteria) was the first CSF approved for the treatment of granulocytopenias. Similarly to Lenograstim

differentiation factors as drugs

Table 1 Myeloid differentiation factors, erythropoietin and thrombopoietin

Cytokine	Molecular mass (kDa)	Predominant producer cells	Major function
Stem-cell factor	36	stromal cells	differentiation of stem cells
IL-3	14–28	T-lymphocytes	differentiation and propagation of myeloid progenitor cells
Granulocyte-macrophage CSF	14–35	T-lymphocytes, monocytes, endothelial cells, fibroblasts	differentiation and propagation of myeloid progenitor cells
Granulocyte CSF	18–22	monocytes	propagation and maturation of granulocytes
Macrophage CSF	35–45 18–26	endothelial cells fibroblasts, monocytes	propagation and maturation of monocytes
Erythropoietin	30–32	peritubular renal capillary cells	maturation of erythrocytes
Thrombopoietin	31	liver, kidney	maturation of platelets

CSF, Colony stimulating factor.

Table 2 Indication for cytokines

I. Reconstitution of a compromised immune system (physiological effects)

Cytokine	Target cell	Indication
Epo	erythroid progenitor cells	anemia
Tpo	megacaryocytic progenitor cells	thrombocytopenia
G-CSF	myeloid progenitor cells	granulocytepenia
M-CSF	monocytic progenitor cells	monocytopenia
GM-CSF	myelomonocytic progenitor cells	leukopenia
IL-3	myelomonocytic progenitor cells	leukopenia
IL-2	lymphocytic progenitor cells	lymphopenia
IL-7	lymphocytic progenitor cells	lymphopenia
IL-11	lymphocytic progenitor cells	lymphopenia
IL-1	hematopoietic stem cells?	stem cell deficiency?
IL-6	hematopoietic stem cells?	stem cell deficiency?

therapeutic effects of G-CSF

(human recombinant G-CSF from eukaryotic cells), it promptly and selectively increases up to 100-fold the number of functionally active neutrophils, for instance in patients with cytotoxic drug-induced granulocytopenias. Treatment with G-CSFs may markedly reduce the incidence and severity of infections leading to hospital admissions in patients receiving chemotherapy for malignant tumors. So far, however, the therapy has not led to an increase in life expectancy. GM-CSF (Molgramostim) has been approved for similar indications. All other CSFs have been evaluated in clinical trials.

Therapeutically administered CSFs are intended to substitute for the loss of a patient's own differentiation factors. Despite this, they – like all drugs – can cause side effects. For the CSFs these include bone and muscle pain, dysuria, sometimes elevation of liver enzymes and uric acid, and rarely, a drop in blood pressure, eosinophilia, or allergic reactions [5].

differentiation of T- and B-lymphocytes

generation of diversity

Differentiation of T- and B-lymphocytes from stem cells proceeds in a much more complex way. The central process consists of the generation of the huge ($>10^8$) diversity of antigen-specific receptors. The most important element involved is the free combination of a finite number of gene elements at the level of DNA during the differentiation of the cell lineages. For this gene rearrangement IL-7 appears to be indispensible, especially in T-lymphocyte development. Additionally, less well-characterized cytokines are involved in the maturation of T-lymphocytes in the thymus or of B-lymphocytes in the bone marrow, including for instance IL-11 [8]. Both have been tested clinically in patients with lymphopenias.

Activation and growth factors

Each immune response requires the interplay of several cell types. The activation of virgin B-lymphocytes is initiated by binding of the specific antigen to their surface immunoglobulin(Ig) M and IgD receptors. This can lead to secretion of small amounts of IgM. The expansion of the antigen-reactive B-cells and, concomitantly, effective immunoglobulin synthesis requires additional stimuli provided by IL-4, IL-5, IL-6 and IL-13 [9]. These cytokines are synthesized and secreted by a subpopulation of CD4$^+$ T helper lymphocytes, the Th2 cells. These interleukins – so named because of their ability to mediate interactions between leukocytes – not only promote the maturation of immunoglobulin-producing B-lymphocytes to the fully secretory plasma cell but also control switching to synthesis of other Ig-isotypes. This includes IgG, which is important for an effective antibacterial defense, and IgA, which is secreted through mucosal linings and thus exerts an early line of defense before entry of bacteria. For the synthesis of IgE, which is responsible for type I allergic reactions but also for defense against parasites, IL-4 is indispensable (Fig. 2) (see Chapter A5).

expansion of the antigen-reactive B-cells and immunoglobulin synthesis

Activation of T-lymphocytes, too, requires participation of cytokines [9]. To ensure an effective cellular immune defense, antigen reactive T-lymphocytes proliferate and thereby expand clonally: from a single lymphocyte up to 10^7 descendants may originate in this way. The predominant T-lymphocyte growth factor is IL-2, which if absent may be substituted by IL-15. IL-2 is formed by the second CD4$^+$ T helper subpopulation, the Th1 cells, and acts on cytotoxic T-lymphocytes as well as on all T-helper lymphocytes. Cytotoxic T-lymphocytes (carrying the surface marker CD8) can kill antigen-bearing target cells, most importantly virus-infected cells. Activated Th1 cells, by secreting interferon (IFN) γ (and other mediators such as tumor necrosis factor (TNF) β), initiate inflammatory reactions (see below). It should be noted that by secreting IL-3 and GM-CSF these T-cells also stimulate the formation of monocytic and myeloid cells in the bone marrow which are required for inflammatory reactions. Interleukins which have been defined so far at a molecular level are summarized in Table 3.

participation of cytokines in activation of T-lymphocytes

interleukins

It is possible that the number of interleukins discovered will increase in the future. On the other hand, some more "novel" interleukins exhibit strikingly similar properties to those which have been known for a longer period. For example, IL-13 exhibits similar properties to IL-4; it even binds to the IL-4 receptor as well as to its own receptor [10]. IL-15 is biologically similar to IL-2. This shows that for important regulatory

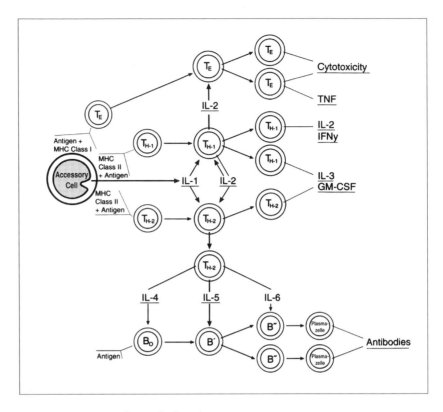

Figure 2 Activation of T- and B-lymphocytes
GM CSF, granulocyte-macrophage colony-stimulating factor; IFN, interferon; IL, inter-leukin; TNF, tumor necrosis factor.

interleukins surrogate molecules exist which take over the function of the former when it is synthesized in sufficient amounts. This redundancy indicates the importance of a functioning immune system for the survival of a species.

Mediators of inflammation

In response to their specific antigen, B-lymphocytes secrete antibodies and antigen-reactive T-lymphocytes expand clonally. Antibodies and cytotoxic T-lymphocytes may immediately deal with antigens, or antigen-bearing cells, for example by neutralizing poisons or killing invaded cells. The major proportion of the defense, however, is generally provided by secondary inflammatory mechanisms. To a large extent, these consist of

secondary
inflammatory
mechanisms

Table 3 Interleukins

Cytokine	Molecular mass	Predominant producer cells	Major functions
IL-1α IL-1β	17	monocytes, many other cells	activation of T-lymphocytes and inflammatory cells
IL-2	15	T-lymphocytes	activation and proliferation of T-lymphocytes, promonocytes, NK-cells
IL-3	14–28	T-lymphocytes	differentiation and propagation of early myeloid progenitor cells
IL-4	15–20	T-lymphocytes	activation and proliferation of T-cells, B-lymphocytes, inhibition of macrophage activation
IL-5	45–60	T-lymphocytes	proliferation of B-lymphocytes, maturation of eosinophils, inhibition of macrophage activation
IL-6	26	T-lymphocytes, many other cells	activation of B-, T-lymphocytes and other cells
IL-7	25	stromal cells	maturation of T- and B-lymphocytes
IL-8	10	monocytes	chemotaxis and activation of granulocytes, chemotaxis of T-lymphocytes
IL-9	37–40	T-lymphocytes	propagation of mast cells, megocaryocytes
IL-10	17–21	T-lymphocytes	propagation of mast cells, inhibition of cellular immune reactions
IL-11	23	stromal cells	maturation of lymphocytes, proliferation of myeloid progenitor cells
IL-12	p35/p40 dimer	monocytes	activation of T-lymphocytes, NK-cells
IL-13	17	T-lymphocytes	activation and proliferation of B lymphocytes, inhibition of cellular immune reactions
IL-14	60	T-lymphocytes	activation of B-lymphocytes
IL-15	14–15	epithelial cells, T-lymphocytes	activation and proliferation of T lymphocytes, NK-cells
IL-16	14	T-lymphocytes	chemotaxis of T-lymphocytes

the infiltration and activation of nonspecific leukocytes, mononuclear phagocytes and various granulocytes. These are recruited by antibodies as well as by mediators formed by Th1 cells. As a typical example, the activation of monocytes/macrophages is depicted in Figure 3. Besides GM-CSF, which not only induces the differentiation of monocytes and granulocytes, but also activates mature cells, IFNγ and TNFβ constitute

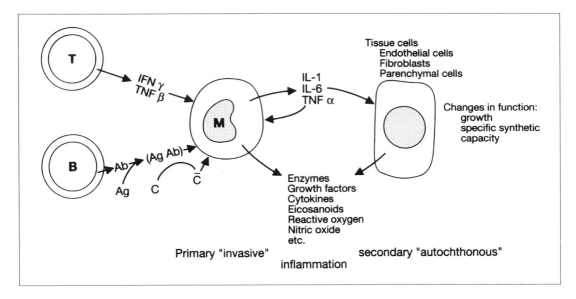

Figure 3 Immune reactions and inflammation

Ag, antigen; Ab, antibody; B, B-lymphocyte; C, complement C-activated complement components; IFN, interferon; IL, interleukin; M, macrophage; TNF, tumor necrosis factor.

macrophage activation

the most important macrophage-activating factors. IFNγ, generated by T-lymphocytes, is a member of the protein family of interferons, IFNαs being formed mainly by monocytes and IFNβ by fibroblasts (Table 5) [11]. In addition to their antiviral activity, all interferons can activate cells, most notably the nonspecific cells of the immune system, i.e. macrophages and granulocytes, to a varying extent. Together with TNFβ, TNFα – which is synthesized mainly by monocytes – is a member of the small family of TNFs (Table 6) [12]. These cytokines possess antitumoral activity against some malignant tumors, an activity which gave them their name. This property is shared with other cytokines of the interleukin group, including IL-1 and IL-6.

"inflammatory cytokines" as mediators of inflammation

More important, IL-1, TNF and to a less extent IL-6 effectively activate many cells, including endothelial cells and parenchymal cells [13]. In this way, these tissue cells are stimulated to contribute to an inflammatory reaction. In addition, these cytokines also enhance the activities of the mononuclear phagocytes and other leukocytes, in an autocrine and paracrine way, thereby amplifying the inflammatory reaction. These dual properties give the "inflammatory cytokines" a central role as mediators of inflammation. In addition to their direct effects, the boosting of inflammatory defense mechanisms against infectious agents and tumors

Table 4 Interferons

Cytokine	Molecular mass	Predominant producer cells	Major functions
IFNs α 15 proteins	19–26	monocytes	induction of antiviral activity
			inhibition of tumor cell growth
IFN β	23	fibroblasts	activation of cells
IFN γ 17–25	T-lymphocytes		induction of antiviral activity activation of macrophages immunoregulation

Table 5 Tumor necrosis factors

Cytokine	Molecular mass	Predominant producer cells	Major functions
TNFα	17	monocytes, many other cells	activation of many cells
			induction of apoptosis
TNFβ	17	T-lymphocytes	cachexia, shock

Table 6 Indications for cytokines
II. Activation of normal cells of the immune system (pharmacodynamic actions)

Cytokine	Target cells	Indication
IFNα	virus-infected cells, tumor cells	viral infections, malignant tumors
IFNβ	virus-infected cells	viral infections
TNFα,β	monocytes/macrophages, tumor cells	malignant tumors
IL-1	monocytes/macrophages, tumor cells	malignant tumors
IL-2	T-lymphocytes, monocytes, NK-cells	malignal tumors bacterial, viral infections (AIDS)
IL-4	B-lymphocytes	parasitic infections (?)
IL-5	B-lymphocytes, eosinophils	parasitic infections (?)
IL-6	monocytes/macrophages, tumor cells	malignant tumors

constitutes the basis for attempts to positively modulate infectious diseases or malignant tumors by the administration of cytokines (Table 6) (see Chapters A11 and C5).

indications for interferons

Approved indications for IFNα and β include severe virus infections, such as recurring varizella zoster-infections, herpes simplex infection of the eye and especially chronic hepatitis B and C. IFNβ has been approved for some forms of multiple sclerosis. IFNα is indicated for the treatment of some malignant tumors, including hairy cell leukemia or chronic myeloid leukemia. It is effective against some other tumors, such as non-Hodgkins lymphoma, cutaneous T-cell leukemia, malignant melanoma, hypernephroma or bladder carcinoma, but against the majority of carcinomas it is ineffective. Antitumor effects of IFNβ and γ in humans are less certain. Clinical side effects of interferons include the common "flu-like" syndrome (fever, fatigue, shivering, muscle and joint pain), paresthesias, disturbances of the central nervous system, gastrointestinal disturbances, cardiac symptoms, granulocytopenia, thrombopenia and anemia.

TNF, IL-1 and IL-2 for the treatment of malignant tumors

The cytokines TNF, IL-1 and IL-2 are currently the subjects of many clinical trials for treating malignant tumors [14–16] (see Chapters A11 and C5). Despite some positive results – such as with IL-2 in metastasizing kidney carcinoma – the overall outcome so far has been rather disappointing. The major reason for this appears to be the limitation of severe toxicity, which arises when these cytokines are administered systemically. This has prompted attempts to increase cytokine concentration locally in the tumor by perfusing it, for instance with TNF. As experiments in animal models have been encouraging, this strategy is being followed in clinical trials with limb tumors or hepatocarcinomas. Another

clinical trials

strategy which is being followed is to transfect either tumor cells or tumor infiltrating cells in a way that they constitutively secrete high amounts of a cytokine such as IL-2 or TNF. After reinfusion and subsequent redistribution to sites of the tumor, a high local concentration of the cytokines in the tumor may be achieved, which supports sufficient antitumoral activity but is accompanied by tolerable systemic effects. First clinical trials of cytokine gene therapy have been initiated.

Infection with HIV leads to progressive and preferential loss of CD4$^+$ T helper cells. Death results from opportunistic infections or, less often, malignant tumors. In combination with effective antiviral treatment strategies (double or triple combinations such as zidovudin, didanosin and sequinavir) first clinical trials report a dramatic amelioration of immunodeficiency by IL-2.

Regulatory factors

While it is desirable during infectious diseases or malignant tumors to augment immune and subsequent inflammatory reactions, in other situations, such as autoimmune, chronic inflammatory or allergic diseases, they are pathogenic. Under physiological conditions, immune reactions are tightly controlled, and immunological diseases may therefore be regarded as failures of immunoregulation. In the recent years, the balance between the activity of Th1 and Th2 cells has emerged as the central control mechanism (Fig. 4, see also Fig. 2) [17, 18].

control of immune reactions

Th1 cells secrete the cytokines IL-2, IL-15 and IFNγ, which as described above promote cellular defense and inflammatory responses. Th2 cells, on the other hand, synthesize those cytokines which regulate the activation of B-lymphocytes, IL-4, IL-5, IL-6, IL-10 and IL-13. Both Th subpopulations develop from common CD4⁺ precursors, Th-p. IFNγ promotes differentiation into Th1 cells, whereas IL-4, IL-10 and IL-13 are responsible for Th2 differentiation. Simultaneously, subpopulation-specific cytokines block development of the opposite Th subpopulation. This implies that if one subpopulation gains a developmental advantage, this is reinforced, whereas the corresponding subpopulation is suppressed.

Th1 and Th2 cells

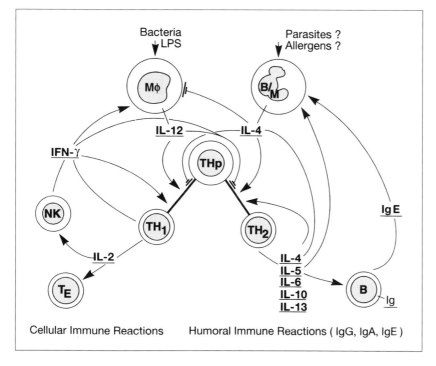

Figure 4 Regulation of immune responses

B/M, basophilic granulocytes/mast cells; B, B-lymphocytes; IFN, interferon; Ig, immunoglobulin; IL, interleukin; M, macrophage; NK, natural killer cell; TH, T helper cell; TH-p, T helper cell precursor; TE, T effector cell.

63

differentiation into a Th subpopulation

Since no Th1 or Th2 specific antigens or epitopes have been detected as yet, the initial channelling of preferential differentiation into a specific Th subpopulation – and thereby the type of immune reaction – must be directed by other cells. For Th1 cells, this is a function of monocytes and macrophages, which following interaction with bacteria or their components (e.g. lipopolysaccharide) release IL-12, which in turn initiates differentiation to this subpopulation. For Th2 cells, it is likely that basophilic granulocytes or mast cells play a similar role, since they contain vast amounts of IL-4, although direct experimental proof so far is limited.

antiinflammatory effects of IL-4, IL-10 or IL-13

It is obvious from these data that IL-4, IL-10 or IL-13 should exert antiinflammatory effects in nonallergic situations. Indeed, this is supported by many *in vitro* experiments and more relevant, experimental animal models. In these studies, it was found that not only development of Th1 cells was inhibited but also the activation of macrophages, the predominant "chronic" inflammatory cells. All these cytokines, therefore, are presently undergoing clinical evaluation in several chronic inflammatory diseases, including rheumatoid arthritis.

infiltration of leukocytes

Nearly all inflammatory – as well as allergic – diseases are confined to certain organs. This implies that all cells of the immune system which participate in the underlying pathomechanism must escape from the bloodstream and penetrate into the respective tissues. The very complex infiltration of leukocytes, which proceeds in several defined steps, is also controlled by various cytokines (Table 7) [19]. Among these, the protein family of chemokines – with molecular masses between 7 and 15 – is steadily increasing in size, as new members are discovered (Table 8) [20].

function of chemokines

According to their structure, at least three groups can be discerned by the relative position of cysteine residues. CXC chemokines (X stands for an arbitrary amino acid) are predominantly chemotactic for neutrophils and T subsets, whereas CC chemokines mostly attract monocytes and lymphocytes and C chemokines, lymphocytes. In addition to their chemotactic properties, chemokines are also potent activators of their target cells, thereby contributing to local inflammation. Chemokines bind to seven transmembrane-spanning (heptahelical) G protein-linked receptors, CXCR 1 to 5 and CCR 1 to 5. CCR 3 and CCR 5 have recently raised great interest as coreceptors (in addition to CD4) for human immunodeficiency virus (HIV) entry into macrophages and CXCR 4 (also termed fusin) for HIV entry into T-lymphocytes. Chemokines effectively blocked *in vitro* entry of macrophage-tropic or lymphotropic HIV strains by binding to their receptor, which raises hope for new therapeutic strategies in acquired immunodeficiency syndrome (AIDS).

Table 7 *Participation of circulating leukocytes in local inflammation*

Reaction step	Cytokines	Main target T-cells
Chemotaxis	IL-8	neutrophils
	eotaxin	eosinophils
	MCP-1	} monocytes
	RANTES	
	RANTES	monocytes
Emigration from the blood	IFNγ	endothelial cells (expression of cell adhesion molecules such asadhesion ELAM-1, ICAM-1, VCAM-1)
Activation	IFNγ	monocytes, granulocytes
	IL-1	
	TNF	
	CSFs	
	IL-8	granulocytes
Expansion	CSFs	myeloid precursor cells

Table 8 *Chemokines*

CXC chemokines:	IL-8
	growth related oncogenes α, β, γ
	platelet factor 4
	granulocyte chemotactic protein-2
	platelet basic protein and derivatives, e.g. neutrophil-activating protein-2
	others
C-C chemokines:	macrophage chemoattractant proteins 1, 2, 3 and 4
	RANTES
	macrophage inflammatory protein-1α and β
	eotaxin
C chemokines:	lymphotaxin

Inhibition of cytokines

target for therapeutic intervention

Because of their multiple functions in the inflammatory process, cytokines offer a useful target for therapeutic intervention. Inhibition of cytokines may be achieved by several mechanisms. Some have already led to approved drugs, whereas other less-advanced approaches are undergoing evaluation in clinical trials.

cytostatic drugs and noncytotoxic immuno-suppressants

Cytostatic drugs such as azathioprine and monoclonal antibodies against T-lymphocyte epitopes (e.g. CD3) are examples of effective drugs used for the treatment of autoimmune diseases (e.g. lupus erythematosus) or for preventing transplant rejection. The same indication is met by noncytotoxic immunosuppressants, including cyclosporin A or tacrolimus (F506) which very selectively block the synthesis of cytokines in T-lymphocytes, especially their growth factor IL-2 (see Chapter C8).

Table 9 Approaches to inhibition of cytokines

I.   **Inhibition of synthesis**

Reduction of the number of cytokine-producing cells
    cytostatic drugs
    monoclonal antibodies to cells

inhibitory cytokines
    TGFβ
    regulatory cytokines

inhibitors of signal transduction
    cyclosporin A and related drugs
    CSAIDs

regulation of gene expression
    glucocorticoids
    STAT molecules?

inhibitors of release
ICE (IL-1 converting enzyme) inhibitors

II. **Decrease of the concentration in active (free) form**

monoclonal antibodies against cytokines

soluble cytokine receptors

III. **Receptor blockade**

monoclonal antibodies against cytokine receptors

cytokine antagonists

In a similar way corticosteroids are also immunosuppresive. They exert their antiinflammatory properties by downregulating the synthesis of the inflammatory cytokines IL-1, IL-6, IL-8 or TNF. Very recently, a new group of experimental drugs, termed cytokine suppressive antiinflammatory drugs (CSAIDs), have been described with striking selectivity for inhibition of IL-1 or TNF synthesis by interfering with a critical signal transduction step [21]. Numerous other attempts at inhibiting cytokines have been made as an attempt to treat autoimmune, chronic inflammatory or allergic diseases [22]. They can only be summarized briefly (Table 9).

corticosteroids

cytokine suppressive antiinflammatory drugs

Antibodies can block the action of secreted cytokines. Thus, an antibody against TNF proved to be efficacious in rheumatoid arthritis resulting, at least in some patients, in long-lasting remission [23]. Similarly, antibodies against cytokine receptors have shown positive effects in animal studies. Illustrating the principle of self-limitation, the extracellular sections of many cytokine receptors are released during immune or inflammatory reactions. As these "soluble receptors" contain the cytokine binding site, they behave like receptor antagonists. Administration of soluble receptors for IL-1 or TNF has been found to ameliorate inflammation in some animal models; in clinical studies the requirement for very high concentrations has so far limited their use.

antibodies against cytokines and cytokine receptors

As a unique example, a natural antagonist for IL-1, IL-1ra, has been cloned. In initial clinical studies, administration of IL-1ra produced positive effects, although again the high doses necessary limited efficacy [13]. Several cytokine mutants with antagonistic properties called "muteins" have been produced by gene technology. Considerable thera-

antagonists of cytokines

Table 10 Potential indications for inhibitors of cytokines

Cytokine	Indication
IL-1	chronic inflammatory diseases
IL-2	autoimmune diseases, transplantation
IL-4	allergic (type I) diseases
IL-5	allergic asthma (?)
IL-6	chronic inflammatory diseases, some hematological tumors
IL-8[*]	chronic inflammatory diseases, autoimmune diseases
TNFα,β	septic shock, chronic inflammatory diseases
IFNγ	autoimmune diseases

[*] *and other chemokines*

peutic hope has been engendered by the use of IL-4 antagonists for the treatment of IgE-dependent allergy. Table 10 summarizes some important diseases in which inhibition of specific cytokines is expected – or has been shown – to be of clinical value.

cytokines as drugs

It was not long after their discovery and subsequent molecular characterizations that cytokines were tested for their therapeutic potential. This was only made possible by gene technology, which allowed sufficient amounts to be produced in good quality. Some of them – interferons or the CSFs – subsequently became established as drugs with great medical and even economic importance. Not all high-flying hopes, however, have come true, especially with regard to the treatment of malignant tumors. Thus, after a period of setbacks, new strategies have begun to evolve which allow high local concentrations to be selectively generated, the most sophisticated approach involving the use of genetically altered cells [24].

On the other hand, cytokines are now know to be crucial participants in the pathogenesis of many diseases. The realization that long-known and valuable drugs, such as the glucocorticosteroids, act predominantly by suppressing the synthesis of certain cytokines, has prompted a search for mechanisms by which the synthesis or function of individual cytokines can be blocked more selectively. Even though cytokines or their inhibitors have developed into indispensable drugs in important indications, it is certain that this is only the beginning. This assumption is based on the growing evidence that these molecules contribute to many more diseases than those anticipated originally; important examples are atherosclerosis, congestive heart failure and neurodegenerative diseases.

A5 Antibody-mediated immunity

Ger T. Rijkers

Towards the end of the 19th century, Koch and Ehrlich discovered that the serum of immunized animals contained substances (antitoxins) with the ability to neutralize the toxins of diphtheria and tetanus. At Christmas 1891 a group of children received diphtheria antitoxin, which cured them from this otherwise fatal disease. These experiments demonstrated that immunization can induce the formation of humoral substances which have the ability to protect against infectious diseases. Half a century later, in 1952, Bruton described a patient with (predominantly bacterial) severe and recurrent respiratory tract infections and an agammaglobulinemia. This milestone demonstrated the significant role of immunoglobulins in defense against infections. Later on, through the pioneering work of Max Cooper and others it was shown that B-lymphocytes are the cells that produce antibodies, and that patients such as the one described above (X-linked agammaglobulinemia or XLA) fail to produce antibodies because they lack B-lymphocytes; B-lymphocyte development in the bone marrow stops at the pre-B-cell stage. In 1993 the molecular basis for this disease was found: XLA is caused by structural defects in the gene encoding an enzyme that is now called Bruton's tyrosine kinase (Btk).

B-cell receptor and signal transduction

B-lymphocyte activation is initiated by specific recognition of antigen by the antigen receptor, i.e. membrane-bound immunoglobulin (mIg). Resting, primary B-lymphocytes express two isotypes of mIg: mIgM and mIgD. Both mIgM and mIgD (as well as other mIg isotypes; see below) are expressed on the cell surface in association with Igα and Igβ molecules; collectively such a complex is called the B-cell receptor complex (BCR). Igα (CD79a) and Igβ (CD79b) are the protein products of the *MB-1* and *B29* genes, respectively, and both belong to the Ig superfami-

B-cell receptor complex

Igα and Igβ

ly. Igα and Igβ fulfill at least three different functions: they are required for expression of membrane Ig on the B-cell surface, they act as transducer elements coupling the antigen receptor to intracellular signalling molecules by virtue of the ITAM motif (see below) and they contain sequences for efficient internalization of antigen.

One of the first signs of cellular activation after antigen-induced ligation of the BCR is the increase in the activity of protein tyrosine kinases. Because the cytoplasmic domains of mIgM and mIgD consist of only 3 amino acids, it could be assumed that Igα (cytoplasmic domain of 61 amino acids) and Igβ (48 amino acids) serve a role in signal transduction. Of crucial importance for signal transduction is the ITAM motif

immunoreceptor tyrosine-based activation motif

(immunoreceptor tyrosine-based activation motif), present in the cytoplasmic domain of Igα and Igβ (Fig. 1). This amino acid motif resides in a 26-amino acid sequence and consists of a tyrosine (Y) followed two residues later by a leucine (L) or isoleucine (I), a submotif that is repeated once after six to seven variable residues. The complete ITAM motif also contains two aspartate (D) or glutamate (E) residues at characteristic positions (Fig. 1). The ITAM motif is found in Igα and Igβ, in the CD3γ and

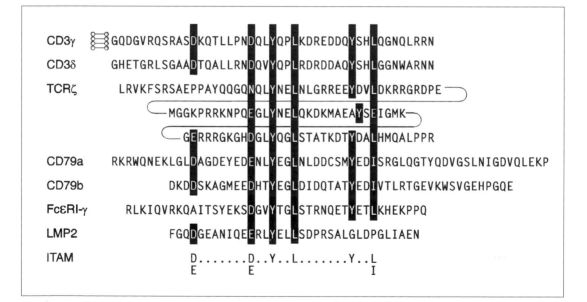

Figure 1 The immunoreceptor tyrosine-based activation motif

The amino acid sequence (given in the single letter code) of the cytoplasmic domains of human CD3γ, CD3δ, the TCR ζ chain, Igα (CD79a), Igβ (CD79b), the γ chain of the type I Fcε receptor (FcεRI-γ) and of the EBV encoded LMP2 protein. Note that the cytoplasmic domain of TCR ζ is depicted in three interconnected parts in order to allow the alignment of the three copies of the ITAM within the sequence. See text for further explanation.

CD3δ chains of the T-cell receptor (TCR) complex, and in the γ chain of the Fcε receptor type I. ζ chains of the TCR contain three copies of the ITAM motif. More or less truncated forms of ITAM are present in CD22 and Fcγ receptor type II. Also a viral encoded protein, LMP2 from Epstein-Barr virus, contains an ITAM. The central role of ITAM in cellular signalling through the BCR complex (as well as through the TCR complex) has become apparent from studies in which single amino acid substitution receptor mutants and chimerical receptor molecules have been used.

Upon triggering of mIg, a number of cytoplasmic tyrosine kinases become associated with the BCR. These include kinases of the src family, such as lyn, fyn and blk as well as the syk tyrosine kinase. The binding is mediated by the interaction of the src-homology 2 (SH2) domain within the tyrosine kinase with phosphorylated tyrosine residues within the ITAMs of Igα and Igβ. Note that this model suffers from a "chicken and egg" problem: if binding of SH2 domains is on phosphorylated ITAM tyrosines, how do ITAM tyrosines become phosphorylated initially? It has been found, however, that an alternative interaction is possible, not depending on phosphotyrosine: the 10 N-terminal residues of src kinases can interact with a specific sequence within the ITAM of Igα (DCSM).

cytoplasmic tyrosine kinases

src-homology 2 (SH2) domain

Binding of src and syk kinases to (phosphorylated) ITAMs triggers a series of downstream signalling events. These include activation of phospholipase Cγ2, GTPase activating protein, MAP kinase (all through the N-terminal regions of lyn, fyn and blk), of phospholipase Cγ1 (through syk), of the guanine nucleotide releasing factor Vav, of p85 PI-3 kinase (through the SH3 domains of fyn and lyn). Thus, originating from the BCR, several src family kinases and the syk kinase are activated, resulting in the initiation of several distinct cell-signalling pathways (Ras, phospholipase C (PLC), PI-3 kinase). These signalling pathways result in the activation of a set of protein kinases, which in turn phosphorylate cytoplasmic and nuclear substrates, and ultimately activate transcription (Fig. 2).

src and syh kinases and downstream signalling events

B-lymphocyte costimulation

Whereas the events described above are causally linked to B-lymphocyte proliferation and differentiation into antibody-secreting plasma cells, in only a few cases is triggering of the BCR by specific antigen sufficient to ensure subsequent B-cell activation and differentiation. In all other instances, involving the vast majority of naturally occurring antigens, the process of B-cell activation and differentiation depends on activation of

receptors on B-lymphocytes

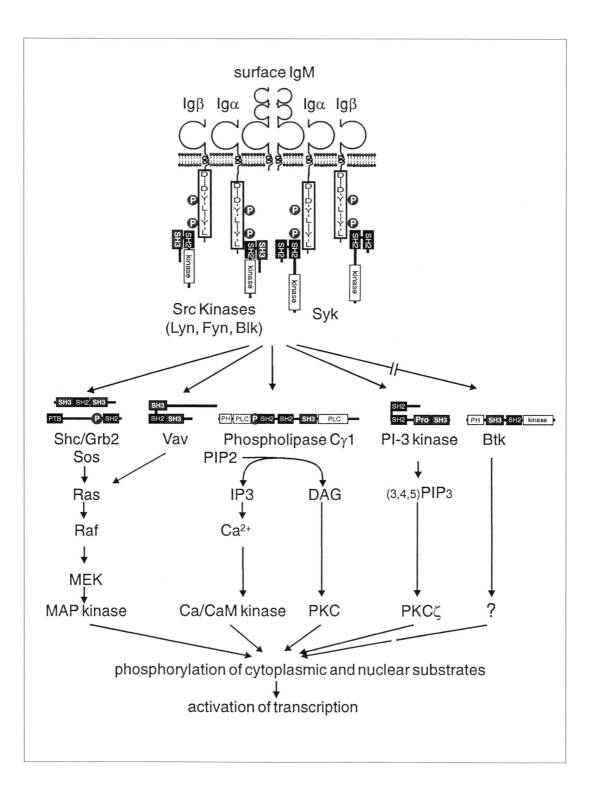

additional receptors on the B-lymphocyte. A number of these receptors interact with counter-receptors on T-lymphocytes, thus providing the structural basis for the interaction between these two cell types in the process of antibody formation. Other receptors on B-lymphocytes have ligands that are expressed on other cell types (such as monocytes, endothelial cells etc.) or have soluble ligands.

A major coreceptor on B-lymphocytes is CD40. This 50-kDa glycoprotein is a member of the so-called TNF receptor superfamily and is expressed on all mature B-lymphocytes. The counterreceptor for CD40 is the CD40 ligand (CD40L), which is expressed on activated T helper cells. The role of CD40 and CD40L for the process of B-lymphocyte activation is depicted schematically in Figure 3. Antigen that is bound to the BCR is internalized and processed, and peptide fragments are expressed on the B-lymphocyte surface by class II major histocompatibility (MHC) molecules. Thus presented, peptides can be recognized by specific T-cells, leading to T-cell activation and expression of CD40L, a 39-kDa cell surface glycoprotein. The interaction of CD40L with CD40 results in progression of the B-cell activation process, including acquisition of the capacity to proliferate in response to soluble cytokines produced by the activated T-cell. The signal received through CD40 is also important for the process of class switching, the mechanism through which antibodies of immunoglobulin classes other than IgM are pro-

coreceptor DC40

class switching

Figure 2 Signalling through the BCR complex

The membrane immunoglobulin is composed of disulphide-linked heavy- and light-chain molecules (only partially shown in the figure) flanked by noncovalently associated dimers of Igα and Igβ. Ovals in membrane immunoglobulin, Igα and Igβ indicate homologous domains of immunoglobulin superfamily members. The cytoplasmic domains of Igα and Igβ contain the ITAM. Phosphorylation (P) of the tyrosine residues (Y) in the ITAMs allows src kinases (lyn, fyn, blk) and syk to associate with the BCR. Activated kinases lead to further phosphorylation of ITAMs, autophosphorylation as well as phosphorylation of a number of cell-signalling molecules. The latter include Shc and Grb2 (initiating the MAP kinase-signalling pathway), Vav (activating Ras and thus also leading to activation of MAP kinase), phospholipase Cγ1 [catalysing the hydrolysis of phosphatidyl inositol bisphosphate (PIP2)], PI-3 kinase [leading to generation of phosphatidyl inositol trisphosphate (PIP3)] and Btk. PIP2 hydrolysis generates inositol trisphosphate (IP3) and diacylglycerol (DAG). IP3 causes the release of Ca^{2+} from intracellular stores and the subsequent activation of Ca^{2+}/calmodulin-dependent protein kinase (Ca/CaM kinase). DAG, in the presence of phosphatidyl serine and high Ca^{2+}, activates protein kinase C (PKC). PIP3 activates the ζ isoform of PKC. Downstream signalling events from Btk are not known at present. All kinases described above phosphorylate cytoplasmic and nuclear substrates (including transcription factors) leading to activation of transcription and thus B-lymphocyte activation.

duced. The biological significance of the interaction between CD40 and CD40L is illustrated in a human immunodeficiency disease, the so-called X-linked hyper-IgM syndrome. Affected patients carry mutations in the CD40L gene resulting in the inability to produce antibodies other than IgM.

X-linked hyper-IgM syndrome

Additional costimulatory receptor-counterreceptor pairs contribute to successful interaction between B-lymphocytes and T-lymphocytes, such as CD28 (on T-cells) and B7 (CD80) on B-cells.

Cytokine regulation

The full stimulatory effect of the interaction between T-lymphocytes and B-lymphocytes depends not only on binding of cell surface receptors and counterreceptors but also on production of T-cell cytokines that promote (various stages) of B-lymphocyte proliferation and terminal differentiation into plasma cells. The soluble cytokines should not be considered merely as endocrine hormones, because they are secreted at the sites of direct cell-cell contact, and therefore the particular B-lymphocyte engaged in cellular interaction with the relevant T-lymphocyte benefits most from these growth and differentiation factors.

IL-4

IL-5

The cytokines that regulate B-lymphocyte growth and differentiation predominantly include interleukin (IL)-4, IL-5, IL-6 and IL-10. IL-4 acts as a costimulator for signals received through the BCR and CD40 in promoting B-lymphocyte growth. Both IL-4 and the related cytokine IL-13 can cause switching to IgE and IgG4 production. IL-5 primarily regulates the differentiation of an activated B-lymphocyte into an antibody-secreting cell. IL-6 and IL-10 have prominent effects on B-lymphocyte differentiation and immunoglobulin secretion.

T-cell independent B-lymphocyte activation

T-cell-independent antigens capsular polysaccharides

In the above section the important role of interaction with T-lymphocytes for the process of B-lymphocyte activation has been emphasized. There is however a category of antigens that is unable to activate T-lymphocytes, whereas B-lymphocyte responses and induction of antibodies can be readily demonstrated. These types of antigens are called T-cell-independent antigens, and major representatives are bacterial capsular polysaccharides from encapsulated bacteria such as *Streptococcus pneumo-*

niae, Haemophilus influenzae type b and *Neisseria meningitidis*. Until now, neither processing and antigen presentation in the context of class II MHC molecules nor specific T-lymphocyte activation has been demonstrated for polysaccharides. This means that, because CD40/CD40L interaction in the case of T-cell-independent antigens is highly unlikely to take place, polysaccharide specific B-lymphocytes should receive an alternative costimulatory signal. Indirect evidence points towards a role for the CD19/CD21 receptor complex in this respect. CD19 is a 95-kDa glycoprotein of the immunoglobulin superfamily that is expressed throughout B-lymphocyte development. A specific ligand for this molecule has not been identified as yet, although purified CD19 protein does bind to bone marrow stromal cells. Activation of CD19 by specific antibodies provides a costimulatory signal for B-lymphocyte activation through the BCR. Indeed, the cytoplasmic domain of the CD19 molecule contains the consensus motifs for binding of src kinases lyn and lck, for binding of PI-3 kinase and for interaction with the protooncogene Vav. On mature B-lymphocytes, CD19 is expressed in a molecular complex that includes CD21, the TAPA-1 protein (CD89) and the Leu-13 molecule. The prevailing model is that in this complex CD19 acts as the signal-transducing moiety for CD21. CD21 is a 145-kDa glycoprotein of the complement receptor family which is expressed on mature B-lymphocytes (and also on follicular dendritic cells and at a low level on a subpopulation of T-cells). CD21 is the receptor for the complement component C3 split products iC3b, C3dg and C3d. CD21 also serves as the cellular receptor for the Epstein-Barr virus, and as an interferon α receptor. Furthermore, CD21 can interact with CD23. The (chemical) coupling of C3d to protein antigens lowers the threshold for antibody induction 100–1000-fold. Bacterial polysaccharides, through the alternative pathway of complement activation, can generate C3 split products, which become deposited on the polysaccharide. Natural complexes of polysaccharide and C3d, thus formed, can cross-link mIg and CD21 on polysaccharide-specific B-lymphocytes. This mechanism may bypass the need for engagement of CD40/CD40L in B-lymphocyte activation (Fig. 3). Compatible with this mechanism is the finding that children up to the age of 2 years who are unable to respond to polysaccharide antigens have a reduced expression of CD21 on B-lymphocytes.

CD19/CD21 receptor complex

CD21; C3d receptor

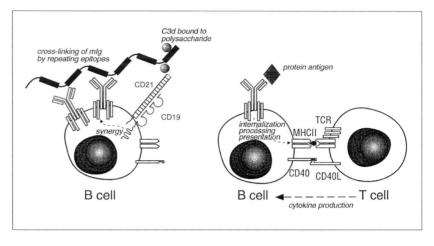

Figure 3 B-lymphocyte activation by T-cell-independent and by T-cell-dependent antigens

Left panel: A polysaccharide antigen with repeating epitopes cross-links mIg on the surface of the B-lymphocyte. Deposited C3d is bound by CD21, which provides a synergistic signal for B-lymphocyte activation. Right panel: A protein antigen is bound and internalized by mIg; following intracellular processing, peptide fragments are expressed in class II MHC molecules. Specific T-lymphocytes recognize these peptides, become activated and express CD40L. Upon interaction of CD40L with CD40, cytokine production is initiated (see text for further information).

Distribution and function of antibodies

The structure and physicochemical characteristics of immunoglobulin classes and subclasses were described in Chapter A1.

Primary and secondary antibody response

primary (antibody) response plasma cells

The first contact of the immune system with a given antigen will induce what is called a primary (antibody) response. B-lymphocytes become activated and differentiate into plasma cells (along routes as described above). Plasma cells are highly differentiated cells which maximally produce 10^4 antibody molecules per second, equalling 40% of the total protein-synthesizing capacity of the cell. The lifetime of a plasma cell is 3–4 days. A second contact with the same (protein) antigen elicits a secondary antibody response, which differs in a number of aspects from a primary response. The latency period (time between contact with antigen and start of antibody production) is shorter in a secondary response, and antibody levels attained are much higher (1–2 orders of magnitude). While during a primary antibody response predominantly IgM, and to a lesser extent IgG, antibodies are produced, IgG, IgA and IgE antibodies are the major classes during a secondary response. The affinity of antibodies produced increases during the response; there may be a 100–1000-fold difference in affinity between antibodies produced at the start of a primary response and at the end of a secondary response. This process (affinity maturation) is the combined effect of somatic hypermutation of CDR1 and CDR2 regions during B-lymphocyte proliferation (see Chapter A1) and the selection of the B-lymphocytes with the highest affinity.

secondary response

affinity maturatrion

A primary antibody response takes place in follicles and the marginal zone of spleen and lymph nodes. During a secondary response, bone marrow is the major site of antibody production. Antibodies which are secreted in mucosal tissue of the respiratory and gastrointestinal tract are produced locally by the bronchus-associated lymphoid tissue (BALT) and gut-associated lymphoid tissue (GALT), respectively (Fig. 4).

organs of antibody response

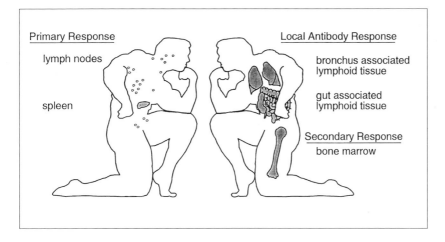

Figure 4 Sites of antibody production

During the primary immune response, a fraction of antigen-specific B-lymphocytes do not differentiate into plasma cells but into so-called memory B-cells. It should be noted that the term *memory cell* is largely conceptual; actual differences between naive and memory B-lymphocytes are found in the isotypes of mIg and affinity of mIg. Naive primary B-lym-

memory B-cells

phocytes express mIgM and mIgD; memory B-lymphocytes have lost mIgD and express mIgG or mIgA, with or without mIgM. Because of the above-described affinity maturation, the affinity of mIg for antigen on memory B-lymphocytes is higher than on primary B-lymphocytes.

All characteristics of a primary and secondary antibody response as described above hold true only for protein antigens. For polysaccharide antigens, a second contact with antigen induces an antibody response that is identical in kinetics and magnitude as a primary response. Affinity maturation does not occur, and isotype distribution of antibodies does not change. Moreover, anti-polysaccharide antibodies use a restricted number of V_H and V_L genes, whereas anti-protein antibodies are more heterogeneous. Finally, IgG anti-protein antibodies to the vast majority of antigens are of the IgG1 subclass; IgG anti-polysaccharide antibodies in adult individuals are predominantly IgG2.

anti-polysaccharide antibodies

Biological functions of antibodies

The biological function of antibodies can be discerned in binding of antigen (through variable V_H and V_L domains) and effector functions mediated by the constant domains (in particular C_{H2} and/or C_{H3} domains). The bacterial toxins mentioned at the beginning of this chapter are neutralized when bound by antibodies. Clearance of immune complexes and antibody-opsonized microorganisms depends on the functional integrity of the Fc part of the antibody molecule. The Fc part can either interact with soluble biologically active molecules, such as the complement system (see Chapter A6) or bind to Fc receptors which are expressed on a variety of cells of the immune system. Fc receptors expressed on monocytes, macrophages and granulocytes are essential for phagocytosis of immune complexes and opsonized microorganisms. Fc receptors for IgG (Fcγ receptors) are expressed on monocytes and macrophages; neutrophilic granulocytes also express receptors for IgA (Fcα receptors). Depending on the class of antibodies in an immune complex, the complement system becomes more or less efficiently activated. This will enhance phagocytosis by monocytes, macrophages and granulocytes, since these cells also express complement receptors in addition to Fc receptors.

Fc receptors

Fc receptors for IgE (Fcε receptor) are primarily expressed by mast cells. In allergic individuals, Fcε receptors have constitutively bound IgE; exposure to allergens causes cross-linking of Fcε receptors, resulting in mast cell degranulation and histamine release. Apart from phagocytosis and degranulation, Fc receptors also mediate cytotoxicity in a process

Fcε receptor

mast cell degranulation

called ADCC (antibody-dependent cellular cytotoxicity). Target-cells (e.g. tumor cells) to which antibodies are bound can be recognized by Fc receptors expressed on cells with cytotoxic potential. The killing process itself is complement-independent. Monocytes, neutrophilic and eosinophilic granulocytes and natural killer (NK) cells display ADCC ac-

antibody-depen-dent cellular cytotoxicity

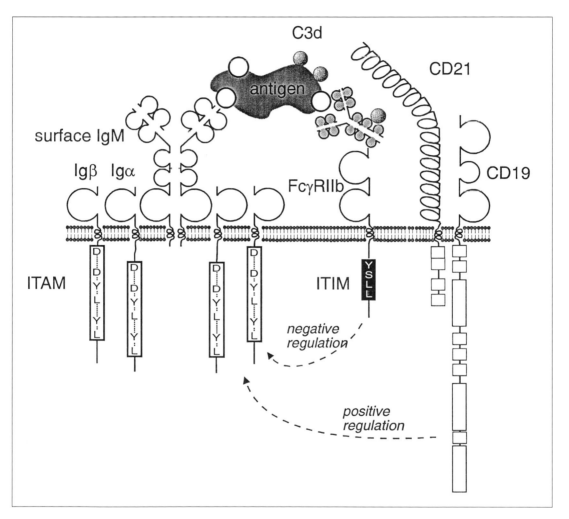

Figure 5 Regulation of BCR activation by coreceptors

Ovals in membrane immunoglobulin (surface IgM), Igα, Igβ, FcγRIIb and CD19 indicate homologous domains of immunoglobulin superfamily members. The cytoplasmic domains of Igα and Igβ contain the ITAM. The Fcγ receptor IIb binds the Fc part of IgG antibodies in immune complexes. The cytoplasmic domain of FcγRIIb contains the immunoreceptor tyrosine-based inhibitory motif (ITIM) YSLL. CD21 (type 2 complement receptor) binds C3d deposited on the antigen or on IgG antibodies. The cytoplasmic domain of CD19 has a positive regulatory effect on signalling through mIg (see text for further explanation).

tivity. ADCC can be a mechanism for removal of tumor cells and has been implicated in tissue damage that occurs in autoimmune diseases.

mechanism of downregulation of B-cell activation

The Fcγ receptor expressed on B-lymphocytes (FcγIIb) plays a role in downregulation of B-cell activation. When high IgG antibody concentrations are reached during an immune response, antigen-IgG complexes will be formed which can cross-link the BCR and FcγIIb on the surface of the B-lymphocyte (see also Fig. 5). The cytoplasmic domain of FcγIIb contains the YSLL motif, which has been termed ITIM for immunoreceptor tyrosine-based inhibitory motif. Tyrosine phosphorylation of this motif causes the association of a protein tyrosine phosphatase. When brought in close proximity to ITAMs, this enzyme causes tyrosine dephosphorylation and therefore inhibits BCR signaling. This mechanism, by which IgG antibodies interact with FcγIIb and co-cross-link with the BCR, is an example of active downregulation of the antibody response. There are other examples of cell surface receptors with either intrinsic (CD45) or associated protein tyrosine phosphatase activity (CD22), but their cellular ligands, and therefore their role in regulation of B-cell activation, are at present unknown.

Clinical relevance and future prospects

The integrity of the humoral immune system is crucial for host defence against bacterial and certain viral infections. Inborn or acquired deficiencies in humoral immunity result in increased susceptibility to potentially life-threatening infections. A dysregulated humoral immune system may result in conditions such as allergy. These and other clinical aspects are discussed elsewhere in this volume (see Chapters A8, A9, C3).

Most of what is known about the cellular and molecular aspects of B-lymphocyte activation and regulation has been gathered from experiments performed during the last decade. Detailed knowledge of the mechanisms that govern the regulation of expression of cell surface receptors and signalling mechanisms allows pharmacological intervention in antibody-mediated immunity. Intervention is possible at three levels: outside the B-lymphocyte, at the cell surface and intracellularly.

polysaccharide-protein conjugate vaccines

The coupling of polysaccharides to protein carriers changes the nature of the anti-polysaccharide antibody response from T-cell independent into T-cell-dependent. These polysaccharide-protein conjugate vaccines bypass the selective unresponsiveness to T-cell independent antigens early in life and thus constitute novel and effective tools in prevention of infectious diseases. Specific targeting of antigens to FcγIIb can be a very efficient way to induce B-lymphocyte unresponsiveness.

A second level of intervention is regulation of cell surface receptor expression. Substituted guanosines like 8-mercaptoguanosine cause increased expression of CD21 and thus could potentiate B-lymphocyte activation. The third level is intracellular intervention. Drugs with the ability to redirect intracellular signalling pathways are potentially powerful tools for enhancement or inhibition of B-lymphocyte activation.

Innate immunity: phagocytes, natural killer cells and the complement system

Dirk Roos, Hergen Spits and C. Erik Hack

In the second half of the 19th century Eli Metchnikoff discovered that bacteria can be ingested (phagocytosed) by leukocytes present in the blood of many different animals, including very primitive ones. At about the same time, Paul Ehrlich found that certain agents dissolved in blood had bactericidal potential. The scientific discussion on the importance of cellular versus humoral factors in our defence against bacteria came to an end when it was recognized that both components enforce each other's effect. In 1908, these scientists shared the Nobel Prize for physiology and medicine.

Further investigation about the nature and the working mechanism of the cells and proteins that consitute our immunological defence system showed that each of these components is made up of several different constituents. In its turn, this led to the insight that a functional differentiation must be made between the adaptive and innate branches of the immune system. The adaptive branch is executed by lymphocytes, i.e. white blood cells capable of generating antibodies against structures foreign to the body and of killing virus-infected cells. Lymphocytes are able to differentiate between structures that belong to the body and those that are alien. Moreover, these cells display immunological memory: once they have encountered foreign material previously, they will recognize and eliminate this material quicker upon subsequent encounters. This elimination is mainly the task of the innate immune system. This branch consists of phagocytes, natural killer cells and the complement system. Phagocytes are white blood cells capable of uptake (phagocytosis) and intracellular killing of microbes, especially after binding of antibodies and complement proteins to the surface of the microbes (Fig. 1). Natural killer (NK) cells are lymphocytes with cytotoxic potential against virus-infected and certain tumor-transformed cells. NK cells differ from cytotoxic T-lymphocytes in their human lymphocyte antigen (HLA)-independent manner of target-cell recognition. The complement system consists of a series of proteolytic enzymes capable of lysing microorganisms, often in an antibody-accelerated fashion. The activities of these in-

adaptive and innate immunology

phagocytes NK cells

complement system

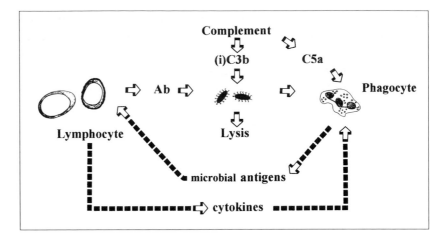

interactions

Figure 1 Interactions between the adaptive and the innate immune system
Microorganisms coated with antibodies and/or complement activation products are ingested, killed and degraded by phagocytes. Fragments of microbial proteins are presented to lymphocytes, which may lead to enhanced antibody production and release of cytokines that activate phagocytes. Other complement activation products (see Table 1) induce lysis of microorganisms and attraction of phagocytes to infected areas.

nate systems are tightly regulated because they are in principle also harmful to the host. This chapter will give a short description of each of the innate systems, their clinical relevance and the potential for therapy in case of failure.

Phagocytes

macrophages
granulocytes

Many cell types are capable – to some extent – of internalizing microorganisms, which sometimes leads to growth inhibition or even killing of the microbes. However, macrophages and granulocytes are the only "professional" phagocytes, because these cells are equipped with a motile apparatus for actively moving to sites of infection (except for organ-localized macrophages, the so-called histiocytes), with surface receptors to bind microorganisms, granules loaded with cytotoxic proteins and with an enzyme that can generate toxic oxygen radicals. Macrophages and granulocytes are formed in the bone marrow from pluripotent hematologic precursor cells, under the influence of growth and differentiation hormones. Macrophages are released into the blood, after about 10 days of development, as immature monocytes. These cells then move to the various tissues and organs, where they further differentiate into macrophages with site-specific characteristics. Granulocytes take about 14 days to develop, and are released as mature cells. Most granulocytes differentiate into neutrophilic granulocytes, cells with a high antimicrobial potential. Other granulocyte types are eosinophilic granulocytes, involved in antiparasite defence, and basophilic granulocytes, which lack the ability to phagocytose but can release histamine in inflammatory reactions. These cells also move into the tissues and organs. Macrophages have an estimated life span in the tissues of several months; neutrophilic granulocytes survive only 4–6 days after release from the bone marrow. Thus, neutrophilic granulocytes (neutrophils) need to be formed in much larger amounts than macrophages for efficient surveillance against microorganisms. Indeed, in healthy adults about 10^{11} neutrophils are released each day from the bone marrow, and this figure can increase 10-fold during infections. Macrophages are formed at not more than 10^9 per day. Phagocytes end their life either through necrosis as a result of phagocytosis and release of toxic mediators (pus formation) or through apoptosis (programmed cell death) and removal by macrophages.

neutrophils

turnover

The importance of phagocytes for host defence against microorganisms can be concluded from the recurrent, life-threatening infections of patients with a genetic or acquired shortage or deficiency of these cells. Patients with a shortage of phagocytes may be treated with growth factors, such as granulocyte colony-stimulating factor (G-CSF), at least when the receptors for such factors are present on the precursor cells. Complete cure may be obtained by bone marrow transplantation.

phagocytopenia

Movement

Neutrophils and monocytes have the ability to actively move to the site of an infection. This is caused by the release of so-called chemotaxins in these areas, small molecules of bacterial or host origin that diffuse into the surroundings and are bound to specific receptors on the phagocytes. The phagocytes are able to "sense" the concentration gradient of the chemotaxins and to move into the direction of the source of these agents until they have reached the site of infection. However, phagocytes in the blood must first pass the blood vessel wall before moving into the tissues. This process of diapedesis is initiated by reversible interaction of L-selectin, an adhesion protein on the surface of leukocytes, to sugar structures on endothelial blood vessel cells. Under normal conditions, this "rolling" of phagocytes over the endothelium leads to stable adhesion, spreading of the phagocytes on the vessel wall, diapedesis

chemotaxis

diapedesis

integrins

adhesion proteins

(transendothelial migration) and movement of the phagocytes into the tissues (Fig. 2). In infected or inflamed areas, these processes are strongly increased by the formation of complement fragment C5a, the bacterial tripeptide formyl-methionyl-leucyl-phenylalanine (fMLP), leukotriene LTB_4 and other chemotaxins. These agents cause an increase in expression of adhesion proteins on the surface of the phagocytes, such as β_1 and β_2 integrins. Moreover, the integrins are also "activated" by means of a change in their configuration, which causes stronger adhesion to endothelial structures. In addition, endotoxin, also generated in these areas, induces the local macrophages to produce interleukin-1 (IL-1) and tumor necrosis factor α (TNFα). Endotoxin, IL-1 and TNFα activate the local endothelial cells to upregulate the expression of intercellular adhesion molecule-1 (ICAM-1), E-selectin and vascular adhesion molecule-1 (VCAM-1), which strongly enhances phagocyte adhesion. Endothelial

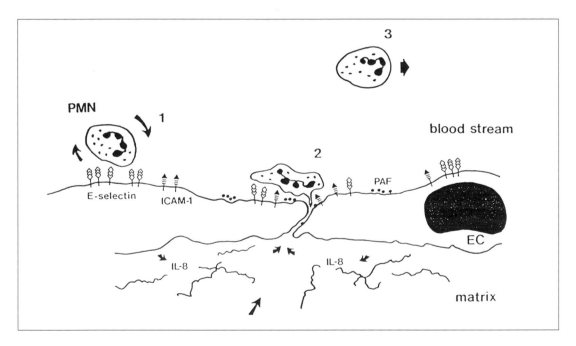

Figure 2 Schematic survey of phagocyte influx in tissues during inflammation [1]

Interaction of L-selectin on the phagocytes with carbohydrate structures on the endothelial cells, and of E-selectin on the endothelial cells with carbohydrate structures on the phagocytes, causes "rolling" of the phagocytes over the blood vessel wall (1). Upregulation and activation of integrins on the phagocytes induces stable binding of these molecules to ICAM-1, VCAM-1 and extracellular matrix proteins, which causes spreading of the phagocytes on the endothelium (2). PAF and IL-8, produced by the endothelium, then induce diapedesis of the phagocytes between two adjacent endothelial cells into the tissues. Phagocytes in the mainstream of the circulation are carried away in the blood (3).

cells also produce platelet-activating factor (PAF) and IL-8 under these conditions, which remain bound to the endothelial cells and stimulate phagocyte migration (Fig. 2). Changes in the composition of the extracellular matrix, induced by transforming growth factor β (TGFβ), and generation of additional chemokines by macrophages, endothelial cells and fibroblasts, add to the influx of phagocytes into inflamed tissues. This influx is phagocyte-specific, because the chemotaxins of the C-C chemokine family, of which monocyte chemotactic protein-1 (MCP-1) is the prototype, have specificity for monocytes and macrophages, whereas chemokines of the C-X-C family, such as IL-8, attract mainly neutrophils and eosinophils. In the tissues, the phagocytes migrate by local attachment to extracellular matrix proteins, propagation of the cell over this fixed area, attachment at another site and dissociation of the first bonds.

PAF

IL-8

chemokines

The biological significance of adherence and migration is clearly demonstrated by the clinical symptoms of patients with leukocyte adhesion deficiency (LAD), namely serious, recurrent bacterial infections, retarded wound healing, persistent leukocytosis and a strong deficiency in the generation of inflammatory reactions. The leukocytes from these patients lack the so-called β2-integrins, adhesion proteins involved in spreading of leukocytes on endothelial cells, in diapedesis and in migration in the tissues. In view of the high incidence of death in LAD patients, aggressive management of infections is indicated. The use of prophylactic treatment with trimethoprim-sulphamethoxazole appears to be beneficial. If a suitable donor is available, bone marrow transplantation is recommended.

LAD

Phagocytosis and killing of microorganisms

Phagocytes are specialized in uptake and intracellular killing of a large variety of bacteria, yeasts, fungi and mycoplasmata. Most microorganisms can only be ingested after being covered with specific antibodies and/or complement fragments (opsonization). Antibodies bind with their Fab regions to microbial antigens, which results in a spacial arrangement of the Fc regions that promotes activation of the classical complement pathway and fixation of fragments such as C3b and iC3b (see below and Fig. 1). The Fc regions of the antibodies and the complement fragments can then bind to Fc receptors and complement receptors, respectively, on the phagocyte surface. This binding of opsonized microorganisms to the phagocytes initiates three reactions in these cells: rearrangement of cytoskeletal elements that result in folding of the plasma membrane around the microbes, fusion of intracellular granules with this phagosome and

opsonization

phagocytosis

degranulation

superoxide

CGD

generation of reactive oxygen species within the phagosome (Fig. 3). The intracellular granules contain an array of microbicidal proteins, such as serine proteases, acid hydrolases, defensins, bactericidal permeability-increasing protein (BPI) and myeloperoxidase, as well as a number of microbistatic proteins, such as metalloproteases, lactoferrin and vitamin B^{12}-binding protein [2]. In neutrophils, these proteins are divided over two distinct types of granule, i.e. azurophil and specific granules, whereas in macrophages only one type of granule seems to be present. The action of these cytotoxic proteins is potentiated by the simultaneous release of superoxide in the immediate surroundings of the ingested microbes. This product of the nicotinamide adenine dinucleotide phosphate, reduced (NADPH) oxidase enzyme is spontaneously converted into hydrogen peroxide, which then reacts with chloride anions in a myeloperoxidase-catalyzed reaction to form hypochlorous acid (HOCl). This last product is very toxic to many bacteria, but is rather unstable. However, it can react with primary and secondary amines to form N-chloramines, which are as toxic as HOCl but much more stable.

The biological significance of the microbicidal apparatus of phagocytes is again illustrated by the consequences of its failure [3]. Patients with chronic granulomatous disease (CGD), whose phagocytes are un-

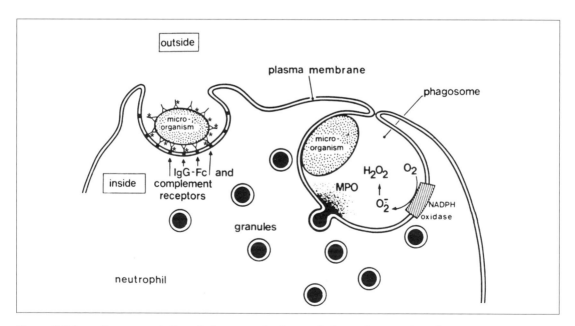

Figure 3 Schematic representation of phagocytosis, degranulation and generation of reactive oxygen products

MPO, myeloperoxidase; *, complement fragments C3b or iC3b.

able to generate superoxide, suffer already at an early age from very serious infections caused by catalase-positive microorganisms (catalase-negative organisms themselves secrete some hydrogen peroxide, which can be used by CGD phagocytes to kill these organisms). Patients with a deficiency of specific granules (a very rare disorder) suffer from recurrent infections with various microbes. Patients with the syndrome of Chédiak-Higashi are characterized by neutropenia and recurrent infections with purulent microorganisms. The phagocytes (and many other cell types) of these patients contain aggregated granules, which decrease cell mobility and degranulation. Infections in CGD and Chédiak-Higashi patients are treated with intravenous antibiotics and surgical drainage or removal of resistant infections. Prophylactic treatment with trimethoprim-sulfamethoxazole is very successful. In addition, prophylaxis with high doses of vitamin C in Chédiak-Higashi patients and with interferon γ (IFNγ) in CGD patients may also be beneficial. bone marrow transplantation, although hazardous, is at present the only curative therapy.

Chédiak-Higashi syndrome

Inflammatory reactions

Phagocytes are also involved in many inflammatory reactions, e.g. by presenting microbial antigens to lymphocytes, by releasing inflammatory mediators (chemotactic peptides, leukotrienes, cytokines) and by removing damaged host cells. Moreover, neutrophils also cause tissue damage, usually limited to the infectious period and intended to give the phagocytes access to the infectious agents. However, in chronically inflamed areas, such as those caused by autoimmune reactions, permanent macrophage activation will occur, and neutrophil influx and activation will continue. This will lead to excessive release of proteases from the neutrophils. Under normal conditions, these proteases are quickly inactivated by serine protease inhibitors (serpins) and α2-macroglobulin, which are abundantly present in plasma and tissue fluids. During neutrophil activation, however, reactive oxygen species and elastase released from these cells will inactivate these protease inhibitors. Moreover, the reactive oxygen compounds will also activate metalloprotease precursors, which will then degrade tissue matrix proteins [4]. When this process is not self-limited, irreversible tissue damage may result. In addition, serpins involved in regulating the complement, the coagulation, the fibrinolytic and the contact system cascades may also be inactivated, which will add to the severity of the clinical symptoms. Well-known clinical conditions in which this may happen are septic shock, gout, rheumatoid arthritis, autoimmune vasculitis, some types of glomerulonephritis,

inflammation

serpins

metalloproteases

adult respiratory distress syndrome, lung emphysema, acute myocardial infarction, burns, major trauma and pancreatitis. At present a number of clinical and experimental studies are being conducted to evaluate the benefit of agents that interfere with neutrophil and/or monocyte infiltration, activation or degranulation. These agents include, amongst others, monoclonal antibodies against adhesion molecules (CD18, CD11b, ICAM-1), oxygen radical scavengers and protease inhibitors.

Natural killer cells

NK cells

Natural killer (NK) cells were described for the first time 20 years ago. Operationally these cells were defined by their ability to kill certain tumor cells *in vitro* without having been in contact with these tumor cells before. Development of NK cells does not require gene rearrangements as is the case for T-cells, but NK cells are nonetheless closely related to T-cells (reviewed in [5]). The site of development of NK cells is still unknown. Cytokines are critical for development of NK cells both in humans and in mice. No NK cells are present in mice with a deficiency of

development

the gamma chain of the IL-2 receptor and in severe combined immunodeficiency patients with mutations in the IL-2R-γ chain. NK cells are implicated in innate immunity against parasites, intracellular bacteria and viruses [6]. They appear to be important in early phases of the immune response in which T-cells do not yet function. There is convincing evidence that, in humans, NK cells are involved in the defence against viral infections, in particular against herpes viruses [7]. The mechanisms by which NK cells mediate their effects in infections have not yet been fully elucidated, but it seems likely that cytokines are involved.

NK cells can mediate acute rejection of bone marrow grafts [8]. This is unlikely to be the "raison d'être" of NK cells; however, this phenomenon has led to the development of the concept that NK cells recognize

major histocompatibility complex (MHC)

cells that lack or have modified one or more self-MHC (major histocompatibility complex) class I antigens, which would explain why normal tissue is protected against NK-cell-mediated lytic activity [8].

Cytokine regulation of NK cells and the role of cytotoxicity mediated by NK cells in immunity against infections

cytokines

NK cells are intermingled in an intricate cytokine network; they respond to and produce cytokines that play a role in immunity against infections

[6, 7, 9]. NK cells respond in particular to IL-12 produced by infected monocytes and dendritic cells. IL-12 induces NK cells to produce IFNγ rapidly after infection [10]. IFNγ not only has antiviral effects itself but is also a strong inducer of IL-12 production. Moreover, it has been convincingly shown that IFNγ-activated macrophages are instrumental in the immune response against certain microorganisms such as *Listeria* monocytogenesis [11]. Furthermore, IL-12 plays an essential role in induction of Th1 cells (producing IFNγ but not IL-4). Thus, a complex interplay between dendritic cells, macrophages, NK and T-cells ensures high levels of production of IFNγ and IL-12, amplified through positive feedback loops. IL-10, a product of macrophages, lymphocytes and other cell types, is a strong negative regulator of IL-12 production by phagocytic cells and of IFNγ production by NK cells. IL-10 may be produced relatively late in an immune response, dampening the strong responses induced by IL-12 and IFNγ.

IL-12

IFNα

Activation of NK cells by viral and microbial infections enhances cytotoxic activity. This is mediated by IFNα/β, which are efficiently induced by viral infections. Some microbial infections, however, activate NK cytotoxicity without IFNα/β induction; this appears to be dependent on IL-12 and IFNγ. It is not clear whether NK cells use their cytotoxic potential in fighting off infections.

Recognition by NK cells

There are two mechanisms of cell-mediated cytolysis. One is mediated through perforin, a protein secreted by cytotoxic lymphocytes that forms pores in the membranes of target cells. Target cells can also be killed by an interaction of the Fas molecule on the target cell and its ligand on the cytotoxic cell. This interaction activates proteases in the target cell, resulting in apoptosis. Clearly NK cells mediate their cytotoxic effects predominantly by a perforin-dependent mechanism, because little NK activity is present in perforin-deficient mice [12]. The remaining NK activity is probably mediated by Fas/FasL interaction [13].

perforin

Fas/Fas ligand

The mechanism of NK cell recognition and the receptors involved have been elusive for a long time. Recent studies, however, have provided some insight into the complex way NK cells recognize their target cells. It is likely that NK cells do not have one single NK receptor that accounts for the biological responses such as cytokine production and cytotoxic activity. Rather, it seems that NK cells utilize a vast array of receptors that induce their effector functions. Monoclonal antibodies against many adhesion, activation or costimulatory molecules on NK

receptors

cells are able to activate these cells *in vitro*. These antigens include CD2, CD16, CD27, CD28, CD44, CD69, NKRP-1, LFA-1, DNAM-1 and others [14, 15]. However, whether NK cells use one or more of these receptors in the responses against infected cells or in graft rejection *in vivo* remains to be determined.

The strong cytotoxic activities of activated NK cells raise the question as to how normal tissue is protected from attack by these cells. A solution to this conundrum came from studies on the phenomenon of hybrid resistance [8]. It was recognized in 1979 that NK cells mediate hybrid resistance to bone marrow or tumor grafts. This is a situation in which bone marrow or tumor grafts of parental origin (either A or B) are rejected by AxB F1 hosts (A and B designate the MHC genotype). This resistance cannot be mediated by T-cells, because these cells are tolerant to the A and B MHC antigens of the parents. It is now clear that NK cells possess a sophisticated system of "inhibiting" receptors that accounts for their ability to reject bone marrow grafts that lack some MHC antigens present on the NK cells themselves. These inhibiting receptors interact with MHC antigens (Fig. 4). This feature of NK cells allows them to efficiently kill MHC class I-negative tumor cells and to remove infected cells with downregulated self-MHC. What is more important, this provides for a mechanism by which normal tissue is protected against cytolytic activity by autologous NK cells. One should assume that all NK cells express at least one receptor for self-MHC class I antigens.

Two groups of these inhibitory MHC binding receptors have now been identified [8]. One group consists of C-type lectin molecules and is exemplified by the Ly49 gene family in the mouse. Ly49A is the best-characterized gene and encodes a disulphide-bonded homodimer that binds to H-2D^k and D^k molecules. As a consequence, target cells that express these MHC antigens are not lysed by Ly49A-positive NK cells. The Ly49 family may comprise around 10 members with different, though overlapping, MHC specificities. Human homologs of Ly49 genes have not yet been identified. However, an inhibitory receptor has been found in humans consisting of a heterodimer of two C-type lectin antigens, namely CD94 and NKG2. Monoclonal antibodies against CD94 affect NK recognition of several human lymphocyte antigen (HLA)-A, -B and -C gene products. Thus, although Ly49 is not a homolog of CD94 or NKG2, both are C-lectin proteins and serve similar functions in rodents and humans.

In humans, a second group of inhibitory receptors appears to function on NK cells that are designated killer inhibitory receptors (KIRs). KIRs are involved in recognition of HLA-A, HLA-B and HLA-C. Unlike the Ly49 receptors, KIRs are type I glycoproteins. They are related to the immunoglobulin gene super-family and are probably encoded by a small

inhibiting receptors

lectins

KIRs

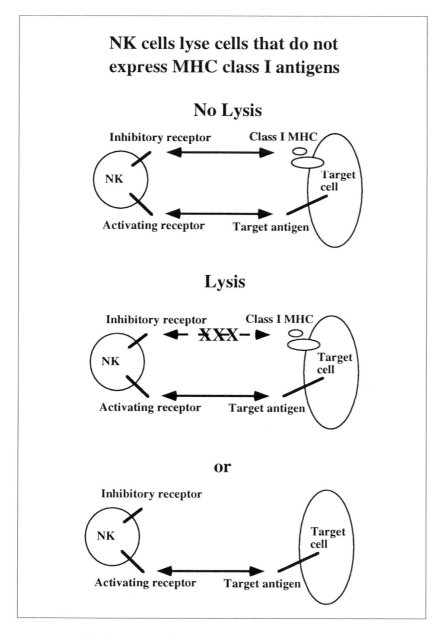

Figure 4 Model of regulation of NK activity by class I MHC-binding receptors
Lysis does not occur when an inhibitory receptor interacts with a class I MHC antigen on the target cell, despite the fact that a cytolysis-activating receptor also interacts with its ligand. NK cells lyse target cells when the interaction between the inhibitory receptor is not triggered, either because the receptor is not specific for the MHC antigen, when this interaction is blocked by antibodies, or when the target cell does not express class I MHC antigens at all.

number of genes. Three different protein isoforms have been described. The KIR recognizing HLA-B are proteins with three immunoglobulin-like domains, whereas HLA-C-binding KIRs have two immunoglobulin-binding domains. Certain KIRs reactive with HLA-A may have three immunoglobulin domains. KIRs with immunoglobulin gene similarity that bind to MHC class I antigens have not yet been found in mice.

The physiological role of these inhibitory MHC class I receptors in conventional immune responses in which NK cells play a role has yet to be elucidated. It is known that certain viruses have the capacity to down-regulate the synthesis of class I MHC antigens on the host cells. This may also hold for certain intracellular bacteria and parasites. It is possible that NK cells are specialized to screen infected cells for diminished levels of class I MHC antigens.

The complement system

complement

cascade

The complement system consists of about 20 proteins. Most of these proteins are synthesized in the liver and circulate in blood as inactive precursor proteins, also known as complement factors. In addition, some complement proteins are expressed as membrane proteins, which serve to dampen undesired activation on cell membranes. During activation, one factor activates the subsequent one by limited proteolysis and so on [16]. Because this activation process resembles a cascade, the complement system is considered to be one of the major plasma cascade systems, the other being the coagulation, fibrinolytic and contact systems. The physiological role of the complement system is to defend the body against invading microorganisms and to help in removing tissue debris.

Activation

classical pathway
alternative
pathway

mannan-binding
lectin pathway

The complement system can be activated via three pathways, namely a classical pathway consisting of the proteins, C1, C2 and C4; an alternative pathway consisting of factors B, D and P and the inhibitor factors H and I; and a so-called mannan-binding lectin pathway, which consists of mannan-binding protein, the recently discovered serine proteinases MASP-1 and MASP-2 (MASP stands for mannan-associated serine proteinase), and C4 and C2 [17]. The three pathways converge at the level of the third complement component, C3, to proceed as the common terminal pathway, which consists of C5, C6, C7, C8 and C9 (Fig. 5). Anti-

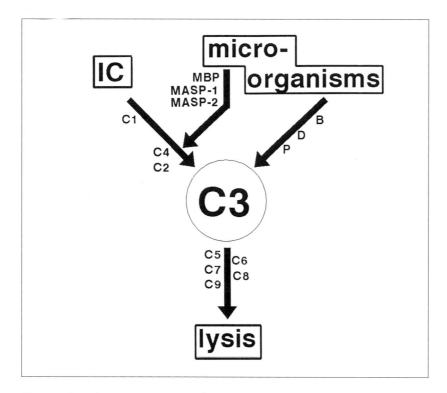

Figure 5 Complement activation pathways
The pathway starting with C1 is the classical pathway, that with MBP is the mannan-bind-
ing lectin pathway and that with factor B is the alternative pathway. Activation of the clas-
sical and mannan-binding lectin pathways is triggered by binding of C1q or mannan-
binding protein (MBP), respectively, to an activator [immune complexes (IC) or microor-
ganisms, respectively]. Initiation of alternative pathway activation is more complex and
involves interaction of a hydrolyzed form of C3 (not indicated in the figure), factors B and
D, factors I and H (not shown in the figure) and the activator. Classical and mannan-bind-
ing lectin pathways converge at the level of C4, which in turn converges with the alter-
native pathway at the level of C3.

gen-antibody (immune) complexes are considered to be the main activators of the classical pathway, and microbial surfaces as the main activators of the mannan-binding lectin and of the alternative pathway. In
addition, recent evidence suggests that also an acute-phase reactant,
C-reactive protein (CRP), may serve as an activator of the classical path-   **C-reactive protein**
way, in particular when bound to necrotic cells or tissue debris. During
activation some complement factors, in particular activated C3, stably
bind to the activator, thereby forming ligands for C3 receptors on phagocytic cells. In the event activation occurs at a cell membrane, the com-

pores

terminal complement complex

mon pathway proteins (C5 to C9) form macromolecular complexes that insert into the membrane as pores. Under normal conditions, the largest part of these transmembrane pores consists of polymerized C9, in addition to C5b, C6, C7 and C8. Insertion of complement pores into cell membranes will allow the exchange of ions and hence lysis of the cell. However, under some conditions complement pores do not lyse cells, but rather lead to signal transduction and hence to an altered activation state of the cell. In addition, complement pores may induce an exchange between phospholipids of outer and inner leaflet of the cell membrane (a so-called flip-flop).

Protection of cells against complement lysis

inhibition

PNH

Membranes of cells near to sites of complement activation may pick up activated complement fragments such as C3b or C5b-C9 complexes, thereby becoming targets of complement activation. To prevent lysis of innocent bystander cells, proteins are present in the membrane that inhibit complement activation at various levels. These proteins include the membrane regulatory protein decay-accelerating factor (DAF), membrane cofactor protein (MCP; not to be confused with the chemokine MCP) and C3b receptor (CR1), as well as homologous restriction factor (HRF) and membrane inhibitor of reactive lysis (CD59). DAF, MCP and CR1 prevent unwanted activation on membranes by inhibiting the assembly of C3 convertases and accelerating their decay. C3 convertases are macromolecular complexes formed during classical or alternative pathway activation that cleave and activate C3. HRF and CD59 inhibit complement lysis by interfering with the formation of C5b-C9 complexes. Several of these proteins, i.e. DAF, CD59 and HRF, are anchored to the cell membrane via a glycan linkage to phosphatidylinositol. This link is defective in the blood cells of patients suffering from paroxysmal nocturnal hemoglobinuria (PNH). Hence, the red cells of these patients have strongly reduced levels of these complement-inhibiting membrane proteins, and are therefore more susceptible to reactive complement lysis, which largely explains the clinical symptoms of PNH. Furthermore, reduction of membrane regulatory proteins has been found locally in the tissues in areas of complement activation, and this is assumed to contribute to complement-mediated tissue damage in inflammation. The mechanism of this reduced expression is not clear.

Biological effects

Activation of complement not only induces fixation of some complement proteins onto the activator, but also results in the generation of biologically active peptides and macromolecular complexes in the fluid phase [18]. Among these are C5a, C3a and C4a, which are released from C5, C3 and C4, respectively, during activation, and – because of their biological effects – are also known as the anaphylatoxins [19]. For example, C5a, the most potent anaphylatoxin, is chemotactic for neutrophils and able to induce aggregation, activation and degranulation of these cells. In addition, the anaphylatoxins may enhance vasopermeability, stimulate adhesion of neutrophils to endothelium, activate platelets and endothelial cells and induce degranulation of mast cells and the production of the vasoactive eicosanoid thromboxane A2 and the peptidoleukotrienes LTC_4, LTD_4 and LTE_4 by mononuclear cells. Moreover, they may stimulate or enhance the release of cytokines such as $TNF\alpha$ and IL-1 and -6 by mononuclear cells. Also the so-called terminal complement complexes (TCC) of C5b, C6, C7, C8 and C9 at sublytic concentrations induce cells to release mediators, such as cytokines, proteinases and eicosanoids. Finally, complement activation products may induce the expression of tissue factor by cells and thereby initiate and enhance coagulation. Thus, complement activation products have a number of biological effects that may induce and enhance inflammatory reactions (Table 1).

active peptides

anaphylatoxins

leukotriens

Table 1 Biological effects of complement activation products

complement activation products

Complement product	Effect
C5a	chemotaxis
C5a; C3a	mast cell degranulation
C5a; C3a	platelet degranulation
C5a	phagocyte degranulation
C5a	stimulation of O_2 metabolism phagocytes
C5a; C5b-9	enhancement of cytokine release
C5b-9; C5a?	expression of tissue factor
C5a; C5b-9	induction of prostaglandin and leukotriene synthesis
C3b; iC3b; C4b	opsonization of microorganisms
C5b-9	cell lysis
C3b	enhanced antibody response

Assays

The functional state of the complement system in patients can be assessed in various ways. The overall activity of the system can be measured by so-called CH50 and AP50 hemolytic assays. In these assays, antibody-sensitized erythrocytes (CH50) or nonsensitized rabbit erythrocytes (AP50) are incubated with dilutions of patient serum. Antibody-sensitized erythrocytes activate the classical pathway, nonsensitized rabbit erythrocytes the alternative pathway. The activity of the serum sample is then expressed in units, which is the reciprocal of the dilution of serum that lyses 50% of the erythrocytes. The CH50 assay measures the overall activity of classical and common pathways, the AP50 assay that of the alternative and the common pathways. A similar assay to assess the mannan-binding lectin pathway is not yet available. These hemolytic assays were the first to be applied in clinical studies. Decreased hemolytic activity of sera may occur during activation of complement in patients because activated complement factors are cleared from the circulation more rapidly than nonactivated (native) complement proteins. However, during an ongoing acute-phase reaction, a decrease in complement protein levels may be masked by increased synthesis. Immunochemical determination of individual complement proteins, for example by nephelometry, has now largely replaced CH50 and AP50 determinations, the more since the pattern of the relative decreases of complement proteins may provide important diagnostic and prognostic information. Nowadays CH50 and AP50 determinations should only be used to screen for the presence of genetic deficiencies. Deficiencies of the classical pathway will yield no activity in the CH50 assay; those of the alternative pathway lead to absence of AP50 activity. Deficiencies of C5 to C9 will yield zero activity in either assay. Activation of complement in patients can best be assessed by measuring levels of specific complement activation products, such as levels of the anaphylatoxins, in particular C3a, C3b, C4b or circulating C5b-C9 complexes. The availability of monoclonal antibodies specifically reacting with neo-epitopes exposed on activation products and not cross-reacting with the native protein has greatly facilitated the development of specific, sensitive and reproducible immunoassays for these activation products, which are now frequently used in clinical practice.

Clinical relevance

Genetic deficiencies of various complement proteins have been described. In general, total deficiencies of the classical pathway are associated with an increased risk for systemic lupus erythematosus (SLE). The reason for this association is not clear, although it has been suggested that classical pathway deficiencies may lead to defective handling of immune complexes, and hence to a greater tendency of immune complexes to become deposited into the tissues, where they may induce inflammatory reactions and tissue damage. Deficiencies of C3 are associated with recurrent infections by pyogenic microorganisms. Finally, deficiencies of C5 to C8 may lead to an increased risk for *Neisseria* infections. Surprisingly, C9 deficiencies are not associated with an increased risk for infections. Hence, opsonization of microorganisms by C3 is apparently essential for defence against pyogenic bacteria, whereas the formation of complement pores contributes to defence against *Neisseria*.

Activation of complement is considered to play an important role in the pathogenesis of a number of inflammatory disorders, including sepsis and septic shock, toxicity induced by the *in vivo* administration of cytokines or monoclonal antibodies, immune complex diseases such as rheumatoid arthritis, systemic lupus erythematosus and vasculitis, multiple trauma, ischemia-reperfusion injuries and myocardial infarction. The pathogenetic role of complement activation in these conditions is probably related somehow to the biological effects of its activation products (Table 1). Inhibition of complement activation may therefore be beneficial in these conditions, which is substantiated by observations in animal models. The availability of clinically applicable complement inhibitors may help in the treatment of these diseases.

As yet, only C1-esterase inhibitor, a major inhibitor of the classical pathway, is available for clinical use. This is largely due to the fact that a heterozygous deficiency state of this inhibitor is associated with the clinical picture of hereditary angioedema (HAE). This disease sometimes leads to the development of life-threatening edema of the glottis, which must be treated with intubation and the intravenous administration of C1 inhibitor. The pathogenesis of angioedema attacks associated with low C1-inhibitor levels is not completely clear but probably involves the generation of C2 peptide and bradykinin. The generation of these peptides results from the unopposed action of activated C1, activated factor XII and kallikrein of the contact system (C1 inhibitor is the main inhibitor of this system as well). Importantly, low levels of functional C1 inhibitor may be caused by a genetic defect but may also be acquired. Acquired C1-inhibitor deficiency is often associated with the presence of autoantibodies against C1 inhibitor, which cause an accelerated consumption of C1 inhibitor. These antibodies are usually produced by a malignant B-cell clone. HAE can be treated by attenuated androgens such as Danazol, antifibrinolytic agents or intravenously administered C1 inhibitor.

SLE

infections

sepsis

C1-esterase

HAE

Inflammatory mediators

Richard J. Gryglewski and Richard Korbut

Inflammation is a protective response of the macroorganism to injury caused by trauma, noxious chemicals or microbiological toxins. This response is intended to inactivate or destroy invading organisms, remove irritants and set the stage for tissue repair. The inflammatory response consists of immunological and nonimmunological reactions. The latter are triggered by the release from injured tissues and migrating cells of lipid-derived autacoids, such as eicosanoids or "platelet-activating factor" (PAF); large peptides, such as interleukin-1; small peptides, such as bradykinin; and amines, such as histamine or 5-hydroxytryptamine. These constitute the chemical network of the inflammatory response.

Eicosanoids

Eicosanoids encompass cyclic prostanoid structure, i.e. prostaglandins (PGs), prostacyclin (PGI$_2$), thromboxane A$_2$ (TXA$_2$) and straight-chain leukotriene structures (LTs), i.e. chemotactic LTB$_4$ and proinflammatory peptidolipids (LTC$_4$, LTD$_4$, LTE$_4$). These biologically active lipids are synthesized by cyclooxygenation (prostanoids) or lipoxygenation (leukotrienes) of a 20-carbon ω-6 polyunsaturated fatty acid (PUFA) – 5,8,11,14-eicosatetraenoic acid (AA, arachidonic acid) (Fig. 1). AA is an important structural constituent of cellular phospholipids, and first must be liberated by acyl hydrolases – directly by phospholipase A$_2$ (PLA$_2$) or indirectly by PLC before it becomes the substrate for the synthesis of eicosanoids.

5,8,11,14-eicosatetraenoic acid (AA, arachidonic acid)

Prostanoids

Prostaglandin H synthase (PGHS) is a dimeric complex which contains cyclooxygenase (COX) and peroxidase (Px). COX cyclizes AA to an un-

Prostaglandin H synthase (PGHS)

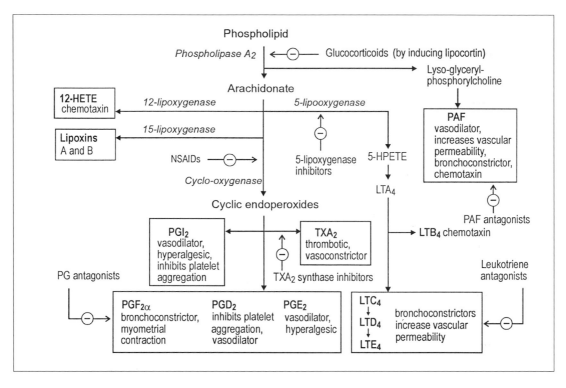

Figure 1 Mediators derived from phospholipids and their actions; the sites of action of antiinflammatory drugs

stable cyclic 15-hydroperoxy prostaglandin endoperoxide (PGG_2), whereas Px converts the 15-hydroperoxy to a 15-hydroxy group, in this way yielding PGH_2. Eventually, the end-product of PGHS (the complex which contains either constitutive COX-1 or inducible COX-2) is an unstable cyclic prostaglandin endoperoxide (PGH_2) which in various types of cells is converted by corresponding isomerases or synthases to stable prostanoids: PGD_2, PGE_2, $PGF_{2\alpha}$ and unstable prostanoids, i.e. PGI_2 or TXA_2. Special biological significance has been ascribed to PGI_2 synthase in vascular endothelial cells and TXA_2 synthase in blood platelets. The transcellular metabolism providing PGH_2 from activated platelets to endothelial cells is the main source of vascular PGI_2 [1]. The biological activity of stable prostanoids is terminated by catabolic enzymes, such as prostaglandin 15-hydroxy dehydrogenase (15-PGDH), Δ^{13}-reductase or α and ω oxidases which are present in high concentration in the lungs. These enzymes also break down inactive TXB_2 and 6-keto-$PGF_{1\alpha}$.

catabolic enzymes

Biosynthesis of prostanoids is initiated by transductional mechanisms in an immediate response to activation of various cell membrane receptors or to various physical and chemical stimuli. These procedures raise cytoplasmic levels of calcium ions $[Ca^{2+}]_i$, and in this way they activate acyl hydrolases which thereby release free AA for metabolism by PGHS. Alternatively, these enzymes can be induced by delayed transcriptional mechanisms which are usually activated by cytokines or bacterial toxins.

Most actions of prostanoids appear to be brought about by activation of the cell surface receptors that are coupled by G proteins to either adenylate cyclase (changes in intracellular cyclic adenosine monophosphate (c-AMP) levels) or PLC (changes in triphosphoinositol – IP_3 and diacylglycerol – DAG levels). The diversity of the effects of prostanoids is explained by the existence of a number of distinct receptors. The receptors have been divided into five main types, designated DP (PGD), FP (PGF), IP (PGI_2), TP (TXA_2) and EP (PGE). The EP receptors are subdivided further into EP_1 (smooth muscle contraction), EP_2 (smooth muscle relaxation), EP_3 and EP_4, on the basis of physiological and molecular cloning information [2, 3]. Subtype-selective receptor antagonists are under development. Only one gene for TP receptors has been identified, but multiple splice variants exist [4]. PGI_2 binds to IP receptors and activates adenylate cyclase. PGD_2 interacts with a distinct DP receptor that also stimulates adenylate cyclase. PGE_1 acts through IP receptors; PGE_2 activates EP receptors but it may also act on IP and DP receptors.

receptors

Products of lipoxygenation of AA

AA can be metabolized to straight–chain products by lipoxygenases (LOXs), which are a family of cytosolic enzymes that catalyze oxygenation of all polyenic fatty acids with two cis double bonds separated by a methylene group to corresponding lipid hydroperoxides [5] (Fig. 1). In the case of AA, these hydroperoxides are called hydroperoxyeicosatetraenoic acids (HPETE's). LOXs differ in their specificity for placing the hydroperoxy group; tissues differ in LOXs that they contain. Platelets have only 12-LOX and synthesize 12-HPETE, whereas leukocytes contain both 5-LOX and 12-LOX producing both 5-HPETE and 12-HPETE. HPETEs are unstable intermediates, analogous to PGG_2 or PGH_2, and are further transformed by peroxidases or nonenzymatically to their corresponding hydroxy fatty acids (HETE's). 12-HPETE can also undergo catalyzed molecular rearrangement to epoxy-hydroxyeicosatrienoic acids called *hepoxillins*. Leukocytes convert 15-HPETE to trihydroxylated derivatives called *lipoxins* (Fig. 1). At present there is preliminary evidence for the existence of conventional receptors for these substances. It is possible that some of these metabolites operate as intracellular second messengers.

**hydroperoxyeico-
satetraenoic acids
(HPETE's)**

**hepoxillins
lipoxins**

Leukotrienes

5-lipoxygenase-activating-protein (FLAP)

In activated leukocytes an increase in $[Ca^{2+}]_i$ binds 5-LOX to 5-lipoxygenase-activating-protein (FLAP), and this complex converts AA to 5-HPETE, which in turn is the substrate for LTA_4 synthase. In the course of transcellular metabolism between leukocytes and blood cells or endothelial cells unstable LTA_4 is converted by corresponding enzymes to stable chemotactic LTB_4 or to cytotoxic cysteinyl-containing leukotrienes – C_4, D_4, E_4 and F_4 (also referred to as sulphidopeptide leukotrienes or peptidolipids) [6] (Fig. 1). Note that the transcellular metabolism of AA

transcellular metabolism of AA

can bring about either "protection" as it is the case during the platelet/endothelium transfer of PGH_2 to make cytoprotective PGI_2 [1] or "damage" as in the case of the leukocyte/endothelium transfer of LTA_4 to make cytotoxic LTC_4 [6].

Consecutive splicing of amino acids from the glutathione moiety of LTC_4 occurs in the lungs, kidney and liver. LTE_4 is already substantially deprived of most of the biological activities of LTC_4 and LTD_4. Also, LTC_4 may be inactivated by oxidation of its cysteinyl sulfur atom to a sulfoxide group. The principal route of inactivation of LTB_4 is by ω-oxidation. LTC_4 and LTD_4 comprise an important endogenous bronchoconstrictor, earlier known as "slow-reacting substance of anaphylaxis" (SRS-A) [7].

receptors for LTs

Three distinct receptors have been identified for LTs (LTB_4, LTC_4 and LTD_4/LTE_4). Stimulation of all of them appears to activate PLC. LTB_4, acting on specific receptors, causes adherence, chemotaxis and activation of polymorphonuclear leukocytes and monocytes, as well as promoting cytokine production in macrophages and lymphocytes. Its potency is comparable to that of various chemotactic peptides and PAF. In higher concentrations, LTB_4 stimulates the aggregation of polymorphonuclear leukocytes (PMNs) and promotes degranulation and the generation of superoxide. It promotes adhesion of neutrophils to vascular endothelium and their transendothelial migration. The cysteinyl LTs are strongly cytotoxic, and cause bronchoconstriction and vasodilation in most vessels except the coronary vascular bed.

Other pathways of AA metabolism

monooxygenase pathway (MOX)

AA can be also metabolized by an NADPH-dependent cytochrome P-450-mediated monooxygenase pathway (MOX). The resulting 19-HETE, 20-HETE and a number of epoxyeicosatrienoic and dihydroxyeicosatrienoic acid isomers show vascular, endocrine, renal, and ocular effects, the physiological importance of which remains to be elucidated [8].

Recently, a nonenzymatic, free radical-mediated oxidation of AA while still embedded in phospholipids has been discovered. Subsequently, acyl hydrolases give rise to a novel series of regioisomers of *isoprostanes* [9]. Formed nonenzymatically, isoprostanes lack the stereospecificity of prostanoids, and consequently the relation between them resembles that of savage Mr. Hyde and his sophisticated prototype – Dr. Jekyll. Highly toxic isoprostanes might contribute to the pathophysiology of inflammatory responses which are insensitive to currently available steroidal and nonsteroidal antiinflammatory drugs. The most thoroughly investigated regioisomer of isoprostanes is 8-epi-$PGF_{2\alpha}$. It has a potent vasoconstrictor action which is mediated by vascular TXA_2/PGH_2 receptors.

isoprostanes

Actions and clinical uses of eicosanoids

Eicosanoids produce a vast array of biological effects. TXA_2, $PGF_{2\alpha}$ and LTs represent cytotoxic, proinflammatory mediators. TXA_2 is strongly thrombogenic through aggregation of blood platelets. LTC_4 injures blood vessels and bronchi subsequent to activation of leukocytes. On a molecular level, their cytotoxicity is frequently mediated by stimulation of PLC or inactivation of adenylate cyclase. Cytoprotective, but not necessarily antiinflammatory actions are mediated by PGE_2 and PGI_2. They are both naturally occurring vasodilators. PGI_2 is the most comprehensive antiplatelet agent which is responsible for the thromboresistance of the vascular wall. PGE_2 through a similar adenylate cyclase-dependent mechanism inhibits the activation of leukocytes. PGE_2 is also responsible for protection of the gastric mucosa. PGE_2 and $PGF_{2\alpha}$ may play a physiological role in labor and are sometimes used clinically as abortifacients. Locally generated PGE_2 and PGI_2 modulate vascular tone, and the imporatnce of their vasular actions is emphasized by the participation of PGE_2 and PGI_2 in hypotension associated with septic shock. These prostaglandins also have been implicated in maintaining of patency of the ductus arteriosus. Various prostaglandins and leukotrienes are prominent components released when sensitized lung tissue is challenged by the appropriate antigen. While both bronchodilator (PGE_2) and bronchoconstrictor ($PGF_{2\alpha}$, TXA_2, LTC_4) substances are released, responses to the peptidoleukotrienes probably dominate during allergic constriction of the airway. The relatively slow metabolism of the leukotrienes in lung tissue contributes to the long-lasting bronchoconstriction that follows challenge with antigen and may be a factor in the high bronchial tone that is observed in asthmatics in periods between attacks. Prostaglandins and leukotrienes contribute importantly to the genesis of the signs and symptoms of inflam-

protection of the gastric mucosa

septic shock

allergic constriction of the airway

vascular permeability

mation. The peptidoleukotrienes have effects on vascular permeability, whereas LTB_4 is a powerful chemoattractant for polymorphonuclear leukocytes and can promote exudation of plasma by mobilizing the source of additional inflammatory mediators. Prostaglandins do not appear to have any direct effect on vascular permeability; however, PGE_2 and PGI_2 markedly enhance edema formation and leukocyte infiltration by promoting blood flow in the inflamed region. PGEs inhibit the participation of lymphocytes in delayed hypersensitivity reactions. Bradykinin, cytokines (tumor necrosis factor (TNF)α, interleukin (IL)-1, IL-8) appear to liberate prostaglandins and probably other mediators that promote hyperalgesia and the pain of inflammation. Large doses of PGE_2 or $PGF_{2\alpha}$ given to women by intramuscular or subcuteneous injection to induce abortion cause intense local pain. Prostaglandins can also cause headache and vascular pain when infused intravenously. The capacity of prostaglandins to sensitize pain receptors to mechanical and chemical stimulation appears to result from a lowering of the threshold of the polymodal

hyperalgesia

nociceptors of C fibers. Hyperalgesia is also produced by LTB_4. When infused into the cerebral ventricles or when injected into the hypothalamus PGE_2 produces fever. The mechanizm of fever involves the enhanced formation of cytokines that increase the synthesis of PGE_2 in circumventricular organs in and near to the preoptic hypothalamic area, and PGE_2, via increases in c-AMP, triggers the hypothalamus to elevate body temeperature by promoting increases in heat generation and decreases in heat loss.

ductus arteriosus

Synthetic PGE_1, acting through IP and EP receptors, is given by infusion to maintain the patency of the ductus arteriosus in infants with transposition of large vessels until surgical correction can be undertaken. PGI_2 (epoprostenol) is occasionally used to prevent platelet aggregation in dialysis machines through inhibition of the thrombocytopenic action of heparin. PGI_2 is also used for the treatment of primary and sec-

pulmonary hypertension

ondary pulmonary hypertension. Stable analogues of PGI_2 (e.g. iloprost) as well as of PGE_1 are used in selected patients with peripheral vascular disease. The PGE_1 analogue, misoprostol is approved in the United States for the prevention of peptic ulcers, especially in patients who are required to take high doses of nonsteroidal antiinflammatory drugs (NSAIDs) for treatment of their arthritis.

Pharmacological interference with eicosanoid synthesis and actions

glucocortico-steroids

PLA_2 and COX are inhibited by drugs which are the mainstays in the treatment of inflammation. We discovered that glucocorticosteroids (hydrocortisone, dexamethasone) inhibit the generation of prostanoids *in vivo* through prevention of the release of AA from phospholipids [10]. This effect is mediated by intracellular steroid receptors which, when activated, increase expression of lipocortins which inhibit phospholipases. Presently, many other actions of glucocorticosteroids on AA metabolism are known, one of them being inhibition of COX-2 transcription.

Aspirin selectively inhibits COX-1, explaining its inhibitory effect on the biosynthesis of TXA_2 in platelets (causing reduced thrombotic tending) of PGI_2 in endothelial cells and of PGE_2 in gastric mucosa (leadins to gastric damage). This action of aspirin is more pronounced than that on the biosynthesis of prostanoids at the site of inflammation, where inducible COX-2 is most active. Consequently, aspirin at low doses seems to be a better antithrombotic than antiinflammatory drug. Aspirin irreversibly acetylates the active centre of COX-1. Unlike endothelial cells, platelets lack the machinery required for *de novo* synthesis of COX-1, and accordingly, aspirin-induced inhibition of TXA_2 synthesis in platelets is essentially permanent (until new platelets are formed), in contrast to the easily reversible inhibition of PGI_2 synthesis in vascular endothelium. The net effect of aspirin is, therefore, a long-lasting antithrombotic action. Unfortunately, most NSAIDs are more effective inhibitors of COX-1 than of COX-2. Meloxicam is the first clinically available drug which is claimed to be a selective COX-2 inhibitor – an antiinflammatory drug with few side effects on the gastrointestinal tract, which causes no bleeding. NSAIDs are usually classified as mild analgesics, and they are particularly effective in settings in which inflammation has caused sensitization of pain receptors to normally painless mechanical or chemical stimuli. NSAIDs do not inhibit fever caused by direct administration of prostaglandins, but they do inhibit fever caused by agents that enhance the synthesis of IL-1 and other cytokines, which presumably cause fever at least in part by inducing the endogenous synthesis of prostaglandins.

Aspirin

antithrombic

Platelet-activating factor (PAF)

PAF (1-*O*-alkyl-2-acetyl-*sn*-glycero-3-phosphocholine) is a specialized phospholipid with an alkyl group (12-18C) attached by an ether bond at position 1 of glycerol and acetylated at position 2. PAF is not stored in cells but it is synthesized from 1-*O*-alkyl-2-acylglycerophosphocholine as required (Fig. 2). Intially, PLA_2 converts the precursor to the inactive 1-*O*-alkyl-2-lysoglycerophosphocholine (lyso-PAF) with concomitant release of AA [11]. Incidentally, in granulocytes, AA produced in this way represents a major source for the synthesis of PGs and LTA_4. In a second step, lyso-PAF is acetylated by acetyl coenzyme A in a reaction catalyzed by lyso-PAF acetyltransferase. This is the rate-limiting step. The synthesis of PAF in different cells is stimulated during antigen-antibody reactions or by chemotactic peptides (e.g. f-MLP), cytokines, thrombin, collagen and autacoids. PAF can also stimulate its own formation. Both PLA_2 and lyso-PAF acetyltransferase are calcium-dependent enzymes, and PAF synthesis is regulated by the availability of Ca^{2+}. The antiinflammatory action of glucocorticosteroids is at least partially dependent on inhibition of the synthesis of PAF by virtue of the inhibitory effect of lipocortin on the activity of PLA_2.

glucocortico-steroids

inactivation of PAF

Inactivation of PAF also occurs in two steps [12] (Fig. 2). Initially, the acetyl group of PAF is removed by PAF acetylhydrolase to form lyso-PAF; this enzyme is present in both cells and plasma. Lyso-PAF is then converted to a 1-O-alkyl-2-acyl-glycerophosphocholine by an acyltransferase. This latter step is inhibited by Ca^{2+}.

PAF is synthesized by platelets, neutrophils, monocytes, mast cells, eosinophils, renal mesangial cells, renal medullary cells and vascular endothelial cells. In most instances, stimulation of the synthesis of PAF re-

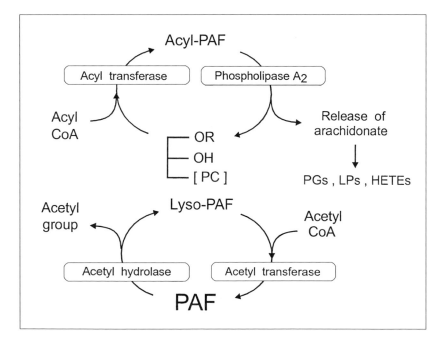

Figure 2 The synthesis and metabolism of PAF
PC, phosphorylcholine.

sults in the release of PAF and lyso-PAF from the cell. However, in some cells (e.g. endothelial cells) PAF is not released and appears to exert its effects intracellularly [13].

PAF exerts its actions by stimulating G protein-linked, cell-surface receptors. High-affinity binding sites have been detected in the plasma membranes of a number of cell types [14]. Stimulation of these receptors triggers activation of phospholipases C, D and A_2, and mobilization of $[Ca^{2+}]_i$. Massive direct and indirect release of AA occurs with its subsequent conversion to PGs, TXA_2 or LTs. Eicosanoids seem to function as extracellular representatives of the PAF message. As its name suggests, PAF unmasks fibrinogen receptors on platelet, leading directly to platelet aggregation. In endothelial cells the synthesis of PAF may be stimulated by a variety of factors, but PAF is not released extracellularly [13]. Accumulation of PAF intracellularly is associated with the adhesion of neutrophils to the surface of the endothelial cells and their diapedesis, apparently because it promotes the expression or exposure of surface proteins that recognize and bind neutrophils. Activated endothelial cells play a key role in "targeting" circulating cells to inflammatory sites. Expression of the various adhesion molecules varies among different cell types involved in the inflammatory response. For example, expression of E-selectin is restricted primarily to endothelial cells and is enhanced at sites of inflammation. P-selectin is expressed predominantly on platelets and on endothelial cells. L-selectin is expressed on leukocytes and is shed when these cells are activated. Cell adhesion appears to occur by recognition of cell surface glycoprotein and carbohydrates on circulating cells by the adhesion molecules whose expression has been enhanced on resident cells. Endothelial activation results in adhesion of leukocytes by their interaction with newly expressed L-selectin and P-selectin, whereas endothelial-expressed E-selectin interacts with glycoproteins on the leukocyte surface; endothelial ICAM-1 interacts with leucocyte integrins.

expression of the various adhesion molecules

PAF also increases vascular permeability. As with substances such as histamine and bradykinin, the increase in permeability is due to contraction of venular endothelial cells, but PAF is 1000-fold more potent than histamine or bradykinin.

Intradermal injection of PAF duplicates many of the signs and symptoms of inflammation, including vasodilation, increased vascular permeability, hyperalgesia, edema and infiltration of neutrophils. Inhaled PAF induces bronchoconstriction, promotes local edema accumulation of eosinophils and stimulates secretion of mucus. In anaphylactic shock, the plasma concentration of PAF is high, and the administration of PAF reproduces many of the signs and symptoms of experimental anaphylactic shock. PAF receptor antagonists prevent the development of pulmonary hypertension in experimental septic shock. Despite the broad implications of these experimental observations, the clinical effects of PAF antagonists in the treatment of bronchial asthma, septic shock and other inflammatory responses have been rather modest.

ginkgoloids from
Ginkgo biloba

PAF receptor antagonists [15] include PAF structural analogues, natural products (e.g. ginkgoloids from *Ginkgo biloba*), and interestingly, triazolobenzodiazepines (e.g. triazolam). The development of PAF receptor antagonists is at an early stage, still leaving the hope that such antagonists may find future therapeutic application.

Cytokines

Cytokines are peptides produced mainly by macrophages and lymphocytes (lymphokines) but also by other leukocytes, endothelial cells and fibroblasts. Cytokines act as regulators of inflammatory and immune reactions; some are involved in multiplication and differentiation of cells and in repair processes. Substances considered as cytokines include interleukins 1 to 12, interferons, tumour necrosis factors (TNF), platelet-derived growth factor (PDGF), transforming growth factor-β, chemokines (chemotactic for leukocytes) and the colony-stimulating factors. Cytokines which are thought to be of particular importance in inflammatory and immune responses include the interleukin-1 (IL-1) family, the interferons and the colony-stimulating factors see (Chapter A4).

Interleukin-1 is the term given to a family of three cytokines consisting of two active, *agonist* agents, IL-1α, IL-1β and an endogenous IL-1-receptor antagonist (IL-1ra) which has been recently cloned. IL-1α remains cell-associated and is active mainly during cell-to-cell contact, whereas the soluble IL-1β is a form predominant in biological fluids. IL-1 is an important inflammatory mediator and it is believed to be implicated in several acute (e.g. systemic inflammatory response syndrome – SIRS – in sepsis) or chronic (e.g. rheumatoid arthritis) inflammatory dis-

immune response

eases. IL-1 is also important in immune responses, facilitating interaction of both B- or T-cells with antigen.

vascular
endothelial cells

In vascular endothelial cells, IL-1 increases synthesis of leukocyte adherence factors, stimulates nitric oxide production, releases PDGF, and activates PLA$_2$, thus inducing the synthesis of prostanoids and PAF. It stimulates fibroblasts to proliferate, to synthesize collagen and to generate collagenase. It regulates the systemic inflammatory response by stim-

systemic inflam-
matory response

ulating synthesis of acute phase proteins, producing neutrophilia, and causing fever by altering a set point of temperature in the hypothalamus.

IL-1 induces the generation of other cytokines such as IL-2, the interferons, IL-3, IL-6 and, in bone marrow, the colony-stimulating factors. It synergizes with TNFα in many of its actions, and its synthesis is stimulated by TNFα [16]. The therapeutic effects of glucocorticoids in rheumatoid arthritis and other chronic inflammatory and autoimmune diseases may well involve inhibition of both IL-1 production and IL-1 activity.

glucocorticoids

inhibition of both IL-1 production and IL-1 activity

TNFα and -β. In endothelial cells those cytokines induce: synthesis of prostacyclin, expression of adhesion molecules and synthesis of cytokines; they are chemotactic for neutrophils and macrophages; TNFα causes fever and releases acute-phase proteins. TNF and IL-1 produce many of the same proinflammatory responses which include induction of cyclooxygenase and lipoxygenase enzymes as well as the activation of B-cells and T-cells

TGFα is a trophic regulator of cell proliferation and differentiation which is important in repair processes; it is involved in angiogenesis and in the organization of extracellular matrix; it is chemotactic for monocytes.

PDGFs cause proliferation of fibroblasts, vascular endothelial cells and smooth muscle; they are implicated in angiogenesis, atherosclerosis and possibly in chronic asthma.

Interferons consitute a group of inducible cytokines that are synthesized in response to viral and other stimuli. There are three classes of interferons (IFNs), termed IFNα, IFNβ and IFNγ. IFNα is not a single substance but a family of 15 proteins with similar activities. The three IFNs (α, β and γ) have antiviral activity, and IFNγ has significant immunoregulatory function. All interferons can be induced by other cytokines such as IL-1, IL-2, TNF and colony-stimulating factors. IFNα and IFNβ are produced in many cell types – macrophages, fibroblasts, endothelial cells, osteoblasts and so on – being strongly induced by viruses, and less strongly by other microorganisms and bacterial products. Interferons induce the expression of MHC class I and II molecules, which are involved in antigen presentation to T-cells. Interferons also stimulate the expression of Fc receptors on granulocytes, promote the differentiation of myeloid cells and modulate the synthesis of cytokines.

GM-CSF (granulocyte-macrophage colony-stimulating factor) regulates hemopoiesis, is chemotactic for neutrophils, and activates neutrophils and macrophages.

MIP-1α (monocyte-inflammatory protein-1α), *MCPs* (monocyte chemotactic proteins) and *RANTES* (regulated upon activation, normal T-cell expressed and secreted!) are members of the family of β-*chemokines*. They are chemotactic for basophils and monocytes, which enter the area several hours after neutrophils. MIP-1α is also chemotactic for lymphocytes. *RANTES* is chemotactic for memory lymphocytes, monocytes and eosinophils.

Neuropeptides

Neuropeptides are released from sensory neurons and in some tissues they contribute to inflammatory reactions. For example, substance P and other tachykinins produce smooth muscle contraction, mucus secretion, cause vasodilation and increase vascular permeability. Calcitonin gene-related peptide (CGRP) is a potent vasodilator, acting on CGRP receptors leading to activation of adenylate cyclase. The overall pattern of effects of tachykinins is similar, though not identical, to the pattern seen with kinins.

Tachykinins

tachykinin receptor

The mammalian tachykinins comprise three related peptides: substance P (SP), neurokinin A (NKA) also called substance K, and neurokinin B (NKB). They occur mainly in the nervous system, particularly in nociceptive sensory neurons and in enteric neurons. They are released as neurotransmitters, often in combination with other mediators. SP and NKA are encoded by the same gene, and they have a similar distribution. Three distinct types of tachykinin receptor are known: NK_1, NK_2 and NK_3. They are selective for three endogenous tachykinins with the following affinity: SP > NKA > NKB for NK_1, NKA > NKB > SP for NK_2 and NKB > NKA > SP for NK_3 receptor. Receptor cloning has shown that tachykinin receptors belong to a family of G protein-coupled receptors. Several potent antagonists of NK_1 and NK_2 receptors have been discovered recently [17], and novel therapeutic agents for various disease states (e.g. pain, asthma, arthritis, headache) may be developed.

CGRP differs from other tachykinins. It is coded for by the calcitonin gene which also codes for calcitonin itself. Differential splicing allows cells to produce either procalcitonin (expressed in thyroid cells) or pro-CGRP (expressed in neurons) from the same gene. CGRP is found in nonmyelinated sensory neurons and it is a potent inducer of neurogenic inflammation.

Kinins

Kinins are polypeptides with vasodilator/hypotensive, thrombolytic, proinflammatory and algesic actions. The two best known kinins are bradykinin and kallidin, and they are referred to as plasma kinins. Since 1980, when Regoli and Barabe divided the kinin-receptors into B_1 and B_2 classes, first- and second-generation kinin receptor antagonists have been developed, leading to a much better understanding of the actions of kinins.

Bradykinin is a nonapeptide; kallidin is a decapeptide and has an additional lysine residue at the amino-terminal position. These two peptides are formed from a class of α-2 globulins known as *kininogens* (Fig. 3). There are two *kininogens*: high molecular weight (*HMW*) and low molecular weight (*LMW*) kininogen which are products of a single gene that arises by alternative processing of messenger RNA (mRNA). The highly specific proteases that release bradykinin and kallidin from the kininogens are termed *kallikreins*. Two distinct kallikreins, formed by different activation mechanisms from inactive *prekallikreins*, act on the kininogens. One of these is plasma kallikrein and the other is tissue kallikrein. LMW kininogen is a substrate only for the tissue kallikrein and the product is kallidin, whereas HMW kininogen is cleaved by plasma and tissue kallikrein to yield bradykinin and kallidin, respectively. Kallidin is similar in activity to bradykinin and need not be converted to the latter to exert its effects. However, some conversion of kallidin to bradykinin occurs in plasma due to the activity of plasma aminopeptides.

bradykinin
kallidin
kininogens

The half-life of kinins in plasma is about 15 s and concentrations of kinins found in the circulation are within the picomolar range. Bradykinin is inactivated by a group of enzymes known as *kininases*. The major catabolizing enzyme in the lung and in other vascular beds is *kininase II*, which is identical to peptidyl dipeptidase – known as angiotensin-converting enzyme (ACE). *Kininase II* is inhibited by captopril, resulting in an increased concentration of circulating bradykinin, which contributes substantially to the antihypertensive effect of captopril. On the other hand, *kininase I* is arginine carboxypeptidase, and it has a slower action than *kininase II*. It removes the carboxyl-terminal arginine residue, producing des-Arg^9-bradykinin or des-Arg^{10}-kallidin, which are themselves potent B_1-kinin receptor agonists.

kininases

There are at least two distinct receptors for kinins: B_1 and B_2. The classical, enestitutive bradykinin receptor, now designated the B_2 receptor, selectively binds bradykinin and kallidin and mediates a majority of the effects of bradykinin and kallidin in the absence of inflammation,

receptors for kinins: B_1 and B_2

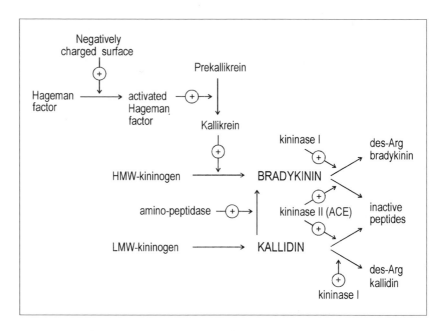

Figure 3 The formation and metabolism of kinins

such as the release of PGI_2 and NO from endothelial cells. On the other hand, inducible B_1 receptors are upregulated by inflammation. They bind des-Arg metabolites of bradykinin and kallidin. In contrast to B_1 receptors, the signalling mechanism of B_2 receptors has been well characterized. The B_2 receptor is coupled to G protein and activates both PLA_2 and PLC. Whereas stimulation of the former liberates AA from phospholipids, with its subsequent oxidation to a variety of proinflammatory eicosanoids, the activation of PLC through IP_3 and DAG leads directly to proinflammatory effects.

During the last decade the existence of other types of kinin receptors (B_3, B_4, B_5) has been suggested. However, recent studies indicate that some of them may actually represent functions of the B_2 receptor [18].

vasodilators

Kinins are among the most potent vasodilators known, acting on arteriolar beds of the heart, liver, skeletal muscle, kidney, intestines and ovaries. They are claimed to play a minor role in the regulation of blood pressure in health individuals, but they play a major vasodepressor regulatory role most likely mediated by arterial endothelium in hypertensive patients [19]. Indeed, kinins contract veins and nonvascular smooth muscle, such as gastrointestinal and bronchial muscle. Bradykinin and kallidin have similar contracting properties. At the level of the capillary circulation kinins increase permeability and produce edema. Stimulation of B_1 re-

hypertensive patients

ceptors on inflammatory cells such as macrophages can elicit the production of the inflammatory mediators such as IL-1 and TNFα [20]. Kinins are also potent pain-inducing agents in both the viscera and skin. In acute pain, B_2 receptors mediate bradykinin algesia. The pain of chronic inflammation appears to involve an increased expression of B_1 receptors.

pain-inducing agents

As in the case of other autacoids, the therapeutic interest in kinins has focused particularly on attempts to modulate their formation or metabolism *in vivo*. Blockade of kinin formation with a kallikrein inhibitor, aprotynin (Trasylol), has been used with some success to treat acute pancreatitis, carcinoid syndrome or Crohn's disease. Experimentally, progress has been made in the development of selective antagonists of kinins. They are not currently available for clinical use; however, recent studies indicate that kinin receptor antagonists might be useful for the treatment of patients with septic shock [21], pancreatitis-induced hypotension [22], bronchial asthma, rhinovirus-induced symptoms and in fighting pain.

blockade of kinin formation

Nitric oxide

In animal tissues, nitric oxide (NO) is generated enzymatically by synthases (NOS). The three NOS isoenzymes (neuronal, endothelial and inducible) are flavoproteins which contain tetrahydrobiopterin and heme, and they are homologous with cytochrome P-450 reductase. Isoenzymes of NOS act as dioxygenases using molecular oxygen and NADPH to transform L-arginine to L-citrulline and NO (Fig. 4). NO formed by endothelial constitutive NOS (ecNOS) is responsible for maintaining low vascular tone and preventing leukocytes and platelets from adhering to the vascular wall. ecNOS is also found in renal mesangial cells. NO formed by neuronal constitutive NOS (ncNOS) acts as a neuromodulator or neuromediator in some central neurons and in peripheral "nonadrenergic noncholinergic" (NANC) nerve endings. NO formed by inducible NOS (iNOS) in macrophages and other cells plays a role in the inflammatory response.

isoenzymes of NOS

nonadrenergic noncholinergic (NANC) nerve endings

NO was discovered by Furchgott and Zawadzki [23] as "endothelium-derived relaxing factor" (EDRF). It soon became obvious that EDRF, like nitroglycerin, activates soluble guanylate cyclase in vascular smooth muscle by binding to its active heme centre. The rise in cyclic GMP achieved is responsible for vasodilation and for other physiological regulatory functions of NO.

The activities of constitutive ncNOS and ecNOS are controlled by intracellular calcium/calmodulin levels. For instance, ncNOS in central

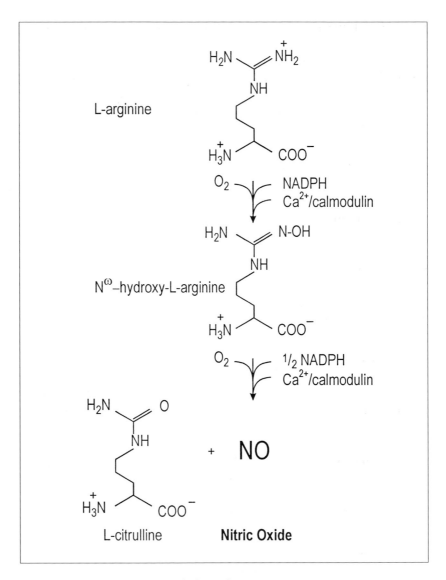

Figure 4 The synthesis and metabolism of NO

neurons is activated by glutamate binding to N-methyl-d-aspartate (NMDA) receptors with a subsequent rise in $[Ca^{2+}]_i$ due to opening of voltage calcium channels, whereas ecNOS is activated by blood shear stress or stimulation of endothelial muscarinic, purinergic, kinin, substance P or thrombin receptors. This triggers an increase in $[Ca^{2+}]_i$ at the expense of the release of Ca^{2+} from endoplasmic reticulum. Calcium ionophores (e.g. A23187) and polycations (e.g. poLy-L-lysine) cause a rise in $[Ca^{2+}]_i$ and activate ecNOS, thereby bypassing the receptor mechanisms.

In contrast to the constitutive isoforms of NOS, iNOS does not require a rise in $[Ca^{2+}]_i$ to initiate its activity. In macrophages, monocytes and other cells the induction of iNOS and the presence of L-arginine are sufficient to initiate the generation of NO. Induction of iNOS can be initiated by IFNγ, TNFα or IL-1β. However, the best-recognized inducer is lipopolysaccharide (LPS) or endotoxin from *Escherichia coli* which is known to be responsible for the development of SIRS in the course of sepsis due to Gram-negative bacteria. Myeloid cells have a receptor for LPS on their cell membrane, m-CD14 protein. LPS, using an LPS binding protein (LBP), is anchored to m-CD14 and then triggers a chain of protein phosphorylation which eventually leads to the activation of the major transcription protein NF-κ-B. This is responsible for transcription of the message: to make iNOS. In cells which lack m-CD14, the induction of iNOS is completed by a complex of soluble s-CD14 with LBP and LPS itself. In a similar manner, LPS can also induce COX-2. Although NO fulfills more paracrine than autoendocrine functions, in the case of iNOS large amounts of locally formed NO may inhibit iNOS itself as well as COX-2 in a negative feedback reaction. Glucocorticosteroids and some cytokines, such as TGFβ, IL-4 or IL-10, inhibit the induction of iNOS.

During the course of an inflammatory response, the large amounts of NO formed by iNOS surpass the physiological amounts of NO which are usually made by ncNOS or ecNOS. The functions of i-NOS-derived NO are also different. In immunologically or chemically activated macrophages, NO kills microorganisms and destroy macromolecules. NO formed by constitutive isoforms of NOS is stored as a nitrosothiol in albumin and acts physiologically as *N*-nitrosoglutathione and *N*-nitrosocysteine. Eventually, within a few seconds, NO is oxidized to nitrites or nitrates. Large amounts of "inflammatory NO" from myeloid cells are usually generated side by side with large amounts of superoxide anion (O_2^-). These two can form peroxynitrite ($ONOO^-$), a "smart bomb" which mediates the cytotoxic effects of NO, such as DNA damage, low density lipoproteins (LDL) oxidation, isoprostane formation, tyrosine nitration, inhibition of aconitase and mitochondrial respiration. The discovery of thin reaction lends new support to the therapeutic use of superoxide dismutase (SOD). Interestingly, overstimulation of NMDA receptors by glutamate may activate ncNOS to such an extent that NO itself exerts neurotoxic properties. NO formed by ecNOS seems to be mostly cytoprotective, possibly due to its unusual redox properties [24].

NO is scavenged by hemoglobin, methylene blue and pyocyanin from *Pseudomonas coereleus*. These last two are also claimed to be inhibitors

m-CD14 protein

N-**nitrosoglutathione**
N-**nitrosocysteine**

peroxynitrite
($ONOO^-$)

glucocorticoids
L-NMMa
L-NAME

of guanylate cyclase. Glucocorticoids selectively inhibit the expression of iNOS. Arginine analogues, such as L-N^G-monomethyl arginine (L-NMMA) and L-N^G-nitro-arginine methyl ester (L-NAME) inhibit inducible and constitutive NOS isoforms nonselectively. Selective iNOS inhibitors (e.g. alkylisothioureas or aminoguanidines) are being intensively investigated in the hope that selective inhibition of iNOS may prevent development of SIRS or MODS (multiple organ disfunction syndrome). Indeed, overproduction of NO by iNOS during septicemia is claimed to be responsible for irreversible arterial hypotension, vasoplegia (loss of responses to noradrenaline), lactic acidosis, suffocation of tissues, their necrosis and apoptosis. However, it is important to remember that NO made by iNOS is of benefit to the host defence reaction by contributing to microbial killing. Moreover, NO generated by ecNOS is essential to maintain tissue perfusion with blood, to offer cytoprotection in the pulmonary and coronary circulation against toxic lipids which are released by LPS and to preserve red cell deformability which becomes reduced in septicemia. Preliminary clinical experience with L-NMMA has been reasonably encouraging, as long as a low dose of the NOS inhibitor is used.

endotoxic shock

In animal models of endotoxic shock, nonselective NOS inhibitors were reported to decrease cardiac output, to increase pulmonary pressure, to decrease nutritional flow to organs, to damage gastric mucosa and to increase mortality rate. On the other hand, inhalation of NO gas (10 ppm) in septic patients has been found to prevent the mismatch of the ventilation/perfusion ratio in their lungs. The exact role of NO in various stages of sepsis, SIRS and MODS still awaits elucidation and evaluation.

Amines

Histamine, 2-(4-imidazolyl)ethylamine, is an essential biological amine in inflammation and allergy. It is found mostly in the lung, skin and in the gastrointestinal tract. It is stored together with macroheparin in granules of mastocytes or basophils (0.01–0.2 pmol per cell), from which it is released when complement components C3a and C5a interact with specific receptors, or when antigen interacts with cell-fixed immunoglobulin E (IgE). These trigger a secretory process that is initiated by a rise in cytoplasmic Ca^{2+} from intracellular stores. Morphine and tubocurarine release histamine by a nonreceptor action. Agents which increase cAMP formation inhibit histamine secretion, so it is postulated that, in these cells, c-AMP-dependent protein kinase is an intracellular restraining mechanism. Replenishment of the histamine content of mast cell or basophil after secretion is a slow process, whereas turnover of histamine in the gastric histaminocyte is very rapid.

Histamine is synthesized from histidine by a specific decarboxylase and metabolized by histaminase and/or by imidazole N-methyltransferase. Histamine exerts its effects by acting on H_1, H_2 or H_3 receptors on target cells. It stimulates gastric secretion (H_2), contracts most of the smooth muscle other than that of blood vessels (H_1), causes vasodilation (H_1) and increases vascular permeability by acting on the postacapillary venules. Injected intradermally, histamine causes the triple response: local vasodilation and wheal by a direct action on blood vessels and the surrounding flare which is due to vasodilation resulting from an axon reflex in sensory nerves, thereby releasing a peptide mediator. Of the many functions of histamine, the stimulation of gastric acid secretion and mediatian of type 1 hypersensitivity, such as urticaria and hay fever, are among the most important. The full physiological significance of the H_3 receptor has yet to be established [16] (see also Chapter A9).

H_1, H_2 or H_3 receptors

5-hydroxytryptamine (*5-HT, serotonin*) was originally isolated and characterized as a vasoconstrictor released from platelets in clotting blood. 5-HT occurs in chromaffin cells and enteric neurons of the gastrointestinal tract, in platelets and in the central nervous system. It is often stored together with various peptide hormones, such as somatostatin, substance P or vasoactive intestinal polypeptide (VIP). The biosynthesis and metabolism of 5-HT closely parallels that of catecholamines, except the precursor for decarboxylase of aromatic amino acids is 5-hydroxytryptophan instead of tyrosine (Fig. 5). 5-HT is inactivated mainly by the monoamine oxidases A or B (MAO A or B) to 5-hydroxyindoleacetic acid (5-HIAA), which is excreted in the urine. Some 5-HT is methylated to 5-methoxytryptamine, which is believed to be involved in the pathogenesis of affective disorders.

biosynthesis and metabolism of 5-HT

The actions of 5-HT are numerous and complex, showing considerable variation between species. For instance, in inflammatory response 5-HT seems to be more important in rats than in humans. 5-HT is known to increase gastrointestinal motility, to contract bronchi, uterus and arteries, although 5-HT may also act as a vasodilator through endothelial release of NO. In some species, 5-HT stimulates platelet aggregation, increases microvascular permeability and stimulates peripheral nociceptive nerve endings. A plethora of pathophysiological functions proposed for 5-HT includes control of jejunal peristalsis, vomiting, hemostasis, inflammation and sensitization of nociceptors by peripheral mechanisms or control of appetite, sleep, mood, stereotyped behaviour and pain perception by central mechanisms. Clinically, disturbances in the 5-HT reg-

actions of 5-HT

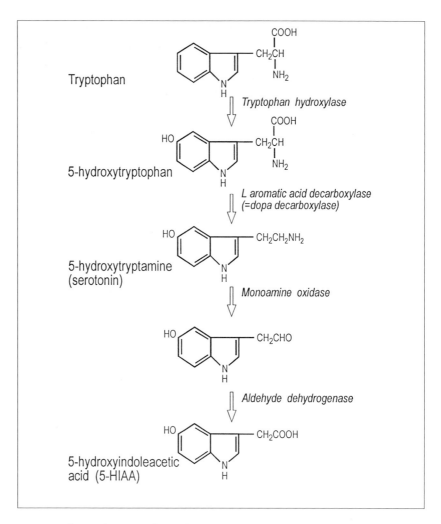

Figure 5 The synthesis and breakdown of 5-HT

ulation system have been proposed in migraine, carcinoid syndrome, mood disorders and anxiety.

5-HT receptor subtypes

These diverse actions of 5-HT are not mediated through one type of receptor. The amino acid sequence for many 5-HT receptor subtypes has been determined by cloning [25], and the transduction mechanisms to which these receptors are coupled have been explained. The basic four types of receptors are 5-HT_{1-4}, 5-HT_1 and 5-HT_2 receptors are further subdivided into A, B and C subtypes. Types 1, 2 and 4 are G protein-coupled receptors; type 3 is a ligand-gated cation channel. 5-HT_1 receptors occur mainly in the CNS (all subtypes) and in blood vessels (5-HT_{1D} subtype). 5-HT_{1B} and 5-HT_{1D} receptors appear to be involved, at least in part, in the modulation of neurogenically induced (following electrical, chemical or mechanical depolarization of sensory nerves) vascular inflamation. 5-HT_2 receptors (5-HT_{2A} subtype being functionally the most important) are more distributed in the periphery than in the CNS, and they are linked to phospholipase C which catalyses phosphatidylinositol hydrolysis. The role of 5-HT_2 receptors in normal physiological processes is probably a minor one, but it becomes more prominent in pathological conditions, such as asthma, inflammation or vascular thrombosis. 5-HT_3 receptors occur particularly on nociceptive sensory neurons and on autonomic and enteric neurons, on which 5-HT exerts an excitatory effect and evokes pain when injected locally.

Catecholamines. It has become increasingly recognized that the release of catecholamines at autonomic nerve endings and from the adrenal medulla may modulate the function of immunocompetent cells. The major lymphoid organs (spleen, lymph nodes, thymus and intestinal Peyer's patches) are extensively supplied by noradrenergic sympathetic nerve fibres. Sympathetic nervous system innervation of these lymphoid organs, as well as the presence of adrenergic and dopamine receptors on immune cells provides the channels for noradrenergic signalling to lymphocytes and macrophages by sympathetic nerves [26]. Catecholamines have a wide range of direct effects on immune cells, particularly on macrophages and lymphocytes. Stimulation of β-adrenergic receptors on LPS-pretreated macrophages prevents the expression and release of proinflammatory TNFα and IL-1, whereas the release of antiinflammatory IL-10 is augmented. On the other hand, α-adrenergic stimulation augments phagocytic and tumoricidal activity of macrophages. Catecholamines acting through β-adrenergic and dopaminergic receptors, which are linked to adenylate cyclase through cAMP, modulate the function of immune cells. An increase in intracellular cAMP inhibits lymphocyte proliferation and production of proinflammatory cytokines. The demonstration of the presence of α_2-, β-adrenergic, D1 and D2 receptors on various immune cells has recently provided the basis for regulation of cytokine production, specifically interleukins and TNF, by these receptors in response to LPS. Vasopressor and inotropic catecholamines seem to have potent immunomodulating properties which, as yet, have not been adequately explored and may contribute to the therapeutic effects of dobutamine or dopexamine in the treatment of septic shock and SIRS.

immunomodulating properties

Immune response in human pathology: Infections caused by bacteria, viruses, fungi and parasites

Jan Verhoef and Harm Snippe

Infections

In the middle of the last century, it was demonstrated that microorganisms are capable of causing disease. At the beginning of this century, the first vaccines were developed against a number of these pathogenic microorganisms in order to prevent the diseases in question (tetanus, diphtheria, pertussis, polio etc.). New infectious diseases and seemingly new pathogens, however, continue to present themselves (e.g. *Legionella*, human immunodeficiency virus (HIV), *Helicobacter*), so that new vaccines must be sought. There is a growing problem of hospital infections, a result of today's intensive medical treatment e.g. catheters, chemotherapeutics and the appearance of microorganisms resistant to many or all available antibiotics. Furthermore, microorganisms hitherto deemed harmless are able to cause opportunistic infections.

pathogenic microorganisms

Humans are surrounded and populated by a large number of different nonpathogenic microorganisms. In the normal – healthy – situation, there is a balance between the offensive capabilities of microorganisms and the defences of the human body. The body's defences are based on vital *nonspecific* and specific immunological defence mechanisms. An infection means that the microorganism has succeeded in penetrating those lines of defence, signaling a partial or complete breakdown of the body's defence system.

immunity vs. infection

Natural resistance

The body's first line of defence comprises the intact cell layers of skin and mucous membrane, which form a physical barrier. The skin's low pH level and bactericidal fatty acids enhance the protection provided by this physical barrier. The defence in the respiratory tract and the gastrointestinal tract is mucous, the "ciliary elevator" of the epithelium, or pro-

first line of defence

**nonspecific
immunity**

vided by motility (small intestine). The presence of normal microbial flora (colonization resistance) in the intestine also plays a role in protection.

The most important humoral natural resistance factors are complement, lysozyme, interferon, collectins and a number of cytokines. Lysozyme, which is found in almost all body fluids, breaks off sections of the cell wall of Gram-positive and – in combination with complement – Gram-negative bacteria. This causes the otherwise sturdy cell wall to leak and the bacterium to burst.

Interferons are glycoproteins which may inhibit the replication of viruses. Within several hours after the onset of a virus infection, interferons are produced in the infected cell and help protect the neighbouring unaffected cells against infection. This protection is brief, but high concentrations of interferons are produced at a time when the primary immunological response is relatively ineffective.

Cytokines, such as IL-2 (interleukin-2), GM-CSF (granulocyte-macrophage colony-stimulating factor) and TNFα (tumour necrosis factor α), stimulate nonspecifically the proliferation, maturation and function of the cells involved in defence (see Chapter A4).

Microorganisms that succeed in penetrating the first line of defence are ingested, killed and degraded by phagocytic cells (leukocytes, monocytes, macrophages), which are attracted to a microbial infection through chemotaxis. The ingestion of the microorganism is enhanced by serum proteins (opsonins), such as antibodies and the C3b component of complement, for which these phagocytes have a receptor. After ingestion, the

phagocytosis

particle is surrounded by the membrane of the phagocyte, forming a vacuole known as a phagosome. The phagosome then fuses with some of the countless lysosomes in the phagocyte, thus allowing the lysosomal microbicidal agents and enzymes to do their work. In the case of leukocytes, the formation of toxic oxygen radicals greatly contributes to the killing and elimination of the ingested microorganism (Fig. 1) (see Chapter A6).

A special role in cellular natural resistance is reserved for the NK (natural killer) cells, which display considerable cytotoxic activity against virus-infected cells. This NK activity is stimulated by interferons and, at a very early stage in the infection, serves to reinforce the nonspecific defence mechanism.

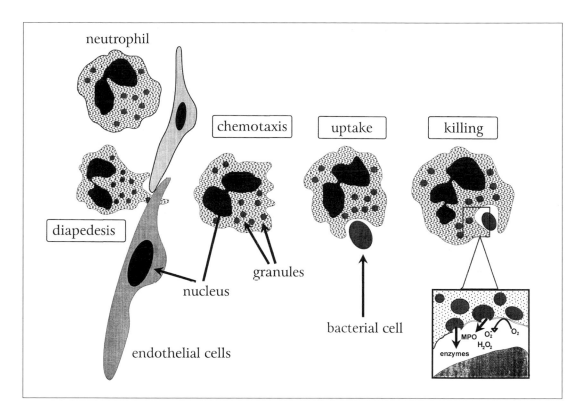

Figure 1 Schematic representation of the progressive steps of phagocytic endocytosis

Specific resistance

In the specific immune response, elements of the natural defence mechanism are directed against a specific enemy. Depending on the microorganism, either the cellular defence mechanism (tuberculosis) or the humoral antibody-dependent defence mechanism (influenza) is of primary importance. In many cases, a joint cellular and humoral response is needed to provide an effective defence (typhus).

specific immunity

Both T-lymphocytes and macrophages play a role in cellular defence. During the first contact with an antigen, macrophages process the antigen and present its protein fragments (T-cell epitopes) to T-cells, which then proliferate and remain present for years in the body as memory cells. When a second encounter occurs, T-cells produce lymphokines, which activate the macrophages. These activated macrophages grow larger, produce more and better degrading enzymes, and are now able to eliminate microorganisms which otherwise would have survived intracellularly (tu-

T-cell immunity

125

berculosis, typhoid fever). Macrophages from non-immune animals are not able to eliminate these microorganisms.

Five different classes of antibodies can be distinguished in humans, namely, immunoglobulin G (IgG), IgA, IgM, IgD, and IgE. They differ from one another in size, charge, amino acid composition and glycosylation (see Chapters A1, C2). In principle, the structure of the antibodies is the same, i.e. two heavy- and two light-chains: it is the variable part of these chains which recognizes the microorganism. The biological function (see below) is determined by the constant part (Fc) of the heavy-chain. With the exception of IgD, all these antibodies are important in antimicrobial activity.

immunoglobulins

– IgA, which is found in all external secretions, reacts with the surface of microorganisms, preventing them from adhering to sensitive cells and mucous membranes.
– IgG neutralizes microbial toxins.
– IgG, IgM and C3b serve as opsonins, which promote phagocytosis.
– IgG, IgM and to a lesser extent IgA activate the complement system after combining with the microorganism. Activation products C3a and C5a ensure that the phagocytes are attracted to the inflammatory response.
– IgG and IgM, in combination with complement and lysozyme, have a lytic effect on bacteria and enveloped viruses.
– IgG and IgM inhibit the mobility of microorganisms by attaching specifically to the flagellum. When this happens the chance of spreading decreases, whereas the chance of phagocytosis increases.
– IgG, together with the killer or K cells, can eliminate infected host-cells which carry viral or other foreign antigens on their surface.
– IgE is of importance in parasite infections. At the site of the infection, mast cells, bearing specific IgE, release large quantities of vasoactive amines which cause the contraction of smooth muscle tissue and increase the permeability of the blood vessels. In the intestine, this results in worms being detached and eliminated.

Defence against bacteria, viruses, fungi, and parasites

Several *noninvasive bacteria*, i.e. those that do not invade the body, cause disease through the production of exotoxins (tetanus, diphtheria,

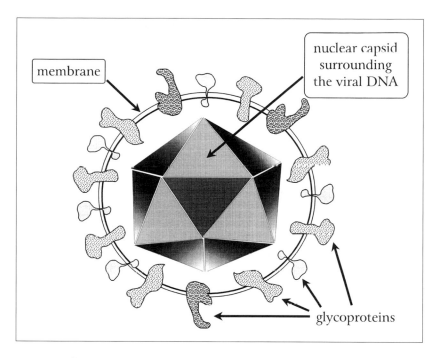

Figure 2 Schematic illustration of an enveloped virus (herpes simplex virus)

cholera). The immune system neutralizes the toxin with the aid of anti- **neutralisation**
bodies (IgG, IgM). If the individual has not been inoculated, the toxin
will act on certain cells in the body directly through a receptor. This bond
is very strong (i.e. has a high affinity), and is difficult to break by the administration of antibodies. In practice, if there are clinical symptoms of
the disease, then large doses of antitoxins must be administered. If one
is trying to prevent the development of the disease, then the presence of
small quantities of specific antibodies (IgG) is sufficient.

The adherence of bacteria to cells is effectively blocked by IgA. Oral **adherence**
vaccination against cholera, for example, is aimed at obtaining sufficient
specific IgA in the intestine so that no colonization of this bacterium can
take place and the cholera toxin can no longer adhere to its receptor.

In general, defence against *invasive bacteria* is provided by antibodies (IgG, IgM) that are directed against bacterial surface antigens. In **invasion**
many cases, these bacteria have a capsule which interferes with effective
phagocytosis. Antibodies against these capsule antigens neutralize the interference, with subsequent elimination of the bacteria by phagocytes.
Antibodies (IgM, IgG, IgA) in combined action with complement kill
bacteria by producing holes in the cell wall of the bacterium.

**intracellular–
cellular immunity**

Although *intracellular bacteria* (tuberculosis, leprosy, listeriosis, brucellosis, legionellosis and salmonellosis) are ingested by macrophages, they are able to survive and multiply. In these cases, cellular immunity alone provides the defence, since antibodies are not effective. Only activated macrophages are capable of killing and degrading these bacteria.

Antibodies neutralize *viruses* (Fig. 2) directly and/or indirectly by destroying infected cells that carry the virus antigen on their surface. The mechanisms of this defence resemble those of humoral defence against bacterial surfaces. The antibody-dependent cellular cytotoxicity reaction is specific for the defence against viruses. Cells which carry on the surface an antigen encoded by the virus are attacked by cytotoxic K cells, bearing antibodies which fit the antigen on the target cell (K cells have Fc receptors for IgG).

cytotoxicity

Not only humoral but also cellular immunity plays an important role in virus infections. People with a genetic T-cell deficiency are highly susceptible to virus infections. In cellular defence, it is primarily the virus-infected cells which are attacked and eliminated. Cytotoxic T-cells recognize MHC-1-presented T-cell epitopes on the surface of virus-infected cells and kill them.

The *fungi* responsible for human diseases can be divided into two major groups on the basis of their growth forms or on the type of infection they cause. Pathogens exist as branched filamentous forms or as yeasts, although some show both growth forms. The filamentous types (*Trichophyton*) form a "mycelium". In asexual reproduction, the fungus is dispersed by means of spores; the spores are a common cause of infection after inhalation. In yeastlike types (*Cryptococcus*), the characteristic form is the single cell, which reproduces by division or budding. Dimorphic types (*Histoplasma*) form a mycelium outside, but occur as yeast cells inside the body. *Candida* shows the reverse condition and forms a mycelium within the body.

**opportunistic
infections**

In superficial mycoses, the fungus grows on the body surface, for example skin, hair and nails (*Epidermophyton*, *Trichophyton*), the disease is mild and the pathogen is spread by direct contact. In deep mycoses (*Aspergillus*, *Candida*, *Cryptococcus*, *Histoplasma*), internal organs are involved, and the disease can be life threatening and is often the result of opportunistic growth in individuals with impaired immunocompetence.

Many of the fungi that cause disease are free-living organisms and are acquired by inhalation or by entry through wounds. Some exist as part of the normal body flora (*Candida*) and are innocuous unless the body's defences are compromised in some way. The filamentous forms grow extracellularly, whereas yeasts can survive and multiply within phagocytic cells. Neutrophils kill yeasts by means of both intra- and extracellular factors. Some yeasts (*Cryptococcus neoformans*) form a thick polysaccharide capsule in order to prevent phagocytic uptake. In addition, many cell-wall components of yeasts cause suppression of cell-mediated immune responses. The role of humoral and cellular immunity in controlling infections caused by fungi is not yet well defined, but cellular immunity is the cornerstone of host defence against (some) fungal infections. As a consequence, HIV infection, which affects the cellular arm of the immune system, results in previously uncommon infections such as those caused by *C. neoformans*.

> capsule = virulence factor

The immunological defence systems against *parasites* are considerably more complex than those against bacteria and viruses. This is due to various factors. In the first place, each parasite has its own life cycle, consisting of various stages with specific antigen compositions. Moreover, parasites are able to avoid the host defence system (mimicry), to combat it (immunosuppression) or to mislead it (antigenic variation). Both humoral and cellular immunity are important for the defence against parasites growing intercellularly, as we have seen in the case of bacteria and viruses. Antibody concentrations (IgM, IgG, IgE) are often elevated. IgE also plays a special role in the removal of parasites (especially worm infections) from the intestine (see above).

Pathogenesis of shock

In Gram-negative (Fig. 3) bacterial infections, the interaction between bacterial endotoxin and various host cell systems has been implicated in the pathogenesis of septic shock. In particular, the release of TNFα (also called cachectin) and interleukin-1 (IL-1) after the activation of host cells by endotoxin induces hemodynamic shock.

> endotoxin

Several lines of evidence support the current hypothesis that the monocyte-macrophage is the principal cellular mediator of endotoxicity. First, C3H/HeJ mice carrying a single gene defect are nonresponsive to lipopolysaccharide (LPS). The transfer of macrophages of a closely related LPS-sensitive strain makes the mice responsive. Second, when the host is challenged with endotoxin, soluble factors are produced by macrophages that mediate fever and an acute-phase response. These factors include the proinflammatory cytokines IL-1, IL-6, IL-8 and TNFα. Together, TNFα and IL-1 stimulate endothelial cells to produce and express proteins on their membrane that have adhesive properties for leukocytes, promoting the margination and passage of polymorphonuclear leukocytes (PMNs) from blood vessels through the endothelial lay-

> cytokines

> PMNs

er, leading to PMN influx into the tissue. Adhesion molecules that mediate the binding of PMNs appear on the endothelium after an inflammatory stimulus, followed by molecules that are specific for adhesion of monocytes or lymphocytes, which may be why neutrophils enter before mononuclear cells. Molecules that are currently known to be involved in leukocyte-endothelium interactions belong to three structural groups: the immunoglobulin gene superfamily, the integrin family and the selectin family.

Concomitant with cytokine release, LPS induces the activation of PMNs, macrophages and many other cells, resulting in the release of toxic oxygen species which lead to tissue damage. At the same time, membrane-associated phospholipases are activated, and products of the arachidonic-acid cascade are released through the cyclooxygenase and/or lipooxygenase pathways (see Chapter A7). Platelet-activating factor (PAF) is also generated, partly in response to the same signals. All these products contribute to a generalized inflammatory state with influx of PMNs, capillary-leak syndrome, disturbances in blood coagulation and myocardial suppression.

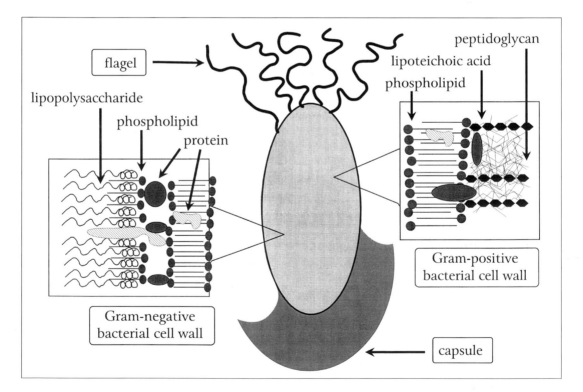

Figure 3 Schematic illustration of the cell envelope of a Gram-negative and a Gram-positive bacterium

Endotoxin and TNFα also produce multiple abnormalities in coagulation and fibrinolysis, leading to microvascular clotting and diffuse intravascular coagulation. They also induce endothelial cells to produce plasminogen activator and IL-6, which is an important modulator of the production of acute-phase proteins by the liver. Interestingly, despite having important structural differences, TNFα and IL-1 have multiple overlapping and few distinct biological activities, act synergistically and mimic the whole spectrum of toxicity caused by LPS (see Chapter A4). IL-8 is an important chemoattractant and activator of neutrophils and is crucial in the early stages of inflammation.

Infusion of endotoxin in healthy humans leads to an early and transient increase in plasma levels of TNFα (detectable after 30 min, peaking after 90 to 120 min and undetectable after 4 to 6 h), which coincides with the development of clinical symptoms and pathophysiological responses encountered in Gram-negative septicemia. TNFα, IL-1, IL-6 and IL-8 levels are also increased in patients with sepsis syndrome, with high levels of these cytokines being correlated with severity of disease.

All these observations support the concept that endotoxin largely acts **shock** by initiating an inflammatory response through the activation of monocytes and macrophages and the subsequent release of cytokines. It also activates the complement system (leading to the generation of C5a, which induces aggregation of PMNs and pulmonary vasoconstriction) and factor XII of the intrinsic coagulation pathway (Hageman factor). Finally, it induces the release of endorphins, which are also involved in the complex interactions of the inflammatory response in endotoxic septic shock.

Gram-positive bacteria (Fig. 3) are frequently and increasingly cul- **gram-positive** tured from blood obtained from patients in shock. Unlike the patho- **bacteria** physiology of shock caused by Gram-negative bacteria, not much is known about the sequence of events that controls the signalling of monocytes and macrophages that leads to the release of cytokines. Cell-wall components, such as peptidoglycan and teichoic acid, are clearly important in the activation of these cells. Exotoxins, however, may also play a role in the pathogenesis of Gram-positive bacterial shock.

HIV infection

HIV is a retrovirus that infects cells bearing the CD4 antigen, such as T-helper (TH) cells, macrophages and dendritic cells. The CD4 molecule, together with other receptor molecules, like chemokine receptor 5, acts

**destruction of
T-cells**

**reduced number
of T-cells**

**opportunistic
infections**

as a binding site for the gp120 envelope glycoprotein of the virus. In an attempt to respond to HIV antigens and concomitant secondary microbial infections, these cells are activated, thus inducing the replication of HIV in the infected CD4 T-cells, which are finally destroyed. In contrast, HIV-1 infection of macrophages is self-sustained and results in an inexorable growth of chronic active inflammatory processes in many tissue compartments including the central nervous system. Infected cells bear the fusion protein gp41 and may therefore fuse with other infected cells. This helps the virus to spread and accounts for the multinucleated cells seen in lymph nodes and brain. As a result of the decreased numbers of $CD4^+$ TH cells and defects in antigen presentation, depressed immune responses in these patients are observed. During the progression of the disease, opportunistic infections by otherwise harmless microorganisms can occur. These include *Candida albicans* esophagitis, mucocutaneous herpes simplex, toxoplasma in the central nervous system and pneumonia caused by toxoplasma and *Pneumocystis carinii*; Kaposi's sarcoma also occurs frequently in these patients. This has been linked to the presence of a previously unknown type of herpes virus (HHV-8). This immune deficiency syndrome is called acquired immune deficiency syndrome (AIDS). It has been suggested that infected monocytes and macrophages carry the HIV virus into the brain where it replicates in microglia and infiltrating macrophages. As a consequence many AIDS patients develop cognitive and motor brain impairments. However, the picture is complicated by the various persistent infections already present in these patients, which give rise to their own pathology in the brain. These include *Toxoplasma gondii*, *Cryptococcus neoformans* and JC virus.

treatment

So far a cure for HIV infection has not been achieved. The main effort in the prevention of HIV infection lies in mass public education programmes. Treatment of infected individuals is possible but expensive. At this moment a triple therapy is being prescribed in Western countries (two reverse transcriptase inhibitors and one protease inhibitor, Fig. 4), each of which interferes with specific steps in the process of HIV replication. One major problem that has arisen is the increasing resistance to these drugs. Blocking of the chemokine receptor 5, a recently described coreceptor on CD4 cells for HIV, may be an alternative treatment for infected persons. This notion is supported by a recent finding that a homozygous defect in this chemokine receptor accounts for resistance of multiple-exposed individuals to HIV-1 infection.

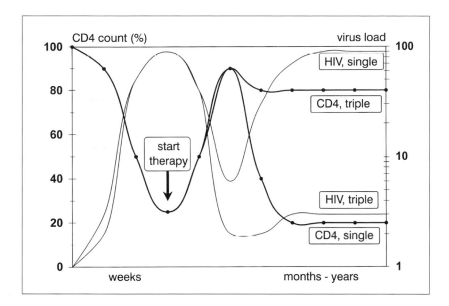

Figure 4 The effect of single and triple therapy on viral load and CD4 cells over time in HIV-infected individuals

Vaccines and vaccination

Pasteur and Koch triggered the stormy development of vaccines (anthrax, rabies, cholera) at the end of the last century. While Pasteur remained faithful to the principle of attenuated microorganisms in preparing his vaccines, Koch employed killed germs (cholera) as a vaccine. Since diphtheria and tetanus cause disease by means of toxins, the next logical step in the development of vaccines was the use of detoxified toxins to induce protection against these diseases (diphtheria, Von Behring, and tetanus, Kitasato). Von Behring and Kitasato were the first to demonstrate that the source of the protective activity induced by vaccines was present in blood serum. Von Behring was also the first to prove that protective immunity could be passed on via serum. The development of new vaccines had its ups (yellow fever) and downs (tuberculosis). With the arrival of antibiotics, all work on new bacterial vaccines was suspended or severely curtailed, although some researchers continued to work on viral vaccines, such as rubella, measles, polio and mumps.

Since it has proved difficult to consistently develop new antibiotics to combat antibiotic-resistant bacteria, interest in vaccines has gradually increased over the last 15 years (see Chapter C1). Today, thanks to new

attenuated vs. killed microorganisms

133

molecular biology

insights into the immune system and modern molecular biological and chemical techniques of analysis and synthesis, it is possible to produce well-defined vaccines. These contain only those determinants of the pathogenic microorganism which induce protection (epitopes). These epitopes are usually short peptide or oligosaccharide chains, which can be produced synthetically or by means of recombinant DNA techniques. The immunogenicity of these products can be enhanced by coupling it with a carrier (tetanus toxoid, liposomes) or by adding an *adjuvant* (a substance which strengthens the immune response nonspecifically). Recombinant DNA techniques can also be used to obtain attenuated strains of microorganisms, which are fully immunogenic and thus provide protection, but which are no longer virulent. One example of this is the development of a new cholera vaccine based on a bacterium which has all the characteristics of a virulent strain, except the toxin. The bacterium has retained all its adherence factors, which allow it to adhere to the intestinal mucosa; the length of time it spends in the intestine is sufficient to stimulate the local immune system. The newest trend in vaccinology is immunization by introducing plasmid DNA into the host. Success has been attained by this method for hepatitis B vaccination.

therapeutics

Not only are new vaccines being developed, but it is also possible to heighten natural resistance for longer or shorter periods. Various interleukins (IL-2, GM-CSF) and interferons are being studied in order to use them to combat infectious diseases. Monoclonal antibodies (antibodies with one specificity) directed against the endotoxin of Gram-negative bacteria are now being administered to patients with severe Gram-negative sepsis (serum therapy). More work is still necessary, however, to refine this technique, as the therapeutic effect is still limited.

Acknowledgments

We thank Dr. CPM van Kessel of the Eijkman-Winkler Institute for the design and layout of the artwork.

Immune response in human pathology: hypersensitivity

Imran R. Hussain and Stephen T. Holgate

The normal immune response involves the recognition of a specific antigen and subsequent clonal proliferation of B-lymphocytes producing specific antibodies [immunoglobulin (Ig) molecules] against this antigen. In infection, immunity is characterised by the binding of antibodies to the infective agent, leading to the neutralisation of the agent (by opsonisation and initiation of the immune cascade). Evolution of the immune response against various parasitic and helminthic infections has led to the development of IgE activation of this pathway by parasite antigens, which leads to stimulation of mast cells, eosinophils and lymphocytes. The interactions between IgE and cells which bear IgE receptors (e.g. the mast cell) are also central to the abnormal response observed in atopic individuals to various allergens. The initial exposure to a potential allergen in an atopic individual will lead to sensitisation, so that a subsequent exposure results in an immediate-type hypersensitivity response. The allergic response is seen in rhinitis, eczema, hay fever and asthma.

IgE

The mast cell was described by Ehrlich (1878) and was characterised by the distinctive metachromatic cytoplasmic granule staining. Mast cells, together with their constituents and IgE have been the focus of research in trying to understand the complex pathways involved in immediate hypersensitivity reactions.

For many years histamine has been known to have an important role in allergic reactions. Initially this was established by Henry Dale (1910), who showed that the response to intravenous histamine includes vasodilation and bronchoconstriction. Lewis (1927) expanded knowledge about histamine by demonstrating its importance in the wheal-and-flare response, though it took a further 2 decades to localise histamine to mast cells located in the dermis.

histamine

The mast cell

mast cell

The mast cell is found at several mucosal sites (intestine, lungs and skin) (MCT), as well as in connective tissue (MCTC). The differences between the two phenotypes are highlighted in Table 1. All mast cells are rich in histamine (main source of histamine in humans, ~3–8 pg/cell). Mast cells have numerous high-affinity IgE receptors which respond to cross-linking of surface-bound IgE by rapid cell activation via activation of tyrosine kinase and cyclic AMP (cAMP) generation, calcium influx and in turn, via protein kinase C activation, which leads to the release of stored and newly synthesised mediators. Mediators released by activated mast cells are listed in Table 2. Other factors can cause the direct release of mediators. These include anti-IgE antibodies, concanavalin A, substance P, polyamines, opiates and several cytokines (e.g. SCF, MIP-1α) [1].

Table 1 Comparison of differences in mast cell phenotypes

	Mast cell type	
	MC_T	**MC_{TC}**
Predominant site	mucosal surfaces	connective tissue
Neutral protease	tryptase (~10 pg/cell)	tryptase (~35 pg/cell)
		chymase
carboxypeptidase		
Histamine release		
(on IgE stimulation)	~17 000 pmol/10^6cells	~3500 pmol/10^6cells
PGD_2 production	~150 pmol/10^6cells	~85 pmol/10^6cells
LTC_4 production	50 pmol/10^6cells	<6 pmol/10^6cells
Changes in mast cell numbers in allergic disorders	increased	no change

Preformed mast cell mediators

Histamine

The action of histamine on the H_1 receptors leads to contraction of airways (and gastrointestinal) smooth muscle. Stimulation of both H_1 and H_2 receptors is required for the wheal-and-flare response (a combination

Table 2 Mast cell mediators

Mediator group	Individual mediators	Action
A. Preformed mediators		
Histamine		vasodilation and increase in vascular permeability
Neutral proteases	tryptase	increases pulmonary smooth muscle hyperreactivity to histamine, activates C3, stimulates fibroblasts and fibrosis
	chymase	increases mucus secretion, basement membrane injury
	carboxypeptidase	cleavage of C-terminal of angiotensin I
	cathepsin G	
Acid hydrolases	β-hexoaminindase/β-glucuronidase/ β-D-galactosidase/arylsulphatase	act on complex carbohydrate chains
Oxidative enzymes	superoxide dismutase/peroxidase	release of reactive oxygen species
Chemotactic factors	inflammatory cytokines (TNFα/GM-CSF)	TNFα induces increased ELAM-1 E-selectin on endothelial cells
	Th2-type cytokines (IL-4/-5/-6/-13)	increase eosinophil recruitment and activation
	chemokines (IL-8/RANTES/MIP-1α/MCP)	increase lymphocyte recruitment and activation
Proteoglycans	heparin chondroitin sulphate	thought to be involved in packaging and may play a part in modulating effect of neutral proteases
B. Newly formed mediators		
Cyclooxygenase products	PGD$_2$/PGF$_{2\alpha}$/PGE$_2$	bronchoconstriction, increased airway secretion
Lipoxygenase products	LT B$_4$	eosinophil and neutrophil chemoattractant, increases vascular permeability
	LTC$_4$/LTD$_4$	increases mucus production, bronchoconstriction, eosinophil chemoattractant
	LTE$_4$	increases vascular permeability, eosinophil chemoattractant
Platelet-activating factor (PAF)		eosinophil chemotaxis, activation, bronchoconstriction, vascular permeability

of arteriolar vasodilation and postcapillary venule constriction leading to plasma exudation). The stimulation of H_2 receptors leads to downregulation of lymphocyte proliferation, T-cell cytotoxicity, lymphokine production and gastric parietal cell acid secretion.

Chemotactic factors (cytokines and chemokines)

cytokines
chemokines

The mast cell is capable of releasing inflammatory cytokines such as tumour necrosis factor (TNFα) and granulaocyte-macrophage colony-stimulating factor (GM-CSF), the former implicated in the ELAM-1 E-selectin expression on endothelial cells. The mast cell produces a variety of Th2-type cytokines which are involved in eosinophil and lymphocyte recruitment, activation, survival (by reduced apoptosis) as well as B-cell proliferation and isotype switching to produce IgE. Certain CC chemokines (e.g. RANTES, MIP-1α, MCP-1) and CXC chemokines (e.g. IL-8) are released, and these are also eosinophil and lymphocyte chemoattractants.

Newly formed mediators (arachidonic acid-derived mediators)

This group of mediators is crucial to the pathogenesis of the acute phase response and also in instigating the late phase response, with the chemotaxis of eosinophils (see also Chapter A7).

Cyclooxygenase products

PGD_2 and $PGF_{2\alpha}$ are potent bronchoconstrictors and peripheral vasodilators, as well as inhibitors of platelet aggregation.

Lipoxygenase products

LTB_4 is involved in neutrophil chemotaxis, adherence and degranulation (at higher concentrations) and has no effect on bronchial smooth muscle tone. LTC_4 and LTD_4 are the most potent bronchodilators known (more potent than PGD_2 and $PGF_{2\alpha}$) and are also potent inducers of vascular permeability. They are thought to be important in the initial edema formation of the acute allergic response. LTE_4, in contrast, is a weak bronchoconstrictor, but enhances bronchial responsiveness to other agents.

Platelet activating-factor (PAF)

PAF is important in the chemotaxis and degranulation of both neutrophils and eosinophils. It also increases vascular permeability and causes bronchoconstriction.

The eosinophil

The eosinophil is one of the cells that is recruited by the mast cell cytokines (IL-3, IL-5 and GM-CSF) and chemokines (RANTES, eotaxin, MCP-3 and IL-8) and along with lymphocytes is present in the cellular infiltrate of the late phase response (Fig. 1). Activation of the eosinophils leads to further release of cytokines (IL-4, -5, -6 and -8) which will stimulate further eosinophil migration and activation. The eosinophil also releases basic proteins that are toxic to the respiratory epithelium [major basic protein (MBP) and eosinophil peroxidase (EPO)] [3, 4].

eosinophils

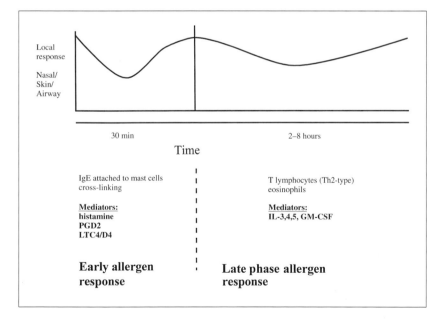

Figure 1 Interaction of mediators involved in the initiation and maintenance of inflammation in immediate type hypersensitivity-type reactions

139

Asthma

**early phase
response**

The pathological changes associated with the early phase response (EPR) to allergen challenge of asthmatic airways include bronchoconstriction (histamine, PGD_2, LTC_4, LTD_4 and chymase); increased mucus secretion (histamine, PGD_2, LTC_4, kinases); vasodilation; increased vascular permeability and protein exudation (histamine, PGD_2, LTC_4). The late phase

**late phase
response**

response (LPR) involves initially a perivascular infiltrate, which is composed of activated eosinophils and lymphocytes. This progresses to be become more generalised. The LPR involves leukocyte priming (IL-3, -4, -5), migration (PAF, IL-5, -6, LTC_4) and activation. Stimulation of Th2-type lymphocytes (IL-4), an increase in IgE synthesis (IL-4) and increased eosinophil survival (IL-5).

Most of the pathological changes of chronic asthma are the consequence of prolonged inflammation. The airways are likely to be plugged with sputum, which is composed of shed epithelial cells, inflammatory cells and mucus. The airway epithelium is disrupted by the action of eosinophil basic proteins (released from activated eosinophils) and the action of toxic oxygen radical species (derived from superoxide dismutase and peroxidase). The epithelial basement membrane shows evidence of thickening, thought to be due to deposition of collagen type III and IV under the action of transforming growth factor β (TGFβ). There is also evidence of an increase in fibroblast and subepithelial fibrosis, under the action of the neutral proteases. The airway smooth muscle is thickened and hypertrophied due to the actions of platelet-derived growth factor, endothelins and histamine. The action of some of the cytokines released by the mast cell (IL-1 and TNFα) is to cause upregulation of adhesion molecules (ICAM-1 and VCAM-1), which will increase the inflammatory cell infiltrate. Narrowed airways due to the smooth muscle thickening and edema will exaggerate any airway lumen narrowing caused by bronchoconstriction and thus have a greater effect on airways resistance. The mast cell, eosinophil and (CD4$^+$) lymphocyte mediators all combine to cause the pathological changes seen.

Contact sensitivity

This differs in pathology from the process described above, and is an example of a type IV (or delayed type) hypersensitivity response; the process is T-cell- rather than IgE-mediated. The allergic sensitisation often occurs against chemicals (e.g. nickel). The chemical is often too small

hapten

to act as an antigen by itself (hapten), and has to combine with skin proteins (carrier) to act as an antigen which is taken up by the skin Langerhans' cells. The hapten-carrier complex is taken to the draining lymph nodes by the Langerhans' cells, where the antigen is presented to T-cells, and T-cell clonal proliferation takes place. On subsequent antigen exposure a T-cell response similar to the late asthmatic response is seen. Initially there is vasodilation of the local blood vessels and a perivascular infiltrate; this is followed by epidermal infiltration of mononuclear cells and interstitial edema. The edema gradually resolves over the next 12 to 24 h, occasionally leaving vacuoles, and there is an increase in the mononuclear cell infiltrate. The mononuclear cell infiltrate is made up predominantly of CD4$^+$ T-cells. There is also an increase in the number of locally present Langerhans' cells.

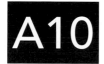

Immune response in human pathology: transplantation

Marcella Sarzotti and Peter S. Heeger

Introduction

The successful transplantation of cells or tissues from one individual to another depends upon the genetic relationship between the transplant donor and the recipient. The histocompatibility antigens (MHC) of each individual determine the fate of the transplant [1]. Tissues transplanted between individuals with identical MHC, such as mice of the same inbred strain or identical twins, are called syngeneic grafts and are accepted by the recipient. Transplants between genetically different individuals of the same species (allografts) or between individuals of different species (xenografts) are normally rejected. The rejection is mediated by antibodies and by thymus-derived immune cells (T-cells) that recognize MHC antigens on the transplanted tissues different from those of the host. In this chapter we will describe the immune responses to tissue grafts and some of the clinical treatments designed to control allograft rejection.

histocompatibility antigens (MHC)

syngeneic grafts

allografts
xenografts
thymus-derived immune cells (T-cells)

Allorecognition

Alloreactive T-lymphocytes (recipient cells reacting to foreign transplants) are found in relatively high frequency when compared with frequencies of nominal antigen-specific T-cells [2, 3]. The reason for this high frequency and the molecular nature of allorecognition have puzzled immunologists for decades. Recent evidence suggests that most allospecific T-cell receptors recognize specific peptides bound to the allogeneic (donor) MHC molecule [4]. Because allogeneic MHC molecules bind and display a universe of donor-derived peptides not previously encountered by the recipient, the recipient's T-cells recognize many of these peptides as foreign. Thus, according to this model, the magnitude of foreign peptides presented on the allogeneic MHC molecules (each of

alloreactive T-lymphocytes

donor-derived peptides "direct allo-recognition"

which stimulates T-cell clones at low frequency) adds up to the high frequency of the alloreactive repertoire. Such recipient T-cell recognition of donor-derived peptides expressed in the context of donor MHC on the surface of the transplanted cells is a process known as "direct allorecognition" (Fig. 1) [5].

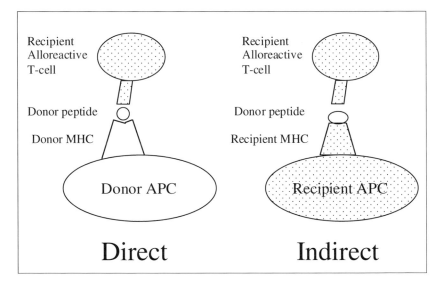

Figure 1 Allorecognition
Recipient alloreactive T-cells recognize donor-derived peptides expressed in the context of donor MHC on the surface of the transplanted cells (direct allorecognition, left panel). Recipient T-cells can also recognize donor-derived peptides processed and presented by "self" (recipient) APCs (indirect allorecognition, right panel).

antigen-presenting cells (APC) "indirect" pathway of allorecognition

In addition to the high-frequency "direct" response, recent studies have demonstrated that recipient T-cells can recognize donor-derived peptides processed and presented by "self" (recipient) antigen-presenting cells (APCs) (Fig. 1) [6, 7]. This so-called "indirect" pathway of allorecognition does not essentially differ from T-cell immune responses to foreign antigens. In the case of transplant rejection, the foreign peptide is derived from the donor MHC molecule. The importance of the indirect pathway in transplantation rejection is underscored by various experimental models in which induction of immunologic tolerance to peptides presented by this pathway totally prevented rejection of an allograft [8]. In addition, it has been hypothesized that T-cells responding to peptides presented by the indirect pathway play a central immunologic role in the development of chronic allograft rejection.

Although allorecognition is essential for activation of effector T-cells, it is not sufficient. Second costimulatory signals, delivered by the APCs are required in order to fully activate the alloimmune T-cells. Costimulation leading to T-cell activation occurs following binding of the B7-1/B7-2 molecules on the APC with the CD28 and CTLA4 molecules on T-cells. Both cardiac and renal allograft survival is markedly prolonged in animals treated with CTLA4-Ig, a soluble fusion protein consisting of the extracellular domain of CTLA4 and an immunoglobulin (Ig) G1 constant region, which has high avidity for the B7-1 and B7-2 molecules and blocks costimulation [9]. Recent studies have also shown that blockade of other costimulatory pathways, including CD2-LFA-1 and the CD40-CD40 ligand interactions, can prolong allograft survival in animal models [10].

costimulatory signals

Effector mechanisms of allograft rejection

Allograft rejection involves both humoral and T-cell-mediated immune responses. Donor-specific antibodies present in the recipient at the time of transplantation cause a prompt reaction called "hyperacute rejection" [11]. These antibodies include anti-MHC antibodies resulting from a previous exposure of the recipient to the donor MHC, anti-blood group antibodies, or antibodies to the vascular endothelial antigens of other species. Following binding of these antibodies to the graft, the complement cascade is initiated, resulting in coagulation, vascular thrombosis and rejection of the graft within hours. Although the role of preexisting antibodies in the hyperacute rejection is well established, it has largely been avoided by cross-matching cells from potential donors with serum from the recipient. Alloreactive antibodies may additionally play a role in some cases of acute and chronic graft rejection.

allograft rejection

"hyperacute rejection"

Alloreactive T-lymphocytes are thought to be the central effectors of allograft rejection [12]. Classic experiments have demonstrated that T-cell-deficient mice readily accept skin allografts, but that adoptive transfer of T-cells into these recipient mice induces rapid rejection of the grafts [13, 14]. Both CD4+ and CD8+ T-cells can mediate allograft rejection. CD8+ T-cells generally have cytotoxic function and directly kill cells expressing foreign MHC. CD4+ T-cells can also exhibit cytotoxic function, but mainly mediate allograft rejection through secretion of cytokines. In a simplified scheme, CD4+ T-cells have been categorized into functional subsets, T helper type 1 (Th1) and type 2 (Th2) cells, based on the type of cytokines that they produce [15]. T-cells, even as early thymus emigrants, can be immunized, tolerized or induced to a type 1/type 2

T helper type 1 (Th1)

type 2 (Th2)

response depending upon the APCs, the dose of antigen and the type of adjuvant they encounter [16-19]. Proinflammatory type 1 immune responses are characterized by the production of interleukin-2 (IL-2), interferon-γ (IFN-γ) and tumour necrosis factor-α (TNF-α). These cytokines promote the differentiation of cytotoxic effector cells and induce the development of complement-binding IgG2a subtype antibody responses, both of which contribute to rejection (Fig. 2). Furthermore, this type of immune response leads to upregulation of the chemoattractant molecules known as chemokines, thus promoting the influx and activation of monocytes, macrophages and additional T-cells. The result is a coordinated type IV delayed hypersensitivity response (DTH) which likely contributes to the destruction of the graft. The activated macrophages themselves may be directly cytotoxic to the transplanted tissue. The macrophages also release toxic mediators such as TNF-α and nitric oxide which, in turn, may promote apoptosis and oxygen radical-mediated DNA damage of the graft and thus contribute to its demise. Studies examining the role of cytokines in transplantation have shown that a type 1 response is manifested during allograft rejection [20]. A specific role for

cytotoxic effector cells

type IV delayed hypersensitivity response (DTH)

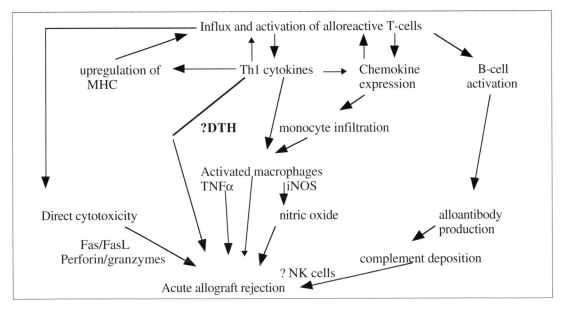

Figure 2 Allograft rejection

T-cells mediate allograft rejection by several mechanisms: they produce cytokines and promote cellular immune responses such as macrophage and cytotoxic T-cell (CTL) activation, and induce the development of complement-binding IgG2a subtype antibody responses. These proinflammatory immune responses may lead to allograft rejection through induction of DTH and through release of macrophage-derived mediators such as nitric oxide.

natural killer (NK) cells has additionally been postulated in some forms of graft rejection (particularly rejection of bone marrow grafts), but this remains an area of controversy.

In contrast, type 2 immune responses are characterized by the production of IL-4, IL-5 and IL-10, and promote allergic immune responses consisting of IgE antibody production and eosinophil infiltration. Type 2 immunity has been shown to inhibit type 1 responses and, in some model systems, has been associated with transplantation tolerance [21], although the distinction between type 1 and type 2 responses in transplantation remains controversial [22–25].

Immunosuppression in human transplantation

An ideal approach to immunosuppression would be to specifically affect the allograft reaction without impairing other immune responses. Present therapies include immunosuppressive agents which affect the immune response nonspecifically and may predispose patients to infectious complications. Despite these problems, the use of immunosuppressive agents has made clinical transplantation a reality. Here we describe some of the immunosuppressive agents presently used in the clinical setting for the treatment of acute allograft reaction and some promising experimental approaches to prevent chronic allograft rejection.

immunosuppressive agents

Present-day therapies result in greater than 90% 1-year allograft survival. The majority of human allograft recipients are treated with some combination of corticosteroids, azathioprine and cyclosporine, all of which are aimed at preventing or downregulating T-cell immunity [26, 27] through inhibition of cytokine or cytokine-receptor gene expression and disruption of cell proliferation (see Chapter C8). Newer medications evaluated in ongoing clinical trials include rapamycin and mycophenolate mofetil [28]. Both of them are touted to be efficacious for the prevention of allograft rejection and may have fewer side effects than the standard immunosuppressive medications. Finally, monoclonal antibodies directed at T-cell surface molecules are being studied as potential regulators of the alloresponse. OKT3, a mouse IgG2a antibody directed at the human CD3ε chain, is the only Federal Drug Administration (FDA)-approved antibody presently available in the United States for use in humans. This reagent effectively blocks T-cell function, induces T-cell depletion, and is clinically used to treat ongoing allograft rejection [29].

allograft survival

Despite the success in the prevention and treatment of acute allograft rejection, we have not been able to effectively prolong allograft survival

acute allograft rejection

chronic allograft rejection

in the long term. For example, the half-life of renal allograft survival, approximately 8 years, has remained unchanged over the last 15 to 20 years. Much of the late allograft loss is due to a poorly understood phenomenon known as chronic allograft rejection [30]. Chronic allograft rejection is characterized histologically by persistent perivascular and interstitial mononuclear inflammatory infiltrates, allograft arteriosclerosis and extensive fibrosis. Immune-mediated mechanisms are central to this process, as persistent mononuclear cells are invariably present in the grafts, and effective costimulatory blockade can totally prevent chronic rejection in animal models. Additional nonimmunologic factors that may be important in the development of chronic rejection include intragraft hypertension, drug toxicity (in particular, cyclosporine toxicity), and the secretion of a variety of growth factors released in response to both ischemic and immunologic injury.

transplantation tolerance

Induction of long-lasting donor-specific tolerance is the optimal strategy to prevent rejection. Transplantation tolerance implies the induction of immunological nonresponsiveness to the graft with preservation of normal responses to other antigens [31]. Several strategies have been designed to induce a state of transplantation tolerance in the host. One promising approach is the blockade of costimulatory pathways, as described above [9, 10]. Central tolerance in the adult is achieved experimentally by eliminating mature T-cells of the recipient, using irradiation or antibody-mediated depletion, and by transplanting donor hematopoietic cells intrathymically [32]. Alternatively, alloantigenic peptides are injected directly into the thymus [8, 33]. These experimental approaches are presently being tested in primate models [34] and represent promising clinical applications.

A better understanding of the factors that lead to chronic rejection, the design of approaches aimed at inducing long-lasting donor-specific tolerance and the development of xenotransplantation for clinical use are the ultimate goals of transplantation immunologists as we move towards the 21st century.

Acknowledgments

This work was supported in part by NIH grant CA65388 to M.S., by NIH Clinical Investigator Award DK02125-05 to P.S.H., and by the Medical Research Service, Department of Veterans Affairs.

A11 Cancer: targets for recognition and elimination of tumor cells by the immune system

Jan W. Gratama, Kees Nooter and Reinder L.H. Bolhuis

Tumor antigens: targets for recognition of tumor cells by the immune system

The discrimination between "self" and "nonself" by the immune system – the 1960 Nobel prize-winning concept of Burnet and Medawar – has been pivotal for modern tumor immunology. Malignant transformation of human cells may result in alterations of their antigenic profiles. Such alterations can include reduction or lack of expression of antigens that are present on the surface membranes of their normal counterparts, but also overexpression of such antigens and/or the appearance of novel antigens that are not expressed by their normal counterparts. Importantly, the latter two alterations provide potential targets for recognition of tumor cells by the immune system. Such *tumor-associated antigens* can be divided into four groups: (1) antigens encoded by viruses; (2) products of oncogenes and tumor suppressor genes; (3) antigens encoded by normal genes, but expressed only by tumor cells; and (4) tissue-specific antigens.

tumor-associated antigens

The advent of the *monoclonal antibody* (*mAb*) technology, yielding its creators, Köhler and Milstein, the 1975 Nobel prize, has greatly facilitated the identification of human tumor antigens by avoiding the limitations posed by the development of tumor-specific conventional antisera. Tumor antigen-specific mAbs are now essential tools for cancer diagnosis, monitoring of disease progression and therapy. Tumor-specific mAbs can be therapeutically effective through direct cytotoxic action (either complement-mediated or, cell-mediated, via immunoglobulin Fc receptors on effector cells); through conjugation with cytotoxic drugs, toxins or radionucleotides; as tools for *ex vivo* removal of tumor cells from hematopoietic stem-cell grafts; through blocking receptors for growth factors on tumor cells; and, as antiidiotypic mAbs, through the induction of specific active immunity to tumor antigens [1].

monoclonal antibody

There is a major difference in the nature of antigens recognized by antibodies and by T-lymphocytes. Seminal to the progress in this field of immunology was the work of 1987 Nobel prize winner Tonegawa, who discovered the genetic principle for generation of antibody diversity, and the discovery of major histocompatibility complex (MHC) restriction by the 1996 Nobel laureates Zinkernagel and Doherty. Antibodies detect specific epitopes on antigenic molecules; the interaction of these molecules with the variable region of the antibody results in recognition. In contrast, antigens recognized by T-cell receptors recognize processed peptides on the surface of the tumor cell, or on an antigen-presenting cell, presented by molecules of the MHC. CD4$^+$ (mostly helper) T-lymphocytes recognize such peptides bound to class II MHC molecules, whilst CD8$^+$ (mostly cytotoxic) T-lymphocytes recognize peptides attached to class I MHC molecules. As a rule, (m)Abs do not detect the small processed peptides associated with MHC molecules. Hence, the nature of the antigens recognized by (m)Abs and T-lymphocytes is very different.

Antigens encoded by viruses

DNA viruses

Several DNA viruses are associated with human cancer. For example, the vast majority (~90%) of cervical and nasopharyngeal carcinoma cases are positive for human papilloma virus (HPV) and Epstein-Barr virus (EBV), respectively. Viral gene products expressed on the surface membrane of the tumor cells provide MHC-restricted targets for T-cell recognition, but are poor targets for mAbs. Examples of sources for MHC-restricted viral tumor antigens are the HPV-transforming proteins E6 and E7 [2] and the EBV latent membrane proteins (LMPs) 1 and 2 [3].

Products of oncogenes and tumor suppressor genes

oncogenes
tumor suppresssor
genes

Oncogenes and tumor suppressor genes are important regulators of cellular division, differentiation and programmed cell death (see below). The transforming potential of oncogenes can be activated by mutations or translocations of their normal counterparts, the protooncogenes. Such mutations or translocations may lead to novel protein sequences and peptide epitopes capable of being presented by MHC molecules to T-lymphocytes (e.g. mutated p21 *ras* in ~10% of solid tumors [4]). Overexpression of otherwise normal proteins and their derived peptides may result in immunogenicity by exceeding the minimum MHC-peptide density threshold required for T-cell recognition and induction of Ab responses (e.g. HER-2/*neu* in breast and ovarian cancer [5]). To the contrary, the inactivation of tumor suppressor genes by mutations or deletions may predispose for cancer development. Mutants of the p53 protein, detectable in ~50% of solid tumors, are a good case in point [6].

Antigens encoded by normal genes, but expressed only by tumor cells

The prototype for this group is melanoma antigen-1 (MAGE-1), expressed by melanoma cells but not by normal melanocytes, and belonging to a family of at least 12 genes with hitherto unknown function. Peptides derived from MAGE proteins are recognized by MHC-restricted T-lymphocytes [7]. Examples of antigens in this group recognized by therapeutically used mAbs are MOv18, the folate receptor overexpressed by ovarian carcinoma cells [8], and the ligand recognized by mAb G250 on renal cell carcinoma cells but not on normal kidney cells [9].

melanoma antigen-1 (MAGE-1)

Tissue-specific gene products

Prototypes of gene products that are expressed in both normal and malignant cells of the same histological type are tyrosinase, gp100, TRP-1 (gp75) and MART-1 (or Melan-A), all exclusively expressed by cells of the melanocytic lineage. All are sources of MHC-restricted peptides and have been shown to function as targets for tumor-infiltrating lymphocytes associated with *in vivo* regressions of metastatic melanoma [10]. These proteins probably function as normal differentiation antigens.

Conclusion

The identification of tumor-associated antigens that are (over)expressed on a significant proportion of malignancies is of crucial importance for the design and use of tumor-specific immunological products for diagnosis, disease monitoring and therapy.

Apoptosis: mechanism of lymphocyte-mediated tumor cell kill

Apoptosis versus necrosis

apoptosis
necrosis

Apoptosis and necrosis constitute the major mechanisms of cell death. Apoptosis requires the operation of an internally programmed cell death mechanism, and necrosis results from overwhelming direct injury to cellular components by external factors. Lymphocyte-mediated cytotoxicity [MHC-restricted, NK-receptor-mediated or Fc receptor (antibody)-dependent] is mediated via apoptosis. Also, tumor necrosis factor (TNF), lymphotoxin and some mAbs (without binding complement) can induce apoptosis. Necrosis is induced by the combined effect of antibodies and complement, hypoxia, ischemia, metabolic poisons, hyperthermia and oxidative stress. The "death pathways" of apoptosis and necrosis can be distinguished morphologically (Fig. 1) and cytochemically [11].

Mechanisms of lymphocyte-mediated apoptosis

CD95

perforin
granzyme B

bcl-2, p53

Cytotoxic T-lymphocytes (CTL) induce apoptosis in their target cells either via cross-linking of CD95 (also known as APO-1 or Fas), a member of the TNFreceptor family, with its ligand, or via the concerted action of perforin and granzyme B, which are released from the CTL by degranulation. Trimerization of CD95 initiates the formation of an intracellular death-inducing signaling complex. Both a component of this complex and granzyme B can subsequently activate a downstream cascade of proteases that, in turn, initiate the effector phase of apoptosis. This phase involves the breakdown of several macromolecules including DNA and proteins, fragmentation of organelles and packaging of the cellular debris into apoptotic bodies which are phagocytosed by macrophages or other nearby cells. Other genes involved in the regulation of apoptosis are *bcl-2* and *p53*. The main function of the proto-oncogene product bcl-2 is maintenance of cell survival, and it appears to interfere with activation of the distal proteases in the apoptotic pathway. The tumor suppressor gene product p53 is required for cell cycle arrest in the G1 phase of the cell cycle following DNA damage from ionizing radiation or cytotoxic drugs; in line with that function, p53 seems to initiate a more proximal component of the apoptotic pathway [12].

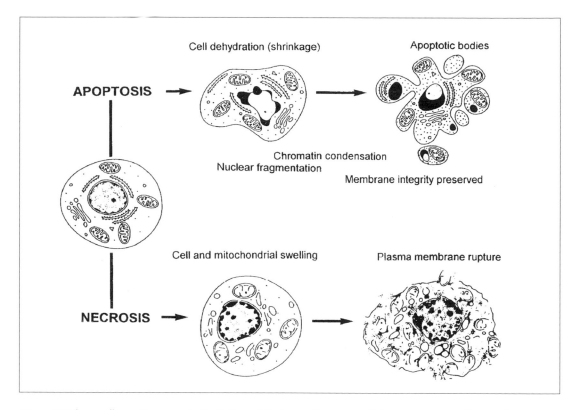

Figure 1 *Scheme illustrating morphological and biochemical changes during apoptosis and necrosis*
Apoptosis: One of the early changes is loss of intracellular water and increase in the concentration of ionized calcium in the cytoplasm. Chromatin condensation, followed by nuclear disintegration and formation of apoptotic bodies represent other typical features of apoptosis. The integrity of the plasma membrane is preserved until the late stages of apoptosis. Activation of endonuclease(s) results in selective degradation of DNA into 50- to 300-kb fragments, and is often followed by internucleosomal DNA cleavage and the orderly breakdown of other macromolecules. Necrosis: Swelling of mitochondria as well as swelling of the whole cell, combined with marginal chromatin condensation, characterize the early stage of necrosis. Rupture of the plasma membrane occurs later, and the content of cytoplasm is released from the cell. Reprinted from [11] with permission of the authors and the publisher.

Conclusion

Research into apoptosis has greatly improved our insight into how cytotoxic lymphocytes kill tumor cells. The discovery of multiple apoptosis receptors and the unraveling of intracellular pathways of the apoptotic process will provide us with new immunopharmacological targets for the induction of apoptosis in tumor cells and, hence, for the immunotherapy of cancer.

153

Neuroimmunoendocrinology

A12

Douglas A. Weigent and J. Edwin Blalock

Historical background

Psychoneuroimmunology refers to the study of the interactions among behavioral, neural, neuroendocrine and immunological processes of adaptation. Although relationships between the brain and the immune system had been suggested for many years, research during the last 25 years has provided mechanisms for how these systems may interact. The current interest in psychoneuroimmunology is sustained by the now widely held belief that it represents a bidirectional system. It is now apparent that the nervous system not only influences immune function but that the immune system modifies the nervous system. Some of the very early observations related to the effects of stress on immune function suggested a psychosomatic-immune axis [1]. Avoidance conditioning was shown to increase virus infection and psychological factors to alter the onset and course of autoimmune disease. Additional results identifying receptors on cells of the immune system, evaluating brain lesions and identifying nerve fibers in compartments of lymphoid organs along with the biological relevance of innervation on immune function supported the idea of a very dynamic interaction between the immune and nervous systems [2]. Over the same time frame, a number of reports appeared indicating the efficacious effects on the immune system of hormone therapy in hormone-deficient animals [3]. Thus it became apparent that the neuroendocrine system could interact with and modulate the immune system by the release of hormones.

The reciprocal situation in which the stimulation of the immune system altered central nervous system function established the bidirectional nature of the communication between these two systems. It was shown that the immune system as a consequence of antigenic challenge altered the firing rate of hypothalamic neurons [4]. Supernatant fluids from activated leukocytes could mimic this phenomenon, and it is now clear that a wide range of lymphocyte products influence the synthesis and secretion or release of neuroendocrine hormones and neurotransmitters [5].

bidirectional communication

shared ligands and receptors

Our own studies reviewed, in part, below discovered that cells of the immune system could be a source of pituitary hormones and that immune-derived cytokines could function as hormones and hypothalamic releasing factors [5]. This evidence suggested a mechanism by which the body's two principle recognition organs, the brain and the immune system, may influence each other, that is they speak the same biochemical language. Collectively, these relationships provide the foundation for behaviorally induced alterations in immune function and for immunologically based changes in behavior. Accumulating *in vitro* and *in vivo* studies indicate that shared ligands and receptors are used as a common chemical language within and between the immune and neuroendocrine systems. Specifically, physical and psychological stimuli may set off patterns of neurotransmitters, hormones and cytokines which bind to receptors on cells of the immune system and alter their function (Fig. 1). In addition, the immune system converts recognition of noncognitive stimuli such as viruses and bacteria into information in the form of cy-

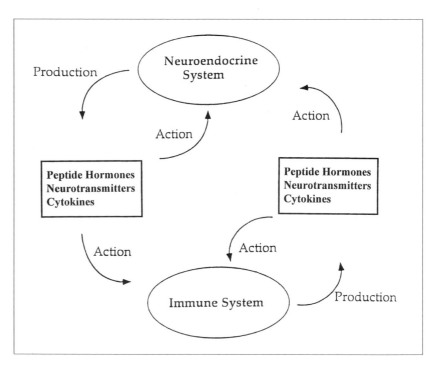

Figure 1

A molecular communication circuit within and between the immune and neuroendocrine systems involving shared ligands and their receptors. (Reprinted with permission from Weigent and Blalock [5] by the Society for Leukocyte Biology.)

tokines, peptide hormones and neurotransmitters, which act on receptors in the neuroendocrine system to alter its function. Therefore, the findings suggest an immunoregulatory role for the brain and a sensory function for the immune system [6]. This chapter will briefly describe the basic and clinical evidence for the role neuroendocrine hormones play in communication between the immune and neuroendocrine system.

Regulation of the immune system by neuroendocrine hormones

A large amount of evidence exists to support both the presence of receptors for neuroendocrine hormones on cells of the immune system as well as the ability of these hormones to modulate specific functions of the various immune cell types (Table 1; [5]). Several examples are discussed below, and the reader is directed to review articles for a further discussion of the topic.

Actions of adrenocorticotropin (ACTH) and endorphins

The receptors for ACTH and endorphins have been identified on cells of the immune system as well as the ability of these hormones to modulate many aspects of immune reactivity. The findings show that B-lymphocytes contain three times the number of ACTH binding sites compared with T-cells and that treatment with a mitogen increases the number of high-affinity sites 2–3-fold on both cell types. The binding of ACTH initiates a signal transduction pathway that involves both cyclic AMP (cAMP) and mobilization of Ca^{2+}. ACTH has been shown to suppress major histocompatibility complex (MHC) class II expression, stimulate natural killer (NK) cell activity, suppress interferon γ (IFNγ) production and function as a late-acting B-cell growth factor. The lymphocyte receptors for the opioid peptides have also been studied and found to share many of the features, including size, sequence, immunogenicity and intracellular signaling as those described on neuronal tissue. Many aspects of immunity are modulated by the opiate peptides including (1) enhancement of the natural cytotoxicity of lymphocytes and macrophages toward tumor cells, (2) enhancement or inhibition of T-cell mitogenesis, (3) enhancement of T-cell rosetting, (4) stimulation of human peripheral blood mononuclear cells and (5) inhibition of MHC class II antigen expression.

T- and B-lympho-cyte ACTH receptor sites

lymphocyte opioid receptor and function

Table 1 Modulation of immune responses by neuroendocrine hormones

Hormone	Cell type with hormone receptor	Modulating effects
Corticotropin	rat spleen T- and B-cells	antibody synthesis IFNγ production B-lymphocyte growth
Endorphins	spleen	antibody synthesis mitogenesis natural killer cell activity
Thyrotropin	neutrophils, monocytes, B-cells	Increased antibody synthesis comitogenic with ConA
GH	PBL, spleen, thymus	cytotoxic T-cells mitogenesis
LH and FSH	–	proliferation cytokine production
PRL	T- and B-cells	comitogenic with ConA induces IL-2 receptors
CRF	PBL	IL-1 production enhanced natural killer cell activity immunosuppressive
TRH	T-cell lines	increased antibody synthesis
GHRH	PBL and spleen	stimulates proliferation
SOM	PBL	inhibits natural killer cell activity inhibits chemotactic response inhibits proliferation reduces IFNγ production

Actions of growth hormone (GH) and prolactin (PRL)

It has been clearly shown that cells of the immune system also contain receptors for GH and PRL and that these hormones are potent modulators of the immune response [7]. The PRL and GH receptors have been

distribution of the PRL receptor

shown to be members of the superfamily of cytokine receptors involved in the growth and differentiation of lymphohematopoietic cells. A systematic survey of PRL receptor expression by flow cytometry showed that PRL receptors are universally expressed in normal hematopoietic tissues with some differences in density, which could be promoted by concanavalin (Con)A treatment. GH receptors from a number of species

GH receptor and IM-9 cells

have been sequenced, and very recently the cocrystallization of human GH with the GH receptor was achieved. GH binding and cellular processing of the GH receptor have been studied in a cell line of immune origin (IM-9) where GH stimulates the proliferation of the IM-9 cell line and the GH receptor is downregulated by phorbol esters. Several lines of evidence indicate that activation of the GH receptor increases tyrosine kinase activity and that the GH receptor is associated with a tyrosine kinase in several cell types, including the IM-9 cell. A role for GH in immunoregulation has been demonstrated *in vitro* for numerous immune functions [7], including stimulation of DNA and RNA synthesis in the spleen and thymus. GH also affects hematopoiesis by stimulating neutrophil differentiation, augmenting erythropoiesis, increasing proliferation of bone marrow cells and influencing thymic development. GH affects the functional activity of cytolytic cells, including T-lymphocytes and NK cells. GH was necessary for T-lymphocytes to develop cytolytic activity against an allogeneic stimulus in serum-free medium. GH has also been shown to stimulate the production of superoxide anion formation from macrophages. It is not clear whether GH directly influences intrathymic or extrathymic development or acts indirectly by augmenting the synthesis of thymulin or insulin-like growth factor-1 (IGF-1). These observations suggest that GH may stimulate local production of IGF-1, which acts to promote tissue growth and action in a paracrine fashion. Likewise, PRL can have modulating effects on the immune system [7]. Recent data show that suppression of PRL secretion in mice with bromocriptine increases the lethality of a *Listeria* challenge and abrogates T-cell-dependent activation of macrophages. Antibodies to the PRL receptor have been shown to abolish PRL-induced proliferation of Nb2 cells.

hematopoiesis and GH and IGF-1

bromocriptine increases lethality of *Listeria*

Actions of hypothalamic releasing hormones

In addition to pituitary hormones, hypothalamic releasing hormone receptors and their effects have been identified on cells of the immune system. A number of similarities have been identified between the pituitary and spleen binding of corticotropin releasing factor (CRF), including affinity and apparent subunit molecular weight. The effects of ACTH and endorphins discussed earlier may be initiated in the immune system via the production of these hormones by cells of the immune system in response to CRF (see below). CRF inhibits lymphocyte proliferation and NK cell activity. The growth hormone-releasing hormone (GHRH) receptor has also been identified on cells of the immune system. The GHRH receptor binding sites are saturable and are found on both thymocytes and splenic lymphocytes. After GHRH binding to its receptor,

lymphocyte CRF binding and function

lymphocyte GHRH receptors

TRH induces TSH

inhibitory effects of somatostatin

there is a rapid increase in intracellular Ca^{2+}, which is associated with the stimulation of lymphocyte proliferation. In addition, leukocytes have been shown to respond to thyrotropin-releasing hormone (TRH) treatment by producing thyrotropin (TSH) messenger RNA (mRNA) and proteins. Recent work has shown the presence of two receptor types for TRH on T-cells. One of these sites satisfies the criteria for a classical TRH receptor and is involved in the release of IFN- from T-cells. Recently, one group has described the existence of distinct subsets of somatostatin (SOM) receptors on the Jurkat line of human leukemic T-cells and U266 immunoglobulin G (IgG)-producing human myeloma cells. The authors speculate that two subsets of receptors may account for the biphasic concentration-dependent nature of the effects of SOM in some systems. Although GH and PRL have immunoenhancing capabilities, SOM has potent inhibitory effects on immune responses. SOM has been shown to significantly inhibit Molt-4 lymphoblast proliferation and phytohemagglutinin (PHA) stimulation of human T-lymphocytes, and nanomolar concentrations are able to inhibit the proliferation of both spleen-derived and Peyer's patch-derived lymphocytes. Other immune responses, such as superantigen-stimulated IFN- secretion, endotoxin-induced leukocytosin and colony-stimulating activity release are also inhibited by SOM.

Neuroendocrine hormone release by immune system cells

There is now overwhelming evidence that cells of the immune system may also produce neuroendocrine hormones. This was first established for ACTH and subsequently for TSH, GH, PRL, luteinizing hormone (LH), follicle stimulating hormone (FSH) and the hypothalamic hormones SOM, CRF, GHRH and luteinizing hormone-releasing hormone (LHRH) [5]. Recent evidence strongly supports the notion that neuroendocrine peptides, endogenous to the immune system, are used for both intraimmune system regulation as well as for bidirectional communication between the immune and neuroendocrine systems. The studies to date show that the structure of these peptides are identical to those

paracrine and endocrine function

identified in the neuroendocrine system and that both similarities and differences exist in the mechanism of synthesis to the patterns previously described in the neuroendocrine system.

At least two possibilities exist concerning the potential function of these peptide hormones produced by the immune system. First, they act on their classic neuroendocrine target tissues. Second, they may serve as endogenous regulators of the immune system. With regard to the latter possibility, it is clear that neuroendocrine peptide hormones can directly modulate immune functions. These studies, however, do not address endogenous as opposed to exogenous regulation by neuroendocrine peptides. A number of investigators have now been able to demonstrate that such regulation is endogenous to the immune system. Specifically, TSH is a pituitary hormone that can be produced by lymphocytes in response to TRH and, like TSH, TRH enhanced the *in vitro* antibody response [8]. This enhancement was not observed with GHRH, arginine vasopressin (AVP) or LHRH and was blocked by antibodies to the β subunit of TSH. Thus it appears that TRH specifically enhances the *in vitro* antibody re sponse via production of TSH. This was apparently the first demonstration that a neuroendocrine hormone (TSH) can function as an endogenous regulator within the immune system. In a similar study, antibody to prolactin was shown to inhibit mitogenesis through neutralization of the lymphocyte-associated prolactin.

antibody response to TSH

Two different approaches have provided further convincing evidence that endogenous neuroendocrine peptides have autocrine or paracrine immunoregulatory functions. First, an opiate antagonist was shown to indirectly block CRF enhancement of NK cell activity by inhibiting the action of immunocyte-derived opioid peptides. Second, we have used an antisense oligodeoxynucleotide (ODN) to the translation start site of GH mRNA to specifically inhibit leukocyte production of GH. The ensuing lack of GH resulted in a marked diminution in basal rates of DNA synthesis in such antisense ODN-treated leukocytes which could be overcome by exogenously added GH [9]. Another group examining SOM found that antisense oligodeoxynucleotides to SOM dramatically increased lymphocyte proliferation in culture.

evidence from antagonist and antisense methodologies

A second major function of GH produced by cells of the immune system is the induction of the synthesis of IGF-1, which, in turn, may inhibit the synthesis of both lymphocyte GH mRNA and protein. Our previous studies also show that both exogenous and endogenous GHRH can stimulate the synthesis of lymphocyte GH. Taken together, these findings support the existence of a complete regulatory loop within cells of the immune system, and they provide a molecular basis whereby GHRH, GH, IGF-1 and its binding protein may be intimately involved in regulating each other's synthesis. Furthermore, data obtained by immunofluorescence techniques suggest that the cells producing GH also produce IGF-1, which suggests that an intracrine regulatory circuit may be important in the synthesis of these hormones by cells of the immune system [10].

IGF-1 synthesis is induced by GH

Functions of leukocyte-derived peptide hormones *in vivo*

lymphocyte mediated steroid response

Although much work needs to be done to fully establish the clinical relevance of leukocyte-derived neuroendocrine hormones, certain experimental models and clinical observations seem to support the view that leukocyte-derived hormones can also act on their classic neuroendocrine targets. The finding that cells of the immune system are a source of secreted ACTH suggested that stimuli which elicit the leukocyte-derived hormone should not require a pituitary gland for an ACTH-mediated increase in corticosteroid. This seemed to be the case, since Newcastle disease virus (NDV) infection of hypophysectomized mice caused a time-dependent increase in corticosterone production which was inhibitable by dexamethasone. Unless such mice were pretreated with dexamethasone, their spleens were positive for ACTH by immunofluorescence [11]. A more recent study has suggested that B-lymphocytes can be responsible for extrapituitary ACTH production. In this report, hypophysectomized chickens were shown to produce ACTH and corticosterone in response to *Brucella abortus*, and the corticosterone response was ablated if B-lymphocytes were deleted by bursectomy prior to hypophysectomy [12]. In children who were pituitary ACTH-deficient and pyrogen-tested, an increase in the percentage of ACTH-positive mononuclear leukocytes was observed. Both the response in hypophysectomized mice and hypopituitary children peaked at approximately 6–8 h after administration of virus and typhoid vaccine, respectively. Such studies have been furthered by a report that CRF administration to pituitary ACTH-deficient individuals results in both an ACTH and cortisol response.

endotoxin shock and lymphocyte ACTH endorphins

Gram-negative bacterial infections and endotoxin shock represent another situation in which leukocyte hormones act on the neuroendocrine system. For example, endorphins have been implicated in the pathophysiology associated with these maladies because the opiate antagonist, naloxone, was shown to improve survival rates and inhibited a number of cardiopulmonary changes associated with these conditions [13]. Further, two separate pools of endorphins have been observed following bacterial lipopolysaccharide (LPS) administration, and it was suggested that one pool might originate in the immune system. Consistent with this idea is the observation that lymphocyte depletion, like naloxone treatment, blocked a number of endotoxin-induced cardiopulmonary changes. Our interpretation of this data is that lymphocyte depletion removed the source of the endorphins, whereas naloxone blocks their effector function. In a different approach, LPS-resistant inbred mice which have essentially no pathophysiologic response to LPS were shown to have a defect in leukocyte processing of proopiomelanocortin (POMC) to endorphins. If leukocyte-derived endorphins were administered to the LPS-resistant mice, they showed much of the pathophysiology associated with LPS administration to sensitive mice [14]. Another exciting new development in the opioid field has come with the demonstration that activation of endogenous opioids in rats by a cold-water swim results in a local antinociceptive effect in inflamed peripheral tissue. This local antinociception in the inflamed tissue apparently results from production by immune cells of endogenous opioids which interact with opioid receptors on peripheral sensory nerves [15]. Another recent study strongly suggests that the immune system plays an essential role in pain control [16]. The findings identify locally expressed CRF as the main agent in inducing opioid release within inflamed tissue. Opioid receptor-specific antinociception in inflamed paws of rats could be blocked by intraplantar α-helical CRF or antiserum to CRF or CRF-antisense oligodeoxynucleotide. This latter treatment reduced the amount of CRF extracted from inflamed paws, as well as the number of CRF-immunostained cells [16]. These observations offer new understanding of the pain occurring in normal and immunosuppressed patients.

lymphocyte CRF and antinociception

In conclusion, the activity of cells of the immune system can be strongly influenced by neuroendocrine-derived and leukocyte-derived neuroendocrine peptides. In many respects, the production and regulation of these peptides by leukocytes is remarkably similar to that observed in neuroendocrine cells. There are, however, a number of noteworthy differences which suggest that rules which apply to pituitary hormone production are not necessarily applicable to the immune system. Once produced, these peptide hormones seem to function in at least two capacities. They are endogenous regulators of the immune system as well as conveyors of information from the immune to the neuroendocrine system. Plasma hormone concentrations do not have to reach the levels required when the pituitary gland is the source, because immune cells are not fixed but are mobile and can locally deposit the hormone at the target site and influence the immune response. It is our bias that the transmission of these molecules along with cytokines to the neuroendocrine system represents a sensory function for the immune system wherein leukocytes recognize stimuli that are not recognizable by the central and peripheral nervous systems [6]. These stimuli have been termed noncognitive and include bacteria, tumors, viruses and antigens. The recognition of such noncognitive stimuli by immunocytes is then converted into information, in the form of peptide hormones and neurotransmitters,

endogenous regulators of immunity

sensory function

lymphocytes and monokines, which is conveyed to the neuroendocrine system, and a physiologic change occurs.

Acknowledgments

We thank faculty colleagues, students and postdoctoral fellows who were pivotal to the studies reported herein. We are also grateful to Diane Weigent for expert editorial assistance. These studies were supported by the Muscular Dystrophy Association to J.E.B. and NIH grants AI37670, MH52527 and NS29719 to J.E.B. and AI41651 to D.A.W.

B   Immunodiagnosis

Antibody detection

Klaus Hermann and Johannes Ring

Introduction

The accurate and reliable determination of biologically active endogenous compounds in plasma, urine and other body fluids for scientific or diagnostic purposes has been a challenge for many decades. In the past, the assessment of such compounds was difficult and tedious because specific and practical analytical tools were not available. In the early days, decisive and convincing conclusions about the significance of a biologically active molecule in disease or health could only be made after purification and isolation of the analyte and identification of its chemical structure. A definite improvement in the analysis of biologically active endogenous compounds was the introduction of bioassays using an intact animal model or *in vitro* tissue preparations. Although the bioassays possessed sufficient sensitivity, there were problems with their lack of specificity. Other analytical procedures such as liquid chromatography, electrophoresis or photometric procedures have also been developed for *in vitro* diagnosis. However, these approaches are either tedious and time-consuming or require expensive equipment and specially trained personal. A landmark in diagnostics was the introduction of immunoassays (IAs) which are inexpensive and easy to perform with high reproducibility, sensitivity and specificity.

immunoassays of biologically active compounds

Basic principle of immunoassays

IAs are based on an antigen-antibody reaction utilizing the exceptional capability of the immune system to produce specific antibodies (Abs) which can recognize and discriminate between a practically infinite number of foreign compounds. The basic requirement for setting up an IA is the production of a specific Ab to a given antigen or hapten by immunizing animals such as mice, rabbits, goats, horses or others. High molecular weight compounds such as proteins are immunogenic and may serve as an antigen which can be injected into the host animal directly to produce Abs. In contrast, low molecular weight compounds such as drugs, amines, peptides or steroids are haptens which do not induce immune responses. They can be rendered immunogenic after coupling to a carrier. The Abs obtained from the serum after several booster injections with the immunogen are heterogeneous polyclonal Abs (pAbs). A more sophisticated approach was the production of monoclonal Abs (mAbs) which was first introduced by Köhler and Milstein in 1975 [1]. This technique allows the production of homogeneous, single Abs in nearly infinite quantities with high specificity for a certain antigen. The method involves the isolation of spleen cells from an immunized animal containing Ab-producing B-cells. The B-cells are then fused with myeloma cells. After selection and screening of the desired Ab-secreting cell line (hybridoma), the Ab can be harvested in the supernatant. These hybridomas can be grown in large volumes for the production of huge quantities of the mAb.

characterization of antibodies

The essentials for the characterization of the Abs produced are high affinity, specificity and sensitivity. The affinity is a measure of the strength of the binding interaction between the antigen and the Ab and can be experimentally determined by the dissociation constant (K_d) of the antigen to the AB. The lower the K_d the greater the affinity. The specificity refers to the specific recognition of the analyte by the Ab without crossreacting with closely related or structurally similar analytes. This in turn is closely related to the ability of the Ab to discriminate between negative and positive samples. The sensitivity describes the detection limit and is defined by the dose-response curve of the antigen to the Ab. The lower the detection limit, the higher the sensitivity.

Antibody structure

Abs, among other serum proteins such as albumins, belong to the gammaglobulin or immunoglobulin (Ig) fraction according to their electrophoretic mobility. They are glycoproteins which are chemically very similar in structure and are constructed of two identical light-chains with an approximate molecular weight (MW) of 50 kDa and two identical heavy-chains with an approximate MW of 110 kDa. Each of the two light-chains are attached to one heavy-chain via disulfide bonds. Likewise, the heavy-chains are bound to each other by disulfide bridging. Two locally distinct binding domains are prominent on Ig molecules. One is

F_{ab}

the antigen binding site (F_{ab}) for the binding and recognition of antigens and the other is the receptor binding site (F_c) for binding to specific receptors on various cells involved in immunological functions such as mononuclear phagocytes, natural killer cells, mast cells or basophil leukocytes (Fig. 1). Although Igs share an overall similarity, they can be divided into different classes and subclasses according to their size, charge, solubility and their behavior as antigens. At present, the classes of Ab molecules in humans can be divided into IgA, IgD, IgE, IgG and IgM. IgA and IgG can be further subdivided into their subclasses IgA_1 and IgA_2 and IgG_1, IgG_2, IgG_3 and IgG_4 (see Chapters A1 and C2).

F_c

classes of Ab molecules

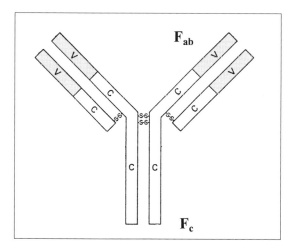

Figure 1 Structure of immunoglobulins
For further details, see text.

Clinical relevance of antibody detection

Initially, the identification and characterization of specific Abs associated with pathophysiological conditions was generally constrained to scientific purposes. However, in many instances the measurement of specific Abs evolved into clinically relevant diagnostic markers in health and disease. Medical conditions in which the determination of specific Abs is used routinely are bacterial and viral infections, infestation with parasites, autoimmune diseases and allergies.

Microbial infections

The determination of Abs in infectious diseases has been known and used for a long time. Bacteria-specific Abs of the IgG and IgM class are rou-

bacteria

tinely detected in the serum of patients infected with different bacteria such as *Borrelia burgdorferi* (lyme disease), *Chlamydia trachomatis* (sexually transmitted infection of the urogenital tract), *Legionella pneumophila* (legionaire disease), *Staphylococcus* and *Streptococcus* and *Treponema pallidum* (lues).

virus

The assessment of IgG and IgM Abs is also a very valuable parameter in the diagnosis of viral infections such as hepatitis, measles, epidemic parotitis and rabies and infections with the Epstein-Barr virus (mononucleosis), herpesvirus (herpes simplex and herpes zoster) and arborvirus (tick encephalitis).

parasites

Infestations with parasites leading to diseases such as leishmaniasis, amebiaisis, malaria, toxoplasmosis, schistosomiasis, echinococcosis, tichinellosis, filariasis or others can induce the formation of Ig molecules of different classes. In the diagnosis of parasitosis it is recommended that the identity of the parasite be ascertained first. In addition, serological methods are available to identify circulating antigens, antigen-Ab complexes or circulating Abs.

Autoimmune diseases

Another area of pathophysiological abnormalities in which the measurement of Abs has predictive and diagnostic value is that of the numerous autoimmune diseases (ADs) in which the self-tolerance of the immune system against its own antigens is abrogated. Examples of an organ-specific AD are Hashimoto's thyroiditis with circulating Abs against thyroglobulin, and myasthenia gravis with auto-Abs against the acetylcholine receptor. Examples of non-organ-specific ADs are Sjögren's syndrome, rheumatoid arthritis, scleroderma and systemic lupus erythematosus affecting the skin, joints and muscles with Abs against nuclear antigens such as DNA, RNA or histones.

Allergy

The most important immunglobulins for the *in vitro* diagnosis of allergic diseases, either immediate-type hypersensitivity reactions such as rhinitis, conjunctivitis, allergic bronchial asthma and anaphylaxis or late phase

IgE

reactions, e.g. allergic contact dermatitis, are Abs of the IgE class [2, 3]. Clinically relevant are the measurement of total IgE or allergen-specific IgE in the patients' serum for the determination of IgE-mediated sensitization. Total serum IgE levels of >100 (Kilo Units) KU/l in adults and children are a good indicator for atopy, a disease characterized by familial hypersensitivity to exogenous environmental agents associated with high IgE Ab titers and altered reactivity against various pharmacological stimuli. However, high total IgE Abs can also be induced by parasitic worm infestations. Extremely high values, higher than 10 000 KU/l are indicative of IgE-producing myelomas. The measurement of allergen-specific IgG Abs as IgE-blocking Abs for monitoring the success of immune therapy with insect venoms in patients with hymenoptera venom allergy has been used tentatively, but with discrepant results.

Antibody detection methods

The detection of Abs in the circulation or in tissue has become a useful analytical tool for the *in vitro* immunodiagnosis of numerous diseases. Several immunological techniques are available for the routine identification of IgA, IgD, IgE, IgG or IgM Ab classes in the clinical chemistry laboratory. The most commonly used methods are discussed briefly.

Immunoprecipitation assay

Immunoprecipitation is a very simple and easy to perform *in vitro* assay for the identification and semiquantitation of soluble Abs. The addition of the antigen to the Ab results in the formation of a three-dimensional, insoluble network of aggregates which precipitate and can be detected with a nephelometer. The assay is very similar to a volumetric acid/base titration. The bulk of precipitate, formed at equivalent concentrations of Ab and antigen, is a measure for the concentration of the Ab. The assay can also be used in reverse to measure the antigen concentration by adding Abs.

in vitro assay

A variation of the immunoprecipitation assay is the hemagglutination test and the complement fixation test. The hemagglutination test allows the identification of Abs to red blood cell antigens or the detection of Abs to antigens which are covalently or noncovalently attached to the red cell surface. The complement fixation test is a three step assay in which the Ab-containing serum is initially incubated with a fixed amount of antigen to form an immune complex. In the second step, complement is added which is firmly incorporated by the immune complexes. Finally, red blood cells are added as indicator cells. Red blood cells will only be lysed if immune complexes have been generated.

hemagglutination test

comlement fixation test

Immunocytochemistry

in situ assay

Immunocytochemistry is a technique for the detection of an Ab *in situ* in tissue slices. Frozen tissue or tissue embedded in various embedding media is cut into thin slices and then immobilized on a slide. After fixation of the tissue with formaldehyde, glutaraldehyde, alcohol or acetone, the tissue is incubated with a specific primary Ab directed against the Ab to be detected. In the direct assay, the primary Ab is chemically coupled to a fluorescent dye (rhodamine, fluorescein), which allows the detection of the analyte by fluorescence microscopy. In the indirect assay, excess primary Ab is thoroughly washed off, and the tissue is incubated with a secondary Ab to form a sandwich. The secondary Ab can be fluoresceinated or coupled to an enzyme, e.g. alkaline phosphatase (ALP) or peroxidase, which allows the visualization of the analyte by fluorescence microscopy or by light microscopy, after addition of a colorless substrate which is enzymatically converted to a colored product. Only cells which contain the analyte will light up under the microscope.

visualization

Immunoblotting

The immunoblot or dot blot technique is similar to the immunoprecipitation assay. However, in immunoblotting the antigen Ab reaction takes place in the solid phase, whereas in the immunoprecipitation assay the Ab reacts with the antigen in solution. The assay utilizes the capability of nitrocellulose membranes to bind antigens. Antigens are applied in small dots, and the membranes are dried. The membranes are treated with ovalbumin, gelatin or milk proteins to prevent nonspecific adsorption. After blocking, the membranes are incubated with the serum and dilutions of the serum which contain the Ab. The membranes are washed to remove abundant Ab. Next, the membranes are incubated with a secondary Ab raised against the Ab of interest which is conjugated with an enzyme. The formation of the antigen-Ab-secondary Ab complex can be visualized by adding a substrate which will be converted by the enzyme of the secondary Ab to yield a colored spot. The intensity of the spots is proportional to the amount of Ab present in the serum samples (Fig. 2A). However, dot blot results alone do not reveal whether the antigen is made up of one or several antigenic components. Further characterization of the Ab can be achieved by separating the antigens electrophoretically. The separated components are transferred from the gel to a nitrocellulose membrane, a process which is called Western blotting. The membranes are then treated like dot blots as outlined above. This methodol-

nitrocellulose
membranes

visualization

Western blotting

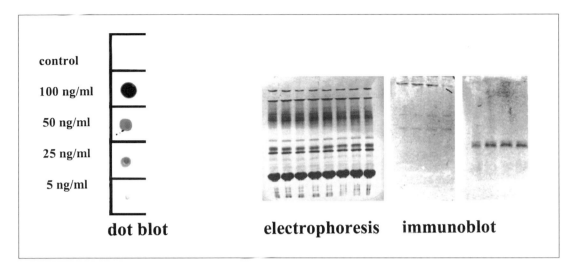

Figure 2 Dot blots and immunoblotting

Specific Abs to an antigen, e.g. an allergen extract, can be detected with the dot blot technique. Further character-ization of the Ab or the antigens present in the allergen extract can be achieved by immunoblotting. For further de-tails see text. Lane 1: MW protein markers; lane 2–8 are different allergen extracts.

ogy combines the high resolving power of electrophoresis and the dis-criminating power of an immunological reaction. Components that are recognized by the Ab show up on the Western blot as colored bands (Fig. 2B).

Immunoadsorbent assays

Immunoadsorbent assay (IAA) techniques are widely used for the mea-surement of serum IgE and IgG Abs. The concept of IAAs is basically very similar to immunoblotting. However, the major difference between immunoblotting and IAA is that the amount of Abs can be quantified. An antigen, e.g. an allergen extract from chicken meat, grass or tree pollen, or house dust mites, is attached to an inert matrix such as the wall of a reaction vial, microtiter plate wells or chemically coupled to a paper disc. The serum of an allergic patient is incubated in a first-step reaction with the allergen-carrying matrix. IgE molecules that recognize the al-lergen are bound. After removal of excess serum, a secondary Ab, in this case an anti-human IgE Ab raised in rabbits, goats or horses, is added which forms an allergen-IgE-anti-IgE Ab complex (second-step reac-tion). Excess of the secondary Ab is also removed by washing. The for-

difference between immunoblotting and IAA

mation of the allergen-IgE-anti-IgE-Ab-complex depends on the amount of specific IgE present in the serum sample. Since the secondary Ab or detecting Ab carries a covalently coupled label or tag, the formation of the allergen-IgE-anti-IgE Ab complex, a sandwichlike structure, can be monitored. Utilizing a standard curve with increasing concentrations of the allergens, the signal obtained with allergen-IgE-anti-IgE Ab complex in the serum sample can be compared with the signal of the standard curve, which permits the quantitation of the IgE Abs. The assay format of an IAA in general is summarized in Fig. 3.

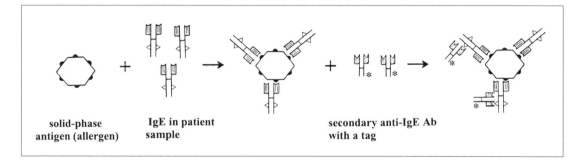

solid-phase
antigen (allergen)

IgE in patient
sample

secondary anti-IgE Ab
with a tag

Figure 3 Immuno-absorbent assay format
Reproduced with permission from DPC Biermann, Germany. For further details, see text.

radio-allergo-sorbent test (RAST)

The radio-allergo-sorbent test (RAST) is a radioimmunoassay (RIA) [4] in which the allergens are chemically coupled to a paper disc and the secondary Ab is radioactively labeled with ^{125}I (Pharmacia Uppsala, Sweden). Similarly, the assay can be performed as an enzyme immunoassay (EIA) in which the secondary Ab is labeled with the enzyme β-galactosidase which can react with a colorless substrate to form a colored reaction product (EAST, Sanofi Diagnostics Pasteur, Chaska, MN, USA). In addition to the RAST or EAST, a RAST or EAST inhibition assay can be performed to confirm and validate the results [5]. The serum samples are first incubated *in vitro* with increasing concentrations of the allergens prior to the RAST or EAST. The binding inhibition of the Ab can be illustrated by a dose-response curve which inversely correlates with the concentration of allergens added; low allergen concentrations still give a high signal in the RAST or EAST, whereas the signal vanishes with high concentrations. The concentration of the allergen at 50% inhibition (IC_{50}) can be calculated from the dose-response curve. A low IC_{50} is a good indicator for a high affinity and specificity of the Ab to the allergens (Fig. 4).

IC_{50}

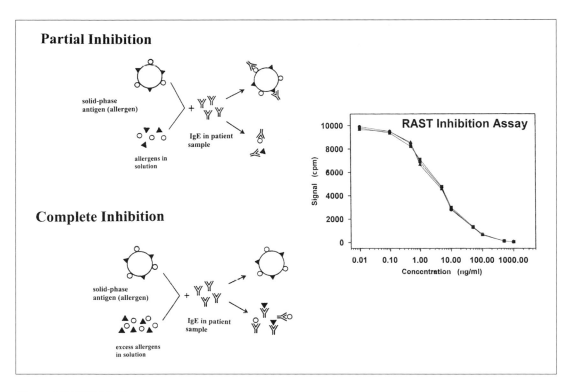

Figure 4 RAST inhibition assay

Reproduced with permission from DPC Biermann, Germany. For further details, see text.

A further development of the RAST or EAST was the introduction of a three-dimensional cellulose sponge instead of the paper disc. This approach is practiced by the Pharmacia-CAP system (Pharmacia Uppsala, Sweden). The Pharmacia-CAP assay is performed in microtiter plates and allows partial automation of the assay. The advantages are higher binding capacity of the cellulose sponges (CAP) and the use of the photometric detection of the allergen-IgE-anti-IgE Ab complex with a microplate reader.

Variations and modifications of this basic assay format have been made with respect to the characteristics of the allergens, e.g. using allergens in liquid phase and replacing the β-galactosidase-labeled secondary Ab with an Ab that is chemically linked to ALP. This unique concept is realized in several recently developed assay formats. The AlaSTAT liquid allergen technology [Diagnostic Product Corporation (DPC), Los Angeles, CA, USA] is based on a four-step reaction. In the first incubation, the biotinylated allergens react with patients' serum IgE. In the second incubation, avidin is added which forms a complex between the

AlaSTAT liquid allergen technology

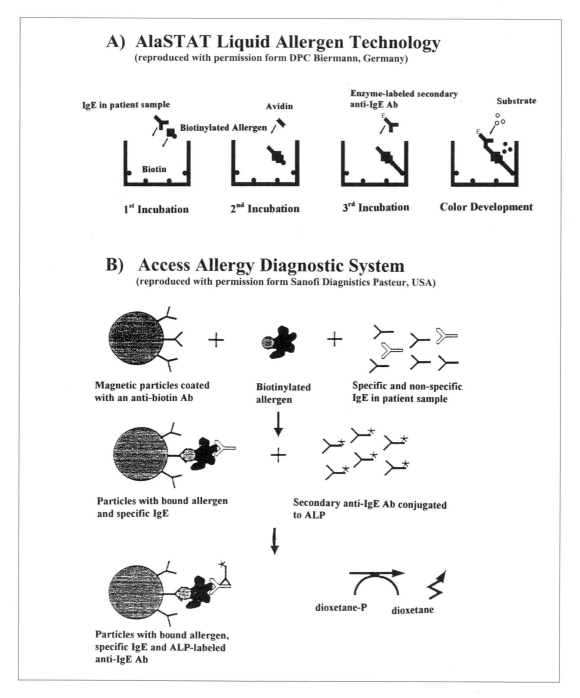

Figure 5 Advanced immunoassay techniques

(A) AlaSTAT liquid allergen technology (reproduced with permission from DPC Biermann, Germany). (B) Access Allergy Diagnostic System (reproduced with permission from Sanofi Diagnostics Pasteur, USA). For further details, see text.

biotinylated allergens and IgE. In the third incubation an enzyme-labeled secondary anti-IgE Ab is added to form a sandwich between the biotin of the reaction vessel, avidin, the biotinylated allergen and the allergen-specific IgE Abs. Finally, the formation of the triple-sandwich complex can be monitored photometrically by the enzymatic conversion of the substrate to a colored product (Fig. 5A). The advantages of this technology are automation with a high sample throughput, increased specificity and reaction kinetic with allergens in liquid phase. Since the allergens are present in a liquid formulation and not immobilized to an insoluble matrix, the same allergens used in the assay are also available for other testing such as skin testing and inhibition experiments.

An even more refined assay technology is realized in the Access Allergy Diagnostic System (Sanofi Diagnostics Pasteur). The assay is also a liquid phase assay using paramagnetic polystyrene beads coated with an antibiotin Ab as a capturing Ab. In a first-step reaction, the biotinylated allergens and the allergen-specific IgE form a triple-sandwich complex between the polystyrene beads, the allergen and the IgE. Excess IgE and allergens are removed in a magnetic field which attracts the paramagnetic polystyrene beads. The second reaction is the incubation with an anti-human IgE Ab (secondary Ab) labeled with ALP, which results in the formation of a quadruple sandwich (paramagnetic polystyrene beads, allergens, IgE and anti-IgE). Excess ALP-labeled secondary Ab is also removed in the magnetic field. Finally, dioxetane-phosphate is added as a substrate which is converted by ALP to a chemiluminescent product which can be quantitated in a luminometer (Fig. 5B). The advantages of the Access Allergy Diagnostic System are similar to the AlaSTAT technology: automation with high sample throughput in a short period of time. Compared with photometric detection, chemiluminescence offers a wide dynamic range for the detection, allowing the determination of low and high IgE concentrations without further sample dilution.

Access Allergy Diagnostic System

Immunohematological identification of leukemia and lymphoma

C. Ellen van der Schoot

Introduction

During the last decades considerable progress has been made in the immunological characterization of proliferative blood diseases [1]. This has become possible by the development of a wide variety of monoclonal antibodies, which were clustered during the six international workshops on leukocyte differentiation antigens as well as by the fast technical improvement of flow cytometers. In connection with these workshops, research groups from all over the world send their antibodies to the organizing workshop committee. The different section leaders select the antibodies, allocate them to different groups and distribute the antibodies as (blind) panels of antibodies to the participants. These groups perform serological, histological, biochemical and functional assays with the antibodies, and the antibodies are tested on transfectant cells that express known antigens. Based on all these results the antibodies recognizing the same antigen are classified into CD-clusters.

CD-clusters

This chapter presents an overview of the present knowledge on the value of immunophenotypic analysis of leukemias and lymphomas.

Indications for immunophenotypic analysis

Indications for immunophenotypic analysis are summarized in Table 1. For several (sub)forms of diseases diagnosis is completely dependent on immunophenotypic analysis, e.g. discrimination between precursor B-acute lymphoid leukemia (ALL) and T-ALL. An important application of imunophenotypic analysis is the discrimination between reactive and monoclonal lymphocytes. However, for most diseases immunophenotypic analysis of malignant cells is used primarily for confirmation of the diagnosis, which has already been suggested by morphological and cytochemical examination, as for the diagnosis of acute myeloid leukemia

Table 1 Indications for immunophenotypic analysis

- Diagnosis of diseases, that cannot be properly diagnosed by other techniques
- Confirmation of diagnosis, thereby enhancing the reliability of the diagnosis
- Identification of clinically relevant subgroups of patients
- Detection of low numbers of malignant cells [staging of B-NHL, detection of minimal residual disease (MRD) in follow up samples]
- Defining target antigens for therapy (purging procedures of autologous stem-cell grafts or *in vivo* immunotherapy)

stem-cell transplantation

(AML) or hairy cell leukemia (HCL). Several studies have shown that immunological characterization greatly enhances the reliability of these diagnoses. Moreover, in these diseases marker expression also can be used to identify subgroups of patients. When the malignant cells express a combination of antigens that is rare in healthy donors, antibodies against these antigens can be used to detect low numbers of malignant cells using double- or triple-colour immunofluorescence assays. Finally, marker analysis can be done at diagnosis to identify the immunophenotype of the malignant cells, thereby defining the antibodies that can be used for therapy. In most cases these antibodies are used to purge autologous stem-cell grafts. The patients are treated with high-dose chemotherapy and/or radiotherapy, and to rescue them from hematopoietic failure, they receive a hematopoietic stem-cell transplantation. In the autologous setting the stem-cell graft is harvested from the patient before the intensified treatment and therefore potentially contaminated with malignant cells. Although it has not been demonstrated to be of benefit to the patient, many clinicians choose to purge the bone marrow graft of tumour cells. This can be achieved by using monoclonal antibodies directed against antigens that are expressed on the clonogenic malignant cells and that are not reactive with the primitive hematopoietic stem cells. Alternatively, hematopoietic stem cells can be purified using an antibody directed against the CD34-antigen, an antigen which is only expressed on hematopoietic progenitor cells, including the most primitive stem cells. Only the CD34-positive cells are given back to the patient, again diminishing the level of tumour contamination. For the most effective depletion of tumour cells, both approaches should be combined. More recently, very hopeful results have been reported for the *in vivo* treatment of non-Hodgkin's lymphoma with monoclonal antibodies belonging to

***in vivo* treatment with monoclonal antibodies**

the CD20-cluster. Especially in the setting of minimal residual disease, this approach may be promising.

Immunophenotypes of the different proliferative blood diseases

Leukemic cells can be regarded as the malignant counterparts of normal cells at different differentiation stages. The expression of various antigens during myeloid and lymphoid differentiation is well described. Therefore, the antigenic makeup of the malignant cells can be used to define the differentiation stage of the malignant cells [1]. In most cases, especially in lymphoproliferative diseases, the differentiation stage of the malignant cell is strictly correlated with the diagnosis. For example, all acute lymphoid leukemias are derived from immature lymphoid cells, whereas all chronic lymphoid leukemias and almost all lymphomas originate from more mature (intermediate) B-cells.

malignant counterparts

Acute leukemias

Classically, the leukemias are ordered according to morphological and cytochemical criteria as defined by the French American British (FAB) group. From a clinical point of view, the subdivision between ALL and AML is the most important one because of the differences in prognosis and response to therapy of these two diseases. A small group of patients could not be classified by the FAB criteria. Some of these morphologically undifferentiated leukemias express at least one myeloid marker, in the absence of the lymphoid specific antigens. Recently, the FAB group has defined this group of leukemias as AML-M0 and thereby employ immunophenotypes in its classification system [2].

In the Netherlands, we have introduced criteria for the immunological characterization of acute leukemia. These criteria are based on the reactivity of a panel of so-called cell-line defining markers, cell-line specific markers and additional markers (Table 2). Cell-line defining markers are reactive with almost all differentiation stages of a particular cell lineage. A positive reaction with at least two of these markers defines the origin of the leukemia. Cell-line specific markers are expressed only by one cell lineage, and all other cell lineages are negative. For subdivision of the leukemia, additional markers have to be used.

criteria

Table 2 Criteria for immunological classification of acute leukemia[*]

Cell-lineage	Cell-line defining markers	Additional markers	
B-cell lineage	CD19 + CD79[†] /CD22[†]	TdT	CD20
		HLA-DR	CD34
		CD10	Cyμ[†]
		SmIg	
T-cell lineage	CyCD3[†] + CD2	TdT	CD5
	and/or CD7	TcR-CD3	CD34
	CD1		
Myeloid cell lineage	MPO[†] + CD13	CDw65	HLA-DR
	and/or CD33	CD14	CD34
		CD15	
Erythroid cell lineage	H-antigen and/or CD36	GpA[†]	
	(CD14, CD41 and HLA-DR-)		
Megakaryocytic lineage	CD41[†] /CD61	CD42[†]	

[*] Criteria as suggested by the Dutch Cooperative Study Group on Immunophenotyping of Leukemias and Lymphoma [11, 12]. [†] Cell-line specific markers.

There is increasing evidence that genetic phenotypes, i.e. subgroups of patients characterized by a common specific genetic aberration, carry the most important prognostic value [3]. Some of these groups can also be recognized by their immunophenotype, as outlined below. However, the relationship between genetic phenotype and immunophenotype is not always consistent.

ALL

ALL is the most frequent malignancy of children, comprising 25% of all cancers. In adults it affect 2 persons per 100 000 annually. ALL is a heterogeneous disease with biological and clinically distinct subsets [4]. The immunological classification is well established and has been shown to be of clinical significance. ALL is initially divided into B- and T-lineages [1, 5].

As can be seen in Table 1, almost all ALL, except the very rare B-ALL, are terminal deoxynucleotide transferase (TdT)-positive. In fact, one should reconsider the diagnosis of ALL, if the leukemic cells are TdT-negative. The enzyme TdT inserts N-nucleotides at the junction sites during the rearrangement of T-cell receptor (TCR) and immunoglobulin (Ig) heavy genes. However, TdT is not lymphoid-specific, because in the majority of AML patients mostly low numbers of weakly TdT-positive blasts can be found. B-precursor ALL is recognized by the expression of the B-cell-specific antigen CD79. CD79a and CD79b are components of the B-cell receptor complex (BCR), Igα and Igβ, respectively. These proteins are structurally and functionally homologous to the CD3 polypeptides, which are associated with the TCR. They play a central role in transmembrane signal transduction upon antigen binding. The expression of cytoplasmic CD3 is specific for T-ALL. Different subtypes of T-ALL also can be recognized. However, these subsets do not seem to be prognostically relevant.

The immunological classification can be used to recognize distinct clinical subgroups of patients (Table 3). Common ALL, which is characterized by the expression of CD10, occurs at a high incidence during early childhood (2–6 years). The prognosis is relatively good. Almost all patients reach complete remission, and 70–80% of patients are completely cured of their disease. Among patients with precursor B-ALL, several specific genetic alterations dramatically affect prognosis. The first of these is t(9;22), the Philadelphia chromosome, which creates the *bcr-abl* fusion gene. This translocation is present in only a few percent of the children, but in 30% of adult patients. Translocations involving 11q23 occur in about 60% of ALL in infants. Both translocations are associated with an unfavorable prognosis, and aberrant expression of myeloid antigens, especially CD15, is often found.

immunological classification

The application of monoclonal antibodies to the detection of minimal residual disease (MRD) in ALL is hampered by the presence of normal cells with the same phenotype as the leukemic cells. However, in some

minimal residual disease (MRD)

Table 3 Immunological classification of ALL

B-precursor ALL	
null-ALL	TdT, CD19, cytoplasmatic-CD79, CD22, HLA-DR, CD34
common-ALL	TdT, CD19, cyt-CD79, HLA-DR, CD22, (CD34), **CD10**
pre-B-ALL	TdT, CD19, cyt-CD79, HLA-DR, CD22, (CD34), **CD10, cyt-IgM**
B-ALL	CD19, **membrane-CD79**, HLA-DR, CD22, (CD10), **membrane Ig**
T-ALL	
	TdT, CD7, CD2, (cyt)-CD3, CD5, (CD4/CD8), (CD10), CD1 (frequently loss of T-cell antigens)

cases, especially in T-ALL, immunofluorescence techniques can be used for the early detection of relapse. The presence of certain phenotypes in blood or bone marrow is indicative for leukemic infiltration, as these cells normally do not circulate outside the thymus. However, for precursor B-ALL the immunological detection of MRD is more complicated. Following induction therapy, high numbers (up to 50%) of TdT+/CD10+ cells can be seen. These cells are normal regenerative bone marrow cells rather than leukemic cells. However, very recently Coustin-Smith et al. showed that it seems to be possible to detect prognostically relevant MRD with multiparameter flow cytometry [6].

AML

FAB classification

The standard classification of AML is still the FAB classification. The immunological characterization of the leukemic cells is primarily used to confirm the morphological diagnosis (Table 4). However, immunophenotypic analysis reveals that AML is a far more heterogeneous disease than the FAB classification suggests [7]. This also explains why it is often very difficult to reproducibly classify a leukemia according to the FAB criteria. No specific phenotypes exist for all the different FAB subclasses, but several membrane antigens are only expressed on the cells of a particular FAB subclass. However, these leukemias can be negative for these markers as well. Leukemias with specific chromosomal translocations tend to have a similar immunophenotype.

prognosis

In several studies, a correlation between immunophenotype and prognosis has been shown. In general, leukemias with a more immature immunophenotype, as reflected by the expression of CD34, CD7, c-kit

Table 4 Immunophenotypic criteria for AML

Minimally differentiated (FAB-M0)	Negative for CD19, CD79, CD3 and MPO Positive for CD13 or CD33
Myeloid (FAB-M1 and M2)	Negative for CD14 Positive for MPO and CD13/CD33/CD65/CD15
Promyelocytic (FAB-M3)	MPO++, CD15–, HLA-DR–
(Myelo)Monocytoid (FAB-M4 and M5)	Positive for CD14 and/or CD11c
Erythroblastoid (FAB-M6)	MPO–, CD36+CD14–, (glycophorin A+)*
Megakaryocytic (FAB-M7)	MPO–, (CD41/CD61+)*, (CD42b+)†

*In most cases but not obligatory; †in some cases.

(CD117) or mdr-1 (multi-drug resistence gene-1), have an unfavorable prognosis [1].

By combining many different antibodies, one can select for each patient a phenotype that is extremely rare in normal bone marrow or peripheral blood. These subpopulations can then be followed during therapy [7]. However, this approach is very laborious and requires trying many combinations. Therapeutic trials, both *in vivo* and *in vitro*, have been carried out with CD33 antibodies.

Chronic lymphoproliferative disorders

Chronic lymphoproliferative disorders are in most cases B-cell malignancies, but also T- and NK-cell proliferative diseases can be found. Except for the lymphoblastic lymphomas these diseases are characterized by the presence of more mature cells. This means for the B-cell diseases that cells carry the complete BCR complex on the membrane, and malignant T-cells a complete TCR complex. Normally, about 65% of B-cells express kappa light-chain, whereas about 35% express lambda light-chain. The normal κ/λ ratio in peripheral blood is between 0.8 and 3.6. Since a B-cell malignancy represents the clonal expansion of a single B-cell, only one type of Ig light-chain is expressed. Therefore, the κ/λ ratio is used for the detection of a mature B-cell malignancy. Most T-cell malignancies are clonal expansions of CD4 cells, although occasionally $CD8^+$ malignant T-cells can be found. Therefore, the CD4/CD8 ratio can be used for the screening of patients with possible T-cell lymphoma. However, in many other circumstances shifts in CD4/CD8 ratios can exist. Therefore, the immunophenotypic analysis can never be used to prove clonality of a T-cell malignancy. For these purposes, Southern blot analysis or polymerase chain reaction (PCR) assays of TCR genes have to be performed.

κ/λ ratio

CD4/CD8 ratio

Mature B-cell malignancies

In analogy to the acute leukemias, the differentiation stage of the malignant cells in mature B-cell malignancies can be determined by the antigenic makeup of the malignant cell. Immunophenotyping of the circulating B-cells in chronic B-cell leukemias can be used to classify the different chronic leukemias [B-chronic lymphoid leukemia (CLL), B-prolymphocytic leukemia (PLL), hairy cell leukemias (HCL) and the leukemic B-non-Hodgkin's lymphomas (NHL)] [8]. Since the introduction of the REAL classification in 1994 for non-Hodgkin's lymphoma,

Table 5

Immunophenotype of chronic B-cell leukemias and leukemic B-non-hodgkin's-lymphoma

Markers	B-CLL	B-PLL	HCL	HCLv	SVL	MCL	FCL
SmIg+CD79	±	++	+/++	+/++	+/++	+	+/++
isotype	μ/μ/	μ/μ	μ/μ/ /		μ/μ/	μ/μ/μ	μ/μ/
CD19	+	+	+	+	+	+	+
CD20	±	+	++	+	+	++	+
CD22	±	++	++	++	++	+	+
CD23	±	±	±	±	±	±	+
CD24	+/++	±	–	–	+	+	+
CD25	–/±	–	+	–	±	–	–
CD5	+	±	–	–	±	+	–
CD10	–	–/±	–/±	–	±	±	±/+
CD11c	–/±	–	+	+	±	–	–
CD103	–	–	+	+	–/+	–	–
FMC7	–/±	++	+	+	+	+	+

CLL, chronic lymphoid leukemia; PLL, prolymphocytic leukemia; HCL, hairy cell leukemia; HCLv, hairy celll variant leukemia; SVL, splenic villous lymphoma; MCL, mantle cell lymphoma; FCL, follicular lymphoma.

immunophenotyping of the lymphoma cells is involved in classification [9]. The immunophenotypes of these diseases are listed in Table 5.

CLL

CLL is the most common adult leukemia in Western Europe and North America. Although the disease is generally indolent, there is a wide range in survival. There is no relationship between immunophenotypic features and prognosis. The major distinction between B-CLL and B-NHL exists in the expression of CD5 and CD23 as well as the weak expression of surface Ig (SmIg) in B-CLL. Mantle cell lymphoma (MCL) may be difficult to distinguish from CLL morphologically. These patients have an unfavorable prognosis and can be recognized by their phenotype (CD5$^+$ CD23$^-$).

hairy cell leukemia

Hairy cell leukemia is characterized by invasion of the bone marrow and spleen by morphologically distinct mononuclear cells with "hairy" cytoplasmic projections. The hairy cells have a characteristic immunophenotype. The expression of CD103 (BLy-7) is, within the B-cell malignancies, specific for HCL. In the variant form of hairy cell leukemia (HCLv), the lymphoid cells resemble hairy cells. This disease is rare. The characteristic difference between the immunophenotype of HCL and HCLv is the lack of expression of CD25 in the latter. This distinction may be important, because the variants do not respond as well to standard hairy cell leukemia therapy. One of the very effective therapies for HCL is cladribine (2-chlorodeoxyadenosine). One complication of this therapy is prolonged suppression of CD4$^+$ T-lymphocytes, which can be monitored by flow cytometry.

Immunophenotyping is a powerful adjunct to cyto- and histomorphology in the diagnosis of lymphoma. However, one should bear in mind that lymphoma classification still greatly depends on histological examination of the involved lymphoid organs. The most characteristic antigen patterns are delineated in Table 5.

lymphoma

The malignant B-cells of Waldenström's macroglobulinemia, heavychain disease and multiple myeloma (= M. Kahler) represent a further step in the maturation of B-cells. Due to the loss of most B-lineage-specific antigens and sIg with maturation to plasma cells, these disorders have been traditionally difficult to assess by flow cytometry. However, the availability of new reagents for membrane permeabilization and the description of plasma cell-specific antibodies (CD138) have made flow cytometric demonstration of monoclonal plasma cells possible. Furthermore, most myelomas express CD56, whereas normal plasma cells are CD56-negative.

multiple myeloma

Mature T-cell malignancies

Chronic T-cell proliferations are much more rare than B-cell malignancies. Quite often skin manifestations can be found. In most cases, the malignant cells are CD4$^+$, but as discussed above, the CD4/CD8 ratio cannot be used to show clonality in any T-cell disorder. Aberrant phenotypes, particularly loss of pan-T-cell antigens, are very common in this group of disorders. The phenotypes are given in Table 6.

Adult T-cell leukemia lymphoma (ATLL) is rare and is caused by a retrovirus, human T-cell leukemia virus (HTLV-1). The disease is almost only found in patients from Japan, the Caribbean and Central Africa. For

adult T-cell leukemia lymphoma

Table 6 Immunophenotype of mature T-cell and LGL-leukemias

T-PLL	CD3-TCR, CD2, CD5, CD7, CD4 (70%) or CD8 (20%)
ATLL	CD3-TCR, CD2, CD5, CD7±, CD4, CD25++
CTLL/Sezary	CD3-TCR, CD2, CD5, CD7– or +, CD4, CD25±
CD3$^+$LGL	CD3-TCR, CD8, CD16, (CD56), CD57
CD3$^-$LGL	CD2, CD7, CD16, CD56

**large granular
lymphocytes**

diagnosis antibodies against HTLV-1 or virus-RNA by reverse transcriptase (RT)-PCR have to be demonstrated. The intense expression of CD25 is characteristic for the malignant cells. The reactivity of the cells with CD7 is relatively low.

Large granular lymphocytes (LGL) are a morphologically recognizable lymphoid subset comprising 10–15% (but in some normal donors more than 30%) of peripheral blood mononuclear cells. Two major lineages can be recognized by CD3 expression. The CD3$^-$ LGLs are natural killer cells (NK) cells that mediate non-major histocompatibility complex (MHC)-restricted cytotoxicity and do not express the CD3/TCR complex or rearrange TCR genes, in contrast to the CD3$^+$ LGLs. These latter cells are thought to represent *in vivo*-activated T-lymphocytes, and they mediate non-MHC cytoxicity. For both cell types, syndromes have been described in which the number of these cells is increased [10]. In most cases, these diseases are associated with neutropenia and other autoimmune features, especially rheumatoid arthritis. However, most patients with increased numbers of CD3$^-$ LGLs do not have clinical features of NK-LGL leukemia and have a relatively benign chronic clinical course. X-linked gene analysis supports polyclonal LGL lymphocytosis in this syndrome.

Immunoassays

Michael J. O'Sullivan

Introduction

For more than 30 years immunoassay has been the method of choice for measuring low analyte concentrations in complex biological fluids. The procedure is equally applicable to the measurement of small molecular weight compounds such as drugs and large protein molecules. The technique combines sensitivity and specificity with ease of use.

Immunoassays are used in basic biological research to investigate the physiological and possible pathological role of a wide range of potent biologically active substances including cyclic nucleotides, prostaglandins, leukotrienes, growth factors and cytokines. Such research often leads to the identification of new therapeutic agents. The assays are also used in the pharmaceutical industry in many aspects of the drug development process. These range from drug screening, toxicological, pharmacological and pharmacokinetic studies through to clinical trials. Immunoassays have perhaps had their greatest impact in the area of clinical diagnostic tests. The technique has been employed for many years in hospital clinical biochemistry laboratories to diagnose disease and metabolic disorders. More recently, applications of this technique have moved out of these core areas into such diverse situations as the biotechnology industry, the food safety industry and even to "over-the-counter" applications such as home pregnancy testing. In fact, it is difficult to think of any area of the biological sciences where immunoassays have not had a significant impact.

The technique was introduced in 1959 by Berson and Yalow [1]. The combination of a signal which could be easily detected and a protein molecule which binds specifically and avidly to the analyte of interest lies at the heart of all immunoassay procedures. Assay designs have proliferated over the last 30 years as have the different types of signal reagents and detection systems. Sophisticated instruments with associated computer hardware have been developed with the aim of increasing sample throughput.

immunoassays: method of choice

immunoassays: clinical diagnostic

Principles of Immunopharmacology, ed. by F. P. Nijkamp and M. J. Parnham
©1999 Birkhäuser Verlag Basel/Switzerland

This chapter will discuss and highlight the main elements of the subject but cannot hope to be an in depth review of the whole field. For the interested reader, *The Immunoassay Handbook*, published in 1994, provides a comprehensive review of the area [2].

Basic principles of assay design

Competitive immunoassays

labelled analyte or limited reagent

In the competitive immunoassay approach (also termed labelled analyte or limited reagent) there is competition between labelled and unlabelled analyte for a limited number of binding sites on an antibody. Antibody-bound analyte is separated from unbound analyte and the proportion of label in either fraction analysed. A curve can then be plotted of the percentage of tracer bound to the antibody against a range of known standard concentrations. The concentration of unknown analyte present in the sample can then be determined by interpolation from the standard curve.

Although an antibody is usually used in these assays, there may be circumstances where it is more appropriate to use a naturally occurring binding protein or receptor. This does not affect the principle of the assay.

This assay format has the advantages that only one antibody is required, and it uses relatively small amounts of the sometimes limited antibody reagent. It has the disadvantages that assay sensitivity is limited by antibody avidity, the assays have a relatively narrow dynamic range and the labelling process may damage the analyte. This format tends to **small analytes** be favoured for small analytes. The principle of a competitive assay is shown in Figure 1.

Immunometric assays

labelled reagents or reagent excess

The immunometric approach (also termed labelled reagent or reagent excess) differs from the competitive approach in a number of ways. It involves two antibodies which are specific for the analyte, one of which is labelled. In its most usual format, one of the antibodies is immobilized on a solid phase, the sample containing the analyte is added and followed by the labelled second antibody. Unbound label is removed by washing. The amount of label bound to the solid phase is related to the amount of analyte in the sample, as both antibodies are present in excess. A standard curve can be constructed using known quantities of analyte, and the

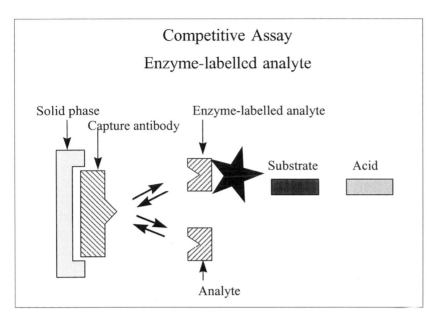

Figure 1 The principle of a competitive immunoassay

concentration of analyte in the sample can be determined by interpolation from the curve.

This method has the advantages that it tends to be more sensitive and precise than the competitive approach. It also tends to have a wider dynamic range, and there is no requirement to label the analyte. The major disadvantages of the technique are the high consumption of antibody and the requirement for two antibodies.

Immunometric assays are the favoured technique for quantitating large molecules. They cannot be applied to small molecules due to the size restraint on binding two large antibodies to one small molecule at the same time. The principle of an immunometric assay, also commonly referred to as a sandwich assay, is shown in Figure 2.

large molecules

These two basic approaches have been the subject of endless permutations, some of which will be touched upon in later sections of this chapter.

Homogenous assays

The assay formats described above suffer from one significant disadvantage, that is the need to separate bound from free tracer. This is a labour-intensive step which is difficult to automate and introduces sig-

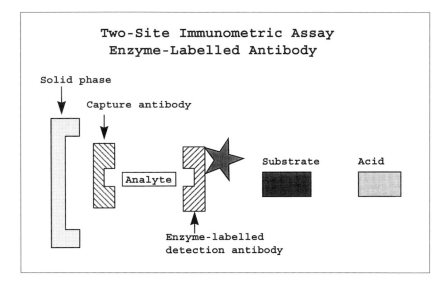

Figure 2 The principle of a two-site immunometric assay

**homogeneous
assays**

nificant imprecision into the assay. In an attempt to overcome this problem, considerable effort, ingenuity and money have been invested in developing homogeneous assays which do not require a separation step. Several successful methods have been developed for the quantitation of small molecular weight analytes, but the methods lack sensitivity and are not generally applicable to the measurement of large molecules. One exception, is the technique [3] termed scintillation proximity which will be discussed later in the chapter.

Components of immunoassays

Tracers

Radioisotopes

iodine 125

For many years after the technique was introduced, radioisotopes were used, virtually exclusively, as the assay tracer. *Radioactive iodine (iodine-125)* was the favoured label, its high specific activity providing good assay sensitivity and a reasonably long half-life giving adequate reagent shelf life. It was also easy in many cases to prepare labelled proteins. The equipment required to measure radioactive decay was also readily available. Finally, the rate and measurement of radioactive decay was not affected by the sample matrix. In most situations iodine-125 remained the label of choice for the next 20 years and is still widely used even today.

Tritium tracers were also widely used for small molecule assays. Such tracers are readily commercially available and have a long shelf life. The tritiated molecule is also virtually identical to the nonlabelled molecule. Many other labelling techniques change the structure of the labelled molecule, which often results in differences in avidity of the interaction of the antibody with the analyte and the label. This can adversely affect assay performance. For these reasons immunoassays for small molecules can often be set up most quickly using tritium tracers. However, tritium tracers do have significant disadvantages. In particular, their relatively low specific activity demands long count times, and their measurement requires the use of organic scintillant cocktails. For these reasons tritium-based assays have a tendency to be replaced by iodine-125 assays if and when labelling problems are overcome.

tritium

Nonisotopic tracers

Radioisotopes are perceived as posing a potential health risk, and there certainly are regulatory problems associated with their use and disposal. In addition, when nonisotopic assays were first being developed, some researchers believed that there would be advantages associated with the use of nonisotopic tracers, although this was hotly disputed at the time by some radioimmunoassay experts. In practice the development of satisfactory labelling techniques [4] and suitable assay designs for nonisotopic tracers did prove difficult. A major breakthrough came with the introduction of 96 well microtitre plates with associated washing and measuring equipment [5].

Today *enzymes* [6] are the most widely used tracers. When used in combination with colorimetric end-points, they provide highly sensitive, robust, precise, accurate and convenient immunoassays. Inexpensive automatic colorimetric multiwell plate readers are readily available. Many commercial kits are on the market which enable relatively inexperienced workers to measure picogram per millilitre levels of biologically active compounds in complex biological fluids with inexpensive, readily available laboratory equipment. Horseradish peroxidase in combination with a ready-to-use formulation of 3,3'5,5'-tetramethlybenzidine has proved extremely popular. Many other nonisotopic tracers have been used, of which *fluorescent* and *luminescent* labels have stood the test of time.

enzymes

In some assays the detection antibody is labelled with biotin rather than an enzyme. The biotinylated antibody is used in combination with a streptavidin/horseradish peroxidase conjugate. Streptavidin has a very high affinity for and binds very quickly to biotin, thus linking the biotinylated antibody noncovalently to the enzyme. This approach tends to label the antibody more consistently and to give a modest two- to four-fold increase in assay sensitivity.

Binding reagent

specificity, avidity

Antibodies are used in the vast majority of assays because they can provide the levels of specificity and avidity required in these binding assays. Binding proteins are used on occasions when suitable antibodies are not available. Antibodies are either *monoclonal* or *polyclonal*. Polyclonal antibodies are produced entirely in animals, particularly rabbits. The animals' immune system generally produces a rather heterogeneous mixture of antibodies. Monoclonal production is initiated in mice, but when an antibody response is observed, their spleens are removed and the suspended spleen cells fused with a myeloma cell line. The fused cell hybridomas are grown in culture. If any culture is positive, it is plated out so that each well contains a single cell. This produces cells that are derived from a single progenitor and gives rise to a single species of antibody.

polyclonal Abs

Polyclonal antibodies tend to be of high avidity and can be very specific. However, their exact composition will vary from bleed to bleed even in the same animal. For this reason it is difficult for commercial kit manufacturers to ensure complete product homogeneity over the lifetime of a commercial immunoassay. Polyclonal antibodies tend to be used in competitive assays, which require high avidity antibodies and do not consume too much antibody.

monoclonal Abs

Monoclonal antibodies tend to be of rather lower avidity but provide a more homogeneous reagent. They also have a more closely defined specificity. These antibodies tend to be used in immunometric assays often in combination with a polyclonal. Finally it should be admitted that antibody production is more of an art than a science.

Standards

standard of immunoassay

Each time the concentration of an analyte is determined in an unknown sample, it is necessary to prepare a standard curve containing known concentrations of the analyte. *The standard is the most important compo-*

nent of an immunoassay. Any error in the standard will produce an error in the estimated analyte concentration. The standard should resemble the analyte as closely as possible. This may seem a rather obvious statement to make, but is often difficult to achieve in practice. For instance, recombinant proteins are often used as standards. Do they have the same conformation and degree of glycosylation as the native molecule? Standards are preferably calibrated against some type of agreed international standard. Commercial companies also have strict internal quality control criteria to ensure that their kit standards do not fall outside tight performance specifications.

Buffer

A multitude of buffers have been employed in immunoassays, although most often phosphate or Tris buffers at near to physiological pH are used. The buffers usually contain a protein additive to reduce nonspecific binding to tube or microtitre plate walls. In addition, buffers contain a bacteriostat to prevent bacterial contamination. One difficult problem often encountered in setting up an immunoassay is related to the different composition of the sample and the standard. This can cause problems during assay validation. Buffers often contain additives such as animal proteins in an attempt to minimize such matrix effects.

additives

Separation systems

Many techniques have been employed to separate antibody-bound analyte from free analyte. Activated charcoal is often used with tritium tracers. The charcoal selectively adsorbs the free tracer but is unable to bind the antibody-bound fraction. The charcoal-bound fraction is separated from the free fraction by centrifugation. Precipitation procedures are popular with iodine-125 tracers. These methods often employ a second antibody specific for the first to form an immune complex which can again be separated from the unbound tracer by centrifugation.

These precipitation techniques have been largely superseded by solid phase techniques, where either the primary or secondary antibody is bound to a solid phase such as finely dispersed particulate suspensions, plastic tubes or microtitre plates. Coated particles are widely used with iodine-125 tracers. These particles are fine suspensions of cellulose, agarose or other material coated with the antibody of interest. Separation of the bound and free fractions can either be achieved by centrifu-

microtitre plates

gation or preferably by using a magnet if a magnetizable component is incorporated into the particle. Coated well techniques have become increasingly popular as the trend away from radioactivity has gained momentum in the immunoassay field. Microtitre plates provide a very convenient format for performing enzyme immunoassays. The antibody is adsorbed to the walls of the plastic wells, and separation of the bound from the free fraction is very readily achieved by washing the plates and decanting off the liquid contents. This is much more convenient than centrifugation methods.

Selected immunoassays

Endothelin-1,2 radioimmunoassay

RIA

This assay has been selected as an example of a competitive assay using an iodine-125 tracer and magnetic separation. Endothelin is a potent vasoconstrictor produced by vascular endothelial cells. It produces a strong and sustained vasoconstriction in most arteries and veins of many mammalian species.

Assay protocol

The assay is performed in polypropylene tubes. One hundred microlitres of standard or sample and 100 µl of antiserum are added and the tubes incubated at 2–8°C for 4 h. Tracer (iodine-125 labelled endothelin-1, 100 µl) is then added and the tubes left overnight at 2–8°C. Two hundred and fifty microlitres of Amerlex-M (magnetizable solid particles coated with a second antibody reagent) is added and left at room temperature for 10 min. The antibody-bound fraction is separated by placing the tubes on a magnetic rack for 15 min and then pouring off the supernatant which contains the unbound iodine-125 labelled endothelin-1. The tubes are then counted for 1 min in a gamma scintillation counter. In these assays, samples and standards are usually assayed in duplicate.

Data presentation and curve plotting

Many approaches have been used for data plotting and curve fitting. One approach is to calculate the binding of tracer in the standard tubes as a

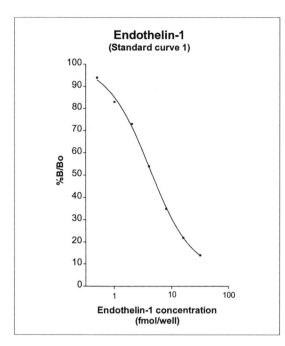

Figure 3 Typical endothelin-1 standard curve

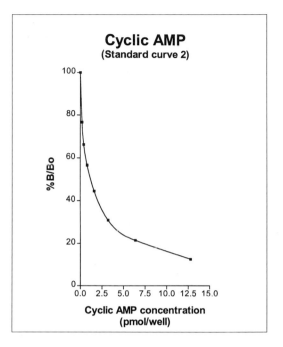

Figure 4 Typical cAMP standard curve

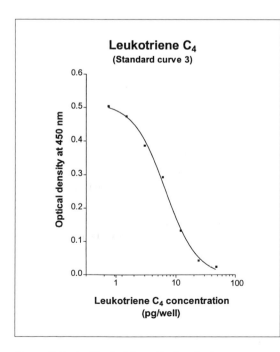

Figure 5 Typical leukotriene C_4 standard curve

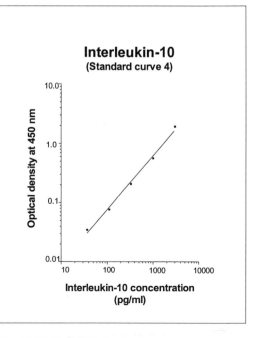

Figure 6 Typical IL-10 standard curve

percentage of the binding in the absence of standard. This is then plotted against the log of the standard concentration. A log plot spreads out the data points and makes manual calculation of sample concentrations easier (see standard curve 1, Fig. 3). A number of alternative curve-plotting methods are illustrated in standard curves 2 to 4 (Figs 4 to 6). The choice of curve fit can generate a lot of discussion. Whatever method is chosen, it is important to plot out the data and demonstrate that the curve does actually fit the data points.

Cyclic AMP scintillation proximity assay

Cyclic AMP is a member of a biologically important class of molecules termed second messengers. This is a term for molecules which are able to transmit intracellularly the biological effects of compounds not able to enter the target cell themselves.

homogeneous competitive immunoassay

This cAMP assay is an example of a homogeneous competitive immunoassay, i.e. an assay in which the bound tracer does not need to be physically separated from the free fraction. This greatly simplifies the assay and makes it more amenable to automation. It is based on the principle that relatively weak beta emitters such as tritium and the iodine-125 Auger electron need to be close to scintillant molecules to produce light; otherwise the energy is dissipated and lost to the solvent. This concept has been used to develop homogeneous radioimmunoassays (RIAs) by coupling second antibodies onto fluomicrospheres containing scintillant. When second antibody-coupled fluomicrospheres are added to a RIA tube, any radiolabelled ligand that is bound to the primary ligand-specific antibody will be immobilized on the fluomicrosphere. This will bring into close proximity the radiolabel and the scintillant, activating the scintillant to produce light. Any unbound radioligand remains too distant to activate the scintillant. The signal is measured in a liquid scintillation counter and is inversely proportional to the concentration of ligand in the sample or standard.

Assay protocol

Fifty microlitres of standard or sample followed by 50 µl of iodine-125 labelled cAMP, 50 µl of antiserum and 50 µl of the scintillant beads are pipetted into each assay tube and incubated at room temperature overnight. The amount of tracer bound to the beads is determined by counting for 2 min in a beta scintillation counter.

A typical cAMP SPA plot is shown in standard curve two. The data are represented as a linear/linear plot.

Leukotriene $C_4/D_4/E_4$ enzyme immunoassay system

The peptido-leukotrienes C_4, D_4 and E_4 comprise the slow-reacting substances of anaphylaxis. They are potent mediators of bronchoconstriction, vascular and nonvascular smooth muscle contraction, and increase vascular permeability and epithelial mucous secretion. They are widely considered to be important mediators in asthma and antagonists to these compounds are being developed as possible antiasthma drugs.

This assay has been selected as an example of a competitive immunoassay using an enzyme label.

competitive immunoassay

Assay protocol

The assay is performed in a 96-well microtitre plate. Fifty microlitres of standard or sample is pipetted into each well and incubated at 4–10°C for 2 h. Fifty microlitres of leukotriene C_4-horseradish peroxidase conjugate is then added and incubated for a further 2 h at the same temperature. The plate is washed thoroughly, and 150 µl of substrate solution is added to each well. The plate is then incubated at room temperature with shaking for 30 min and the reaction terminated with 100 µl of 1 M sulphuric acid. The optical density of each well is determined in an automatic plate reader at 450 nm.

Interleukin-10 (mouse) ELISA system

Interleukin-10 is a glycoprotein that inhibits cytokine synthesis by the TH1 subpopulation of T-cells. The TH1 cytokines are responsible for many aspects of cell-mediated immunity, so IL-10 has immunosuppressive activity. There is considerable interest in investigating the use of IL-10 in transplantation, rheumatoid arthritis and septic shock.

This assay has been chosen as an example of an immunometric assay using a biotin-labelled antibody in combination with a streptavidin-horseradish peroxidase tracer.

immunometric assay

Assay protocol

The assay is performed in a 96-well microtitre plate. Fifty microlitres of assay buffer and 50 µl of either standard or sample are added to each well. The plate is incubated at room temperature for 3 h, and then washed. Fifty microlitres of biotinylated detection antibody is added to all wells and incubated at room temperature for 1 h, and the plate washed. Streptavidin-horseradish peroxidase (100 µl) is then added, incubated for 30 min and the plate washed again. Substrate solution (100 µl) is then added and incubated for a further 30 min. The reaction is finally terminated with 100 µl of dilute sulphuric acid and the optical density measured at 450 nm.

A typical IL-10 log/log plot analysed by linear regression is shown in standard curve 4.

Assay performance and validation

When either developing or evaluating an immunoassay, a number of questions relating to the performance of the assay need to be considered. These include the likely cost of the assay, how easy it is to perform, the equipment required to carry out the assay, what analyte concentration can be measured, how reproducible is the assay and whether or not the assay measures the true analyte concentration. Some of these questions have already been covered. The remainder are discussed in the following sections.

Assay precision

definition

Precision is an index of assay reproducibility and is a guide to how much the determined analyte concentration is likely to vary from measurement to measurement. Within-assay and between-assay precision refers to the reproducibility of measurement in single and multiple assays, respectively. Precision is likely to vary throughout the standard curve range. A precision profile of the assay can be constructed by performing multiple measurements at each standard concentration. It is difficult to state what is acceptable with regard to assay precision as this will vary depending upon the intended application of the assay. A reasonably well designed assay will have a within-assay precision, of <10% at the extremities of the standard curve and <5% over most of the assay. The between-assay precision is usually a few percent higher than the within-assay precision. In a well-designed assay, the sample concentrations will fall within the part of the standard curve having the highest precision.

Assay sensitivity

The sensitivity of an assay is the lowest level of analyte which can be detected. Various ways of calculating assay sensitivity have been used. One common method is to calculate the standard deviation of the zero standard optical densities and express the sensitivity as that value corresponding to two standard deviations from the mean zero standard optical density. However, it is important to be aware that samples cannot be assigned a precise value near to the sensitivity limit of an assay, because the precision at these concentrations will be extremely poor. Samples should only be given values when they fall within the range of the standard curve data points. The range of the data points should be set from the precision profile. Any sample values outside the standard curve range should really be given the value of less than or greater than the lowest or highest standard, respectively.

definition

Assay validation

Before using an immunoassay, it is important to validate the assay. An assay should be validated for each sample matrix such as plasma, serum or cell culture supernatant that will be used in the assay. The *specificity* of an assay is confirmed by testing against related substances. The analytical *recovery* is assessed by adding known amounts of the analyte to the sample matrix under evaluation and measuring the percentage recovery of the analyte. Assay *linearity* is determined by diluting samples and determining whether or not the measured values are in agreement with the nondiluted sample when the dilution factor is taken into account.

specificity

recovery

linearity

In some situations it can prove impossible to develop a valid assay without some kind of sample purification step. Vitamin D metabolite assays, especially the assay for 1 α-25-dihydroxy vitamin D, require such a step because this molecule is present at concentrations ~1000-fold lower than other metabolites such as 25-hydroxy vitamin D. Given the close similarity of these molecules, it has proved impossible to produce an antibody with the specificity to discriminate to the required extent between the metabolites. In such circumstances it is necessary to remove the 25-

dihydroxy metabolite, for example on small silica cartridges, prior to the assay. However, such procedures are time-consuming and should be avoided if at all possible.

The future of immunoassay

cytochrome P-450

It is easy to predict that the range of analytes measured by immunoassays will continue to grow. For example, immunoassays for cytochrome P-450 isoenzymes and metalloproteinases have been recently developed. The way in which the technology will develop is more difficult to foresee. Automation will become even more widespread in the clinical field and high-throughput pharmacological screening. Enzymes may be used with more sensitive detection methods such as enhanced luminescence or fluorescence. It is even possible that labels will be abolished altogether by using biosensors.

C Immunotherapeutics

Vaccines

Wim Jiskoot

Introduction

Vaccines are the most commonly administered immunotherapeutics. Supported by large improvements in sanitation facilities such as safe drinking water, vaccination has been the most effective measure to control a diversity of life-threatening infectious diseases in the 20th century. The most impressive success of vaccination was the global eradication of smallpox in the 1970s. Moreover, the incidence of many other infectious diseases, such as diphtheria, tetanus, pertussis, poliomyelitis, measles, mumps and rubella, has been drastically reduced thanks to extensive vaccination programs.

eradication of smallpox

Upon natural infection with a pathogen, an unprotected person usually falls ill before the immunological defence system is able to respond adequately. Vaccination aims to stimulate the specific immune response against a pathogen by the administration of attenuated or killed organisms, or fractions thereof. If vaccination is successful and the host subsequently comes into contact with the pathogen, the specific immune response will be immediate and sufficiently strong to kill the invading organism before it has the opportunity to multiply and cause disease. Thus, in a strict sense vaccines are immunoprophylactics rather than therapeutics.

aim of vaccination

In most cases, repeated doses of the vaccine are given to boost the immune response. Apart from the number of doses, several other factors determine vaccine efficacy, as summarized in Table 1. If a high enough proportion of a population is immunized, vaccination not only protects the immunized individuals but also may help to protect the community, because it decreases the chance that nonimmunized persons may encounter the pathogen. This is referred to as herd immunity [1].

repeated doses

herd immunity

A brief history of vaccination is given below. Next, current vaccine categories for human use will be addressed. Finally, new developments in vaccinology will be outlined.

Table 1 Factors determining vaccine efficacy

Pathogen-dependent	Host-dependent	Vaccine-dependent	Vaccination schedule-dependent
port of entry	species	nature of antigenic component(s)	route of administration
localization in host	age	antigen content	number of doses
antigenic variation	genetic factors	antigenic presentation form	immunization intervals
mutation frequency	physical state	adjuvants	simultaneous administration of other vaccines (administered separately)
	immune status	combination with other vaccine components (in one vial or syringe)	

Historical background

Vaccination has a long history [1, 2]. The most prominent milestones of vaccinology are listed in Table 2. The first attempts at immunity probably date back to as early as the 7th century, when Indian Buddhists drank snake venom and may thus have become immune against this toxin. Written reports bear witness to the practice of variolation, i.e. the administration of scabs or pustule preparations obtained from patients recovered from smallpox, ever since about 1000 A.D. in various parts of the world, amongst others in China, India, North Africa and England.

Variolation was widely applied until Edward Jenner introduced cowpox vaccination at the end of the 18th century. His practice was based on the recognition that milkmaids were frequently subjected to mild pox infection acquired from the cows they milked, but were spared from disease during smallpox epidemics. The first demonstration that the principle of immunization works was Jenner's anecdotal experiment with an 8-year-old boy who remained healthy when challenged with smallpox virus after he had been immunized with cowpox virus. It was Jenner who introduced the terms *vaccine* for cowpox preparations (derived from the Latin *vacca* = cow) and *vaccination* for the administration thereof. Later, in honor of Jenner, Louis Pasteur generalized the meaning of vaccination to immunization with agents other than cowpox. During the 19th century vaccination with live cowpox virus became common practice. In

variolation

cowpox
vaccination
Edward Jenner

Louis Pasteur

Table 2 Milestones in vaccine history[*]

Year	Event[†]
ca. 1000	Intranasal administration of preparations of scabs from smallpox patients in China
16th–17th century	Parenteral variolation in India by Hindus
17th century	Oral administration of white cow flea pills for smallpox prevention in China
1796	Immunization of 8-year-old boy with cowpox virus and challenging with smallpox virus (Edward Jenner)
1798	Initiation of general cowpox immunization with Jenner's variola vaccine
1870s	Discovery of attenuation of fowl cholera bacteria (Louis Pasteur)
1884	Attenuated *Vibrio cholerae*: the first bacterial vaccine used in humans (Robert Koch)
1885	First administration to humans of attenuated rabies vaccine (Louis Pasteur)
1896–1897	Introduction of the first heat-inactivated vaccines against typhoid, cholera and plague
1923	Introduction of the first subunit vaccine: formaldehyde-treated diphtheria toxin
1927	Introduction of BCG, attenuated tuberculosis vaccine
1955	Introduction of inactivated poliovirus vaccine (Salk): the first vaccine developed with tissue-culture technique
1961	Attenuated poliovaccine (Sabin) as the first licensed oral vaccine
1980	Declaration of the eradication of smallpox by the WHO
1986	Licensing of the first rDNA vaccine: recombinant HBsAg
1987	Licensing of the first conjugate vaccine against Hib: PRP-T

[*] *Sources: [1, 2]*
[†] *BCG, bacille Calmette-Guérin; HBsAg, hepatitis B surface antigen; Hib, Haemophilus influenzae type b; PRP-T, polyribosylribitol phosphate-tetanus toxoid conjugate vaccine; WHO, World Health Organization.*

attenuation

the 20th century, vaccinia virus, which is closely related to cowpox virus [1], became widely used as a live vaccine until smallpox was eradicated.

Pasteur gave a new impetus to vaccinology in the last quarter of the 19th century. He showed that the virulence (i.e. infectivity) of pathogens could be reduced by successive passage in culture. Vaccination with attenuated strains thus obtained could confer protection without causing disease. The efforts of Louis Pasteur and others led to the development of live attenuated vaccines against cholera, anthrax and rabies. Along with the introduction of attenuated vaccines, it became apparent that infection with live material was not essential to induce immunity. The procedure of killing bacteria by heat and subsequent stabilization with phenol was de-

heat inactivation

veloped, resulting in the introduction of heat-inactivated whole-cell vaccines against cholera, typhoid and plague at the end of the 19th century.

live and killed vaccines

At the beginning of the 20th century the development and introduction of new live (tuberculosis, yellow fever) and killed vaccines (pertussis, influenza, rickettsia) followed. Moreover, it was being recognized

subunit vaccines

that some components of a microorganism were more relevant for protection than others, and the concept of subunit vaccines was born. This and the discovery of chemical inactivation of bacterial toxins with formaldehyde led to the introduction of subunit vaccines against diphtheria (1923) and tetanus (1927).

tissue culture

In the early 1950s tissue-culture techniques for virus progagation were developed. This resulted in the licensing of Salk's inactivated polio vaccine (IPV) in 1955. In the same period Sabin developed an oral polio vaccine (OPV) consisting of live attenuated viruses, which became available in the United States in 1961. Several other viral vaccines derived from tissue-cultures followed. Furthermore, several bacterial subunit vaccines based on purified proteins or polysaccharides have been introduced since the 1970s. The first vaccine based on recombinant DNA technology was marketed in 1986.

Current vaccine categories

Classification

The currently available vaccines for human use are either of bacterial or viral origin and can be divided into several categories (see Table 3). These categories are discussed below. For a more detailed description of individual vaccines currently in practice, the reader is referred to the excellent vaccine textbook of Plotkin & Mortimer [1].

Table 3 Classification and examples of current vaccines

Category	Example	Vaccine characteristics
Live attenuated organisms		
viral	poliovirus (Sabin)	attenuated viruses, serotypes 1–3; oral vaccine
	measles virus	attenuated virus
	mumps virus	attenuated virus
	rubella virus	attenuated virus
	yellow fever virus	attenuated virus
bacterial	bacille Calmette-Guérin	attenuated *Mycobacterium bovis*
	Salmonella typhi	attenuated bacteria, oral vaccine
Killed whole organisms		
viral	poliovirus (Salk)	formaldehyde-inactivated viruses, serotypes 1–3
	rabies virus	β-propiolactone-inactivated virus
	hepatitis A virus	formaldehyde-inactivated virus
	Japanese B encephalitis virus	formaldehyde-inactivated virus
bacterial	*Bordetella pertussis*	heat-inactivated bacteria
	Vibrio cholerae	phenol-inactivated bacteria
	Salmonella typhi	heat-inactivated bacteria
Subunit vaccines		
viral	influenza virus	influenza surface antigens
	hepatitis B virus	recombinant hepatitis B surface antigen
bacterial	*Corynebacterium diphtheriae*	formaldehyde-treated toxin
	Clostridium tetani	formaldehyde-treated toxin
	Bordetella pertussis	mixture of purified proteins
	Neisseria meningitidis	purified capsular polysaccharides
	Streptococcus pneumoniae	purified capsular polysaccharides
	Haemophilus influenzae type b	polysaccharide-protein conjugates

Live attenuated vaccines

Attenuation through serial passage and selection of less virulent and less toxic variants has been applied to obtain safe vaccine strains. Once a suitable strain has been obtained, master and working seedlots are prepared.

The seedlot system provides the basis for the reproducible production of live (and other) vaccines. The dose of live vaccines is determined on the basis of the number of viable organisms.

live vaccine, advantages

Live vaccines have a number of advantages over nonliving vaccines. Although attenuation generally means reduced infectivity, attenuated strains will replicate to some extent in the recipient. This furnishes a sustained dose of antigens, inducing strong immune responses even after a single dose. In general, live vaccines generate higher cell-mediated immune responses than inactivated vaccines. A single immunization with a live vaccine often provides lifelong immunity.

live vaccine, disadvantages

The major drawback of live vaccines is the risk of reversion to pathogenicity. For instance, the occurrence of vaccine-associated paralytic poliomyelitis after the introduction of OPV has been reported [1, 3]. Furthermore, live vaccines sometimes cause mild symptoms resembling the disease caused by the pathogen. Live vaccines should never be given to immunosuppressed persons, because they lack the ability to respond even to infections by attenuated organisms.

Attenuated viral vaccines

Examples of live viral vaccines are polio, measles, mumps and rubella vaccines. Attenuated polio vaccine is administered orally. Poliovirus is a nonenveloped single-strand RNA virus. Its four structural proteins (VP1-4) form a regular three-dimensional structure with a diameter of 28 nm.

oral polio vaccine

OPV contains the three existing serotypes, which differ from each other in a number of distinct epitopes relevant for protection. The virus is relatively stable, and the thermal stability of the vaccine is further enhanced by additives such as magnesium chloride or sorbitol. OPV is included in

measles-, mumps-rubella vaccine

many childhood immunization programs. It is usually administered to infants in a four-dose scheme and probably provides lifelong protection.

Attenuated mumps, measles and rubella viruses are often combined in one vaccine combination (MMR vaccine). These attenuated RNA viruses vary in size and number of structural proteins. Measles, mumps and rubella vaccines, whether separate or combined, are lyophilized preparations stabilized with sucrose, sorbitol, hydrolized gelatin and/or amino acids. They contain the antibiotic neomycin and have to be kept refrigerated. The three vaccine components have in common that one single subcutaneous administration is probably sufficient for lifelong protection. Nevertheless, in some countries the first dose given at 12–15 months of age is followed by a second vaccination at the age of 4–6 or 11–12 years. Both humoral and cell-mediated immunity are important for protection.

Vaccine efficacy is estimated to be at least 90%, and combining the components does not seem to influence their effectiveness. Side effects are generally mild and usually occur 7–12 days after vaccination. MMR vaccines are not indicated for infants below the age of 1 year, because circulating maternal antibodies impair vaccine efficacy in this age group.

Attenuated bacterial vaccines

The most well-known attenuated bacterial vaccine is tuberculosis vaccine, which was incorporated in many immunization programs as of the 1930s. The vaccine is based on *Mycobacterium bovis* bacteria, which primarily infect cattle but can also infect humans. The vaccine consists of lyophilized attenuated *M. bovis*, known as bacille Calmette-Guérin (BCG), and is administered intradermally to infants and older children. Current vaccine strains vary in the extent of attenuation, and the dosage varies among vaccine suppliers. The immunization schedule varies significantly among nations. The nature of the immune response is not known in detail, but cell-mediated immune mechanisms are probably involved in protection, whereas antibodies do not seem to play a substantial role. Besides strain variations, the lack of reliable tests for immunity and the poorly understood mechanism of action contribute to the fact that estimates of vaccine efficacy vary from 0% to 80% [1].

bacille Calmette-Guérin (BCG)

Oral attenuated *Salmonella typhi* vaccines are indicated for high-risk groups, such as children in endemic areas and travelers, to prevent typhoid fever. The only licensed strain is Ty21a, whose attenuation has been stimulated by using nitrosoguanidine, a chemical mutagenic agent. Strain Ty21a lacks the ability to synthesize capsular polysaccharides, which are essential for virulence. In order to protect the bacteria against peptic digestion, the vaccine is formulated as lyophilized bacteria in enteric-coated capsules. Protection is achieved through 3–4 doses administered every other day. The vaccine provides significant protection by inducing relatively strong intestinal immunoglobulin A (IgA) and cell-mediated responses, and a weak systemic antibody response. Protective antibodies are directed against flagelli and lipopolysaccharides.

Salmonella typhi **vaccine**

Killed whole organisms

Inactivated bacterial and viral vaccines are obtained from virulent strains by heat treatment or by chemical inactivation, usually with formaldehyde. Since killed pathogens are not able to propagate after administration, these vaccines usually are less immunogenic than live vaccines. An advantage over the latter is the inability to revert to virulence. On the other hand, deficient inactivation has caused vaccine-related accidents. For instance, immunization with insufficiently inactivated polio vaccine in 1955 resulted in cases of paralytic disease [1, 2]. Examples of this category include inactivated polio vaccine (IPV) and whole-cell pertussis vaccine, which are discussed below.

IPV

inactivated polio vaccine

IPV is currently used in several countries. The vaccine consists of formaldehyde-inactivated poliovirus and includes the three serotypes. The dose is determined on the basis of antigen contents. Advantages of IPV over OPV are a better temperature stability, the lower risk of vaccine-related disease and the possibility of combination with diphtheria, tetanus and pertussis components in one formulation (DTP-IPV vaccine). In contrast to OPV, IPV does not elicit substantial amounts of secretory IgA antibodies, but its effect relies on the induction of virus-neutralizing serum IgG. A vaccination regimen with both IPV and OPV combines the advantages both vaccines and is applied in Denmark [1].

Whole-cell pertussis vaccine

whole cell *pertussis* vaccine

Pertussis (whooping cough) vaccine consists of heat-inactivated *Bordetella pertussis* cells. The dose is determined on the basis of the opacity of the inactivated cell suspension. The vaccine potency is tested by protection assays in mice. The protective efficacy of whole-cell pertussis vaccines is probably based on antibodies against several pertussis antigens,

pertussis antigens

such as pertussis toxin, filamentous hemagglutinin and lipopolysaccharides. Whole-cell pertussis vaccines are notorious for their frequent side reactions, mostly fever and irritability. Other side reactions include excessive sleeplessness, persistent inconsolable crying and shocklike phenomena. The adverse effects of whole-cell pertussis vaccines are largely

lipopoly-saccharides

due to the lipopolysaccharides present in the outer membrane of *B. pertussis*. The adverse effects are stronger in older children and adults, so that whole-cell pertussis vaccines are not indicated for these age groups, despite the fact that protection is probably restricted to a period of about 10 years. The vaccine contains colloidal aluminum salt as adjuvant and is usually combined with diphtheria and tetanus vaccine components (DTP vaccine). The vaccine is given in 4–5 intramuscular doses.

Subunit vaccines

Subunit vaccines contain one or more selected antigens (subunits) significant for protection against the pathogen they are derived from. Subunit vaccines have better-defined physicochemical characteristics and show fewer side effects than vaccines consisting of attenuated or inactivated organisms. Antigens used for current subunit vaccines include viral and bacterial proteins as well as bacterial capsular polysaccharides.

Proteins

Protection against *Corynebacterium diphtheriae* or *Clostridium tetani* is mainly based on the presence of antibodies directed against the respective toxins. These toxins are water-soluble proteins and form the basis of **toxins** diphtheria and tetanus vaccines. In order to eliminate the toxicity of diphtheria and tetanus toxin, they are incubated with formaldehyde. This **reaction with** process is called toxoidation, and the resulting products are referred to **formaldehyde** as toxoids. Formaldehyde forms covalent bonds with the toxin, which is **toxoids** initiated by a reversible reaction of formaldehyde with the ε-amino groups of lysine residues, followed by an irreversible reaction with other amino acid residues [2]:

$$R\text{–}Lys\text{–}NH_2 + CH_2O \leftrightarrow R\text{–}Lys\text{–}NH\text{–}CH_2OH \qquad (1)$$
$$\leftrightarrow R\text{–}Lys\text{–}N{=}CH_2 + H_2O$$

$$R\text{–}Lys\text{–}N{=}CH_2 + R'\text{–}H \rightarrow R\text{–}Lys\text{–}NH\text{–}CH_2\text{–}R' \qquad (2)$$

where R is the toxin, Lys is a lysine residue and R' can be an amino acid residue of the same or a second toxin molecule, or a free amino acid (e.g. lysine, tryptophan, tyrosine, histidine). Thus intra- and intermolecular cross-links (oligomers) are formed, yielding a heterogeneous product with respect to number and sites of formaldehyde adducts and molecular weight. The degree of toxoidation is highly dependent on the reaction conditions, including formaldehyde concentration, pH, temperature and the presence of other components. The toxoidation process must be a compromise between sufficient detoxication and preservation of relevant epitopes. To enhance the relatively poor immunogenicity of toxoids, they are adsorbed to aluminum salt suspensions.

Recently, a solution to the risk of residual toxicity and loss of immunogenic sites has been found by the introduction of genetic toxoidation, **genetic** which has been applied to pertussis toxin, a crucial component in recent- **toxoidation** ly developed subunit vaccines against pertussis. Genetic toxoidation of pertussis toxin was achieved by site-directed mutagenesis of the site responsible for toxicity. The resultant toxoid is devoid of toxicity and well defined, does not bear the risk of reversal to toxicity and is more immunogenic than chemically detoxified pertussis toxin [4]. Curiously, genetically obtained pertussis toxoid is stabilized with low concentrations of formaldehyde.

acellular pertussis vaccines

Acellular pertussis vaccines were introduced in Japan in the early 1980s as alternatives to the whole-cell vaccines and recently in the United States for the immunization of older children. Although pertussis toxoid alone may be sufficient for protection against whooping cough, most acellular pertussis vaccines contain at least two proteins important for the virulence of *B. pertussis*, including (inactivated) pertussis toxin, filamentous hemagglutinin, fimbriae and pertactin. Recent field trials indicate that the efficacy of these vaccines is comparable to that of whole-cell vaccines, whereas the acellular vaccines induce virtually no adverse effects [5]. This makes them suitable for immunization of older children and adults. Acellular pertussis vaccines are likely to be introduced in many national immunization programs in the next coming years, combined with diphtheria and tetanus components (DTaP vaccine).

recombinant hepatitis B vaccines

Hepatitis B subunit vaccine was the first marketed recombinant vaccine, which has replaced conventional hepatitis B vaccines obtained from plasma of infected humans. Recombinant hepatitis B vaccines are composed of hepatitis B surface antigen (HBsAg) derived from yeast or mammalian cells. Introduction of the genes for HBsAg in eukaryotic cells has been accomplished by inserting the protein gene into a plasmid, which was then used to transform the host cells. Purified HBsAg self-assembles to 22 nm particles identical to those excreted by cells infected with the native virus. Advantages of the recombinant DNA (rDNA) vaccine when compared to the plasma-derived product are safety, high yields and consistent quality. The ease of production has made the vaccine available worldwide. In most countries the vaccine is only given to at-risk individuals (e.g. drug abusers, homosexuals, newborns of HBsAg-positive mothers) in a multidose schedule [1].

Capsular polysaccharides

Many bacteria have a capsule consisting of high molecular weight polysaccharides, which act as virulence factors. Capsule-forming species include both Gram-positive (e.g. pneumococci) and Gram-negative bacteria (e.g. meningococci). The polysaccharides of the different species are composed of linear repeat oligosaccharide units that vary in sugar composition and chain length. The host defence against encapsulated bacteria relies on anti-polysaccharide antibodies interacting with complement to opsonize the organisms and prepare them for phagocytosis and clearance. Licensed capsular polysaccharide vaccines include meningococcal (serogroups A, C, W-135, Y), pneumococcal (up to 23 serotypes) and *Haemophilus influenzae* type b (Hib) vaccines.

capsular polysaccharide vaccines

The main disadvantage of capsular polysaccharide vaccines is their T-cell independency, which implies that they do not elicit immunological memory. Moreover, infants up to 2 years of age show very weak, non protective immune responses, whereas they belong to the highest risk groups for infections with the encapsulated bacteria mentioned above.

immunological memory

Polysaccharide-protein conjugate vaccines

The poor immunogenicity of plain polysaccharides can be overcome by covalent coupling to carrier proteins containing T-cell-epitopes. These helper epitopes make them T-cell dependent and permit the induction of strong immune responses and immunological memory in all age groups, including infants. The only conjugate vaccines licensed so far are Hib vaccines. The Hib polysaccharide consists of repeat units of ribosyl(1-1)ribitol phosphate. An effective *H. influenzae* vaccine is relatively easy to produce because – in contrast to the diversity of pathogenic meningococcal and pneumococcal strains – Hib is responsible for about 95% of infections with *Haemophilus* species, so only one polysaccharide type has to be included in the vaccine. Table 4 shows that the four licensed Hib conjugate vaccines vary in composition, owing to differences in polysaccharide length, carrier protein, coupling procedure and polysaccharide-to-protein ratio. As a result, these vaccines differ with respect to immunogenicity and efficacy [6]. The vaccines are incorporated in many childhood immunization programs and are normally administered intramuscularly in a multidose schedule with DTP, either separately or as a combined DTP-Hib vaccine. Other conjugate vaccines being developed are meningococcal and pneumococcal vaccines.

conjugate vaccines

Hib conjugate vaccines

Pharmacological effects of vaccination

The efficacy of a vaccine is difficult to estimate, because the relationship between immune response and degree of protection is not straightforward. Seroconversion, i.e. the increase in the level of specific circulating antibodies, is commonly determined as a measure for the immunogenic-

seroconversion

Table 4 Characteristics of licensed Haemophilus influenzae type b conjugate vaccines[*]

Property	Vaccine[†]			
	PRP-D	HbOC	PRP-OMP	PRP-T
Polysaccharide size	medium	small	medium	large
Polysaccharide content (µg)	25	10	15	10
Carrier protein	diphtheria toxoid	diphtheria toxin mutant	meningococcal group B outer membrane proteins	tetanus toxoid
Protein content (µg)	18	20	250	20
Linkage	via spacer	direct	via spacer	via spacer
Formulation	aqueous solution	aqueous solution	lyophilized, reconstituted with alum salt suspension	lyophilized, reconstituted with aqueous buffer

[*] Source: [1]

[†] PRP, polyribosylribitol phosphate; PRP-D, PRP-diphtheria toxoid conjugate vaccine; HbOC, Haemophilus type b oligosaccharide conjugate vaccine; PRP-OMP, PRP-outer membrane protein conjugate vaccine; PRP-T, PRP-tetanus toxoid conjugate vaccine

ity. Moreover, the protective quality of these antibodies can be measured with assays for bactericidal activity, i.e. their ability to kill bacteria in the presence of complement (e.g. meningococcal vaccines), virus-neutralizing activity (e.g. polio vaccines) or toxin-neutralizing activity (e.g. diphtheria and tetanus vaccines). However, it is hard to correlate the level and persistence of circulating antibodies with their protective efficacy. Moreover, the extent of cell-mediated immunity may in some instances be a better measure for protection, e.g. against tuberculosis, but is more difficult to measure. The effectiveness of vaccination is most clearly demonstrated by the reduction of disease after introduction of a vaccine in national immunization programs. A recent example is the drastic reduction in incidence of Hib infections observed in those areas where routine vaccination in infants was introduced. There is much indirect evidence of vaccine efficacy. For instance, in the Netherlands, where the use of IPV has effectively protected most of the population, two significant outbreaks of poliomyelitis in 1978 and 1992 were restricted to communities which refuse vaccination on religious grounds [3]. Concerns about the safety of whole-cell pertussis vaccines in the 1970s were the cause of a sharp decline in vaccination levels in Great Britain, which in turn resulted in whooping cough epidemics in 1978 and 1982; after renewed public acceptance of the vaccine the incidence of disease dropped again [1].

cell-mediated immunity

Since the target groups of vaccines in many cases include healthy infants and young children, vaccine safety is of particular importance. The occurrence of side effects may be due to the antigenic components (e.g. lipopolysaccharides in whole-cell pertussis vaccine), contaminants derived from the production process, (e.g. chick protein from the cell substrate used for measles vaccine production), or to additives used in a vaccine formulation (e.g. neomycin or gelatin in MMR vaccines, aluminum salts in subunit vaccines). Before a new vaccine candidate is licensed, its safety is investigated in phase I, II and III field trials. Phase I trials include a small number of healthy adults and serve to collect preliminary safety data and to assess vaccine dosage. In phase II studies safety and immunogenicity are determined in a larger number of volunteers. Phase III trials are meant to evaluate safety and efficacy in large target populations.

vaccine safety

field trials

New developments

Notwithstanding the success of vaccination, several infectious diseases remain against which an effective vaccine is still not available. New vaccines against bacterial (e.g. group B meningococci), viral (e.g. human immunodeficiency virus) and parasitic (e.g. malaria) infections are under development. Apart from new prophylactic vaccines, current research is also focused on the development of therapeutic vaccines, especially for the treatment of chronic diseases such as acquired immune deficiency syndrome (AIDS) and cancer. The rationale of administering vaccines to patients already suffering from disease is to specifically boost the immune system weakened by the disease.

therapeutic vaccines

the ideal vaccine

Ideally, a vaccine should provide lifelong protection in any individual of any age, be absolutely safe, easy to produce in unlimited quantities, stable under varying conditions, easy to administer and cheap. The design of a vaccine with all these ideal characteristics combined still remains an important challenge for developers of new and better vaccines.

combination vaccines

The number of vaccines used routinely is expected to increase. This demands that efforts be made to reduce the number of injections. An obvious way to achieve this is to combine separate vaccine components into one vial or syringe, examples of which have been given above. Simply mixing vaccine components, however, may not only pose pharmaceutical problems (e.g. incompatibility of vaccine components and/or excipients), but also bears the risk of immunological interference. A recent example of the latter is the reduced immunogenicity of the Hib component when mixed with DTaP vaccine [7].

Modern technologies

Whereas traditional vaccine development has largely been dependent on empirical methods, a better insight into immune mechanisms and immunogenic structures of infectious organisms has led to a better understanding of what would be the optimal vaccine composition in relation to the desired immunological effect. Moreover, the advent of (bio)technological advances has enabled scientists to translate improved immunological knowledge into the rational design of new vaccines. Several classical and modern approaches to the development of a variety of new vaccines are currently being explored, the most important of which are shown schematically in Figure 1. Approaches not yet addressed pre-

Figure 1 Schematic representation of (A and B) classical vaccine components and (C–G) new generation vaccine components

(A) whole bacterium or virus, live attenuated or killed, with protein antigens (grey objects) containing protective epitope (black semicircle); (B) subunit vaccine: antigen isolated from pathogenic organism; (C) live vector: antigenic proteins derived from pathogenic organism expressed by live, nonpathogenic bacterium or virus; (D) recombinant subunit vaccine:

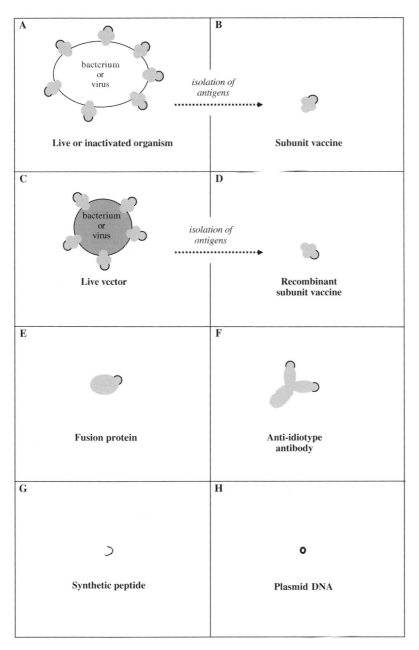

antigenic protein isolated from heterologous expression system; (E) fusion protein: non-toxic protein containing epitope of protein from pathogen isolated from nonpathogenic organism; (F) anti-idiotype antibody: antibody containing antigen binding sites mimicking epitope of antigen from pathogen; (G) synthetic peptide with amino acid sequence mimicking epitope of antigen from pathogen; (H) nucleic acid vaccine: plasmid DNA containing the gene encoding antigenic protein or epitope from pathogen.

viously are discussed briefly below. For more detailed information about modern vaccine technology the reader is referred to specialized textbooks [1, 2, 8, 9].

advantages of modern technologies

Several of the modern technologies (Fig. 1C–H) offer the following common advantages over classical vaccines: (1) relevant epitopes of pathogenic organisms or cancer cells can be obtained by safer means and (2) in greater quantities, (3) the products are better defined, and (4) epitopes of a single or multiple pathogenic agents can be combined easily in one vaccine. The design of many new candidate vaccines against a variety of life-threatening and chronic diseases is based on one of the following categories.

Recombinant live vaccines

viral and bacterial vectors

Nonpathogenic or attenuated organisms can be used as carriers for heterologous protein antigens. Such live carriers are called vectors (Fig. 1C). They are obtained by cloning the desired gene and introducing it in an appropriate carrier organism. Both viral (e.g. vaccinia virus, attenuated poliovirus) and bacterial vectors (e.g. *Salmonella* species, BCG) are being explored as carriers to express a variety of antigens. The properties of recombinant live vaccines are comparable to those of classical attenuated vaccines.

Fusion proteins

fusion proteins

Fusion proteins are nontoxic proteins containing inserted epitopes derived from pathogenic species. They are obtained by the insertion of DNA sequences encoding epitopes in the gene of the carrier protein, such as HBsAg [10]. The recombinant gene is expressed in a suitable organism, and the fusion protein is then purified (Fig. 1E). A drawback of this technology is possible misfolding of the epitope when incorporated in the carrier protein, which would lead to irrelevant immune responses.

Antiidiotype antibodies

antiidiotype vaccines

The concept of antiidiotype antibody vaccines involves the generation of a monoclonal antibody (AB-1) recognizing a relevant epitope of the pathogenic agent, followed by the generation of a second monoclonal antibody (AB-2) directed against the idiotype, i.e. the antigen-binding site of

AB-1. AB-2 thus mimics the original epitope (Fig. 1F) and can be used for vaccination, thereby eliciting protective antibodies (ABs-3). Virtually any desired epitope can be structurally mimicked by antiidiotype antibodies, whether it be continuous or discontinuous epitopes of either protein or polysaccharide nature [1].

Synthetic peptide vaccines

Chemically synthesized peptides are among the best-defined vaccine components presently under investigation. The synthetic peptide technology allows for the design of vaccines consisting of selected epitopes free from irrelevant or unwanted structures. Large amounts of linear peptides resembling T-cell or B-cell epitopes (Fig. 1G) can be prepared by automated methods. The immunogenicity of synthetic peptide antigens is weak, but can be enhanced by conjugation to carrier proteins (analogous to polysaccharide-protein conjugates) or to lipids, or by the construction of multiple-antigen peptides [9]. These options offer the possibility of rendering synthetic B-cell epitopes T-cell-dependent. Furthermore, the conformational freedom of small linear peptides can be restricted by cyclization, which is intended to force them into a conformation which reflects the native structure, an especially important requirement for peptide analogs of B-cell epitopes [11].

linear peptides

cyclization

Nucleic acid vaccines

A recent development of potential clinical use is genetic immunization, i.e. direct administration of naked DNA encoding antigens of interest (Fig. 1H). Upon intramuscular immunization with nonreplicating plasmid DNA, the protein encoded is produced and expressed by the host cell. RNA may also be used, but is less suitable because it is rapidly degraded *in vivo* and more expensive to produce. Nucleic acid vaccines are capable of eliciting both humoral and cellular immunity. A sustained production of antigen after a single immunization is expected to provide long-term protection [12].

genetic immunization

Local immunization

Local immunization is an attractive alternative to parenteral vaccination, not only because of the ease of administration, but also because it induces

local immune response

oral vaccines

both systemic and mucosal (secretory IgA) responses. The latter is advantageous because mucosal surfaces are the common port of entrance of many organisms, and a strong local immune response may hamper entry into the host by preventing adherence to and colonization in mucosal surfaces. However, although local immunization is one of the oldest means of vaccination (see Table 2), the number of vaccines suitable for local immunization is limited to a few oral vaccines. Poliovirus can be given orally because the virus is relatively resistant to low pH, whereas oral typhoid vaccine is protected from gastric breakdown by formulation in enteric coated tablets. Other local administration routes, such as nasal or vaginal delivery, have the advantage that the harsh conditions in the gastrointestinal tract are circumvented. Approaches to augment the immunogenicity of future mucosal vaccines include the use of delivery systems and coadministration of adjuvants (see below) [13–16].

Delivery systems and adjuvants

In general it can be stated that the smaller the size of a vaccine component, the weaker its immunogenicity and, hence, the more important its presentation form. As a result, a lot of effort has been and is being put into enhancing the immune response to subunit vaccine components by suitable presentation forms, including sophisticated delivery systems and adjuvants [8, 9].

delivery systems

Delivery systems are carriers that allow multimeric antigen presentation. Besides antigens, adjuvants are sometimes incorporated into these carrier systems, and many carrier systems have intrinsic adjuvant activity. Carrier proteins and live vectors are delivery systems which have already been discussed. Other delivery systems include particulate carriers, such as biodegradable microcarriers, nanoparticles, liposomes and immune-stimulating complexes (ISCOMs). Most of the carriers function as a depot at the administration site, resulting in sustained delivery and a reduction of the number of doses required. Moreover, they may protect the antigen from proteolytic attack (e.g. in oral vaccine formulations), and enhance humoral and/or cellular immune reactions.

adjuvants

Adjuvants comprise a large number of substances of variable chemistry and origin [9]. Examples are colloidal salts, lipid matrices, surface active compounds and emulsions of mineral, bacterial, vegetable or synthetic nature. Adjuvants have in common that they are not immunogenic *per se*, but enhance the immunogenicity of coadministered antigens. The traditional aluminum phosphate and hydroxide colloid salts, which are the only adjuvants currently used in licensed products for human use, only stimulate humoral immune responses. Many novel candidate adjuvants also augment cellular immune responses and mediate their effect through nonspecific induction of several cytokines. Cytokines such as interleukins and interferons have become of interest as more specific adjuvants, especially in the search for potent vaccines against AIDS and cancer.

Concluding remarks

Paradoxically, the introduction of modern vaccines, which are intended to be more effective and safer than conventional vaccines, is likely to be retarded not because of technological problems but rather because of safety concerns among regulatory authorities. In particular, the safety of rDNA vaccines and the potential risk of incorporation of vaccine-derived DNA into the host's genome is a great concern. Moreover, existing vaccines, some of which would probably not be accepted for registration by present authorities, have impressive safety and efficacy records. Nevertheless, it is expected that vaccines will be marketed in the near future that are based on some of the modern vaccine technologies discussed above and – like the conventional vaccines – will make a significant contribution to the improvement of public health.

safety concerns

Sera and immunoglobulins

Friedrich R. Seiler, Gerhard Dickneite, Ernst-Jürgen Kanzy and Peter Gronski

Humoral immunity

The immune system within the organism of an individual has a broad variety of functions, and these are performed by a number of cellular and humoral defense mechanisms. These may be divided into two functional systems: the nonspecific and the specific. Nonspecific or innate immunity constitutes the first defense cordon against infection, with the specific immune system coming into action should this cordon be overcome. However, this specific immune system must first develop specific functions against attackers before usually eliminating them.

nonspecific immunity

The specific immune system comprises T- and B-lymphocytes and immunoglobulin molecules synthesised from plasma cells derived from B-cells. Whereas the specific immune cells have been well examined and documented, particularly in the past decades, specific humoral immunity was discovered and put to therapeutic use a century ago [1]: in other words, antibody molecules, or immunoglobulins as they have come to be called since the 1930s.

specific immunity

Immunoglobulins are a protein-chemical family of molecules of essentially similar structure yet with variable composition but virtually identical basic components and similar molecular size. Their major task lies in binding and eliminating of substances which are alien to the individual or the species, for instance pathogens such as bacteria and viruses. As we know, the healthy organism is able to produce antibodies against an almost incredible number and variety of alien substances, and these antibodies are able to attach themselves with a high specificity to alien antigen structures, thereby regulating their further elimination and breakdown.

To be able actively to provide specific antibodies against new or still foreign antigens, the organism normally requires a few days. This humoral immune response does not only give rise to one type of antibody which can then be synthesised as a quasi-monoclonal antibody by a single specifically stimulated plasma-cell clone, a situation that rarely arises in the healthy organism (myeloma as degeneration!). Nature normally produces in excess and in variations, and this also applies to the immune response: a considerable number of expanding plasma-cell clones produces, as it were in polyclonal concert, antibodies with related and slightly varying specificities and binding properties and, moreover, against various antigenic sections (epitopes) of a molecule or pathogen. The interaction of these various kinds of antibody usually provides the basis for an effective immunological response (see Chapter A5).

In the case of an existing or induced immune deficiency, the requisite antibodies are either not produced quickly enough or in sufficient amounts, or they are not produced at all. Even a florid infection with a rapidly multiplying pathogen leaves the immune system little time to rally its defenses. It is particularly for such situations that passive immunotherapy with immunoglobulin preparations has continued to be developed since its discovery in 1890 [2]. Nowadays antibodies of various **i.m. or i.v.** origin, preparation and specificity are available for intramuscular or in**substitution** travenous substitution (Table 1).

Homologous preparations for rapid and high-dosage intravenous therapy have been made available for about 35 years. In actual fact, these products vary in production, composition, properties (see Table 2) and

Table 1 Homologous and heterologous sera and immunoglobulin preparations for human use

Antitoxic or antibacterial	Antiviral	Others
Heterologous (animal origin)		
botulism-antitoxin		anti-CD3 murine mab
diphtheria-antitoxin		anti-T-cell immune serum
gas-gangrene-antitoxin		anti-digitalis
immune serum against:		
scorpion venoms		
snake venoms		
Homologous (human origin) i.m. or i.v. immunoglobulin (Ig)		
tetanus-Ig	Cytomegalo-Ig	normal polyvalent Ig
	Hepatitis A-Ig	IgM-enriched polyvalent Ig
	Hepatitis B-Ig	Rh_0 (D)-Ig
	Rabies-Ig	
	Rubella-Ig	
	Tick-borne encephalitis-Ig	
	Varicella zoster-Ig	

Table 2 Various i.v.-immunoglobulin preparations

Method of preparation after cold ethanol fractionation	Excipients	Formulation	pH of solution to be infused	Viral inactivation	IgG-constituents 7S	5S	<5S	IgA (µg/ml)	Manufacturer (selection)
pH4, solvent detergent	maltose, 10% or glycine, 1.6%	liquid, 5% liquid, 10%	4.2	pH 4, solvent detergent	+			up to 270	Bayer
stabilizing, pasteurization	sucrose, 5% albumin, 3%	lyophilized, 5%	6.8	pasteurization 10 h 60 °C	+			≤25	Centeon
PEG, bentonite, ion exchanger, (solvent detergent)	mannitol, 2% or	lyophilized, 5%	6.8	PEG/bentonite	+			10–50	Alpha Therapeutic Corp.
	sorbitol, 5%	liquid, 5%, 10%	5.2–5.8	(solvent detergent)					
ultrafiltration, ion exchanger, solvent detergent	glucose, 2%	lyophilized, 5%	6.8	solvent detergent	+			0.4–3.7	Baxter Hyland, American Red Cross
ion exchanger, solvent detergent	albumin, 5% glucose, 2.4% glycine, 0.4%	lyophilized, 5%	6.8	solvent detergent	+			10–15	Pharmacia
pH4, trace pepsin	sucrose, 5%	lyophilized 3%–6%	6.6	pH4/pepsin		+		up to 720	Novartis
PEG, trypsin	glucose, 5%	lyophilized, 5%	7.0	PEG/trypsin	+		+	10–50	Immuno
aerosil adsorption, β-propiolactone	glucose, 2.75%	liquid, 5%	7.0	β-propiolactone	+			500–1200	Biotest
ion exchanger, S-sulfonation	glycine, 2.25% mannitol, 1% albumin, 0.25%	lyophilized, 5%	6.8	S-sulfonation	+			150	Teijin
S-sulfonation octanol	glycine, 2.25%	lyophilized, 5%	6.8	S-sulfonation, octanol	+			5000–10 000	Centeon
pepsin, pasteurization	glycine, 2.25%	lyophilized, 5%	6.8	pH4.3 + pepsin pasteurization		+	+	no intact IgA detectable	Centeon

Examples of preparations produced by different procedures with emphasis on their formulation, viral inactivation, main IgG constituents (S means coefficient of sedimentation. 7S corresponds to monomeric IgG, 5S to $F(ab')_2$ or Fab/Fc and <5S mainly to Fab, Fc and/or fragments thereof) and IgA-content.

mechanisms of action. The functional elements of immunoglobulin molecules are dependent on particular structural properties of the molecule.

The structure of immunoglobulins

variable part

constant part

The construction of all immunoglobulins reflects their two decisive and major functions: one part is responsible for antigen recognition and varies from molecule to molecule – the variable part. The other covers nonspecific effector functions. This part has a uniform structure – the constant part. The antibody is thus a bifunctional protein molecule, or rather a two-phase molecule; since the bifunctional capability of the antibody, particularly effective in Fc-mediated secondary reactions, only develops subsequent to binding to the antigen (primary reaction). For physicochemical and structural details see Chapter A1.

Fc-mediated reactions

Unlike the variable domains, the constant domains of the heavy-chains are responsible for the Fc-mediated effector functions of immunoglobulins [3]. Such Fc-mediated reactions are (see Table 3): (1) complement activation in the "classic" manner via the binding of Clq; (2) binding to reactive T-lymphocytes via Fc receptors, which enables antibody-mediated cytotoxicity to develop; (3) binding to Fc receptors on the cell surface of macrophages and neutrophil granulocytes (in addition to binding to C3b-receptors, this mechanism is effective in clearing immune complexes); (4) regulation of immunoglobulin G (IgG) synthesis in terms of either negative or positive feedback; (5) control of biological half-life and of catabolism of the immunoglobulin; (6) binding to thrombocytes with ensuing thrombocyte aggregation and activation; and (7) possible binding to other membranes, for instance basement membranes of the lung or the kidney.

Classes and sub-classes of human immunoglobulins

Humans, like most mammals, have five classes of immunoglobulins which are defined by the heavy-chains, that is they may be characterised by specific antigen determinants on the H-chains. These are IgM, IgG, IgA, IgE and IgD with their corresponding H-chains $\mu, \gamma, \alpha, \varepsilon$ and δ. Each of the five Igs can have either kappa (κ) or lambda (λ) as L-chains, for instance $\gamma_2\lambda_2$ or $\gamma_2\kappa_2$. IgG has four sub-classes in humans, IgG1, IgG2, IgG3 and IgG4. IgA has two subclasses: IgA1 and IgA2 (Table 3; Figure 1).

Table 3 Biological functions of the human immunoglobulins

Immunoglobulin	IgG1	IgG2	IgG3	IgG4	IgM	IgA1	IgA2	IgD	IgE
Placental passage	++	+	++	++	–	–	–	–	–
Complement Classical pathway of activation	++	(+)	+++	–	+++	–	–	–	–
Complement Alternative pathway of activation	–	–	–	–	–	+	+	–	–
Binding to FcγRI on monocytes, macrophages, neutrophils	++	(+)	+++	+	–	–	–	–	–
Binding to FcγRII on monocytes, neutrophils, eosinophils, basophils, B–cells, platelets, macrophages, Langerhans' cells	+	+	+++	(+)	–	–	–	–	–
Binding to FcγRIII on NK-cells, neutrophils, eosinophils, macrophages	+++	(+)	+++	(+)	–	–	–	–	–
Binding to FcεRI on mast cells, basophils	–	–	–	–	–	–	–	–	+++
Binding to FcεRII on B-cells, T-cells, follicular dendritic cells, inflammatory cells	–	–	–	–	–	–	–	–	+++
Binding to Staph. protein A	+	+	–	+	–	–	–	–	–
Strept. protein G	+	+	+	+	–	+	–	–	–
Virus neutralization	+	+	+	+	+	–	+	–	–

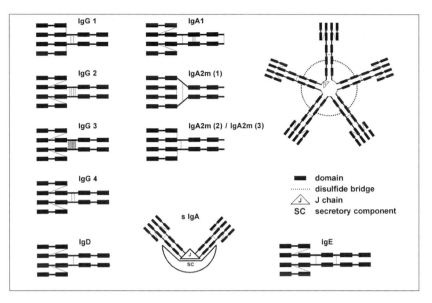

Figure 1 IgG classes and subclasses
Schematic structures of human immunoglobulin classes and of the IgG and IgA subclasses. Dark boxes represent domains, the basic elements of the immunoglobulin structure.

IgM

Serum IgM comprises a pentamer $(\mu_2 L_2)_5$ which is held together by an additional acidic protein of 15 000 Da, the J-chain (junction). This has a molecular weight of about 900 000, and thus here M stands for macroglobulin. Its complement-binding activity is much stronger than that of IgG, for instance one IgM molecule is capable of lysing one erythrocyte. IgM is the natural antibody in the first phase of the immune response, and phylogenically and ontogenetically it is the earliest antibody molecule.

A cell-membrane-bound, monomeric form of IgM is used by early B-lymphocytes as an antigen receptor, sometimes together with membrane-bound IgD. In virus infections, the appearance of IgM in serum is considered a sign of primary infection. IgM antibodies often have specificity for polysaccharides and a particular binding affinity for multimeric antigens (multivalency).

IgG

IgG accounts for approximately 75–80% of all immunoglobulins in the human organism and combines almost all the important characteristics of an antibody molecule. Of the four subclasses known in humans, IgG1 accounts for 60–70%, IgG2 for 14–20%, IgG3 for 4–8%, and IgG4 for 2–6%. IgG1 and IgG3 bind and activate the classic complement pathway via the complement components C1 and Cq particularly well. The binding takes place at the C_H2 domain. IgG is the only immunoglobulin that is capable of passing the placenta and thus of transmitting passive immunity from the mother to the embryo and the child.

To a small extent, IgG also passes kidney filtration and can be found in the urine. IgG is also important for selfregulation in control of IgG synthesis. Above all, IgG1 and IgG3 are primarily involved in binding to Fc receptors on lymphocytes, monocytes, macrophages and other leukocytes, which explains the opsonisation and phagocytosis of IgG-bound antigen or pathogens and antibody-dependent cellular cytoxicity (ADCC).

It does need to be emphasised in this respect that, under normal conditions, immune complex-bound antigen is transported to and bound at the site where elimination and breakdown of antigens can occur. In the case of pathophysiological overload, Fc receptor-mediated reactions can also lead to clinical side effects (see the section on *Side effects of immunoglobulin therapy*).

IgA

IgA is present in the serum predominantly as a monomer with a molecular weight of 160 000 Da, but also as a polymer (dimer to tetramer). Like IgM, the oligomers contain one J-chain per molecule. After IgG, IgA is the second most frequent immunoglobulin at about 15%. The particular clinical significance of secretory IgA lies in its presence in saliva, tear fluid, intestinal secretions, mucous membranes as well as in the colostrum, and in other body fluids. Secretory IgA also contains an additional glycoprotein with a molecular weight of around 60 000 Da, the "secretory piece". It is synthesised locally by the epithelial cells of the mucous membranes and is bound covalently to the IgA-dimer, which it provides with resistance to acids and enzymes. This secretory piece is, moreover, important in the transport of IgA to the surface of mucous membranes, where IgA clearly provides protection for the outer body surfaces against the attachment of microorganisms.

secretory IgA

Serum IgA is able to activate complement via the alternative pathway; secretory IgA can neither bind nor activate complement. Secretory IgA plays an important role in the localisation of infectious processes, for instance in virus infections of the mucous membranes in the intestine or the nose, and it can take part in the neutralisation of bacterial toxins.

serum IgA

IgD

Probably as a result of its low serum concentration of less than 0.2% of human serum immunoglobulins, IgD was only discovered in 1965, as a myeloma protein. It can be found in the serum and membrane-bound as a monomer. It has a molecular weight of 185 000 Da and a biological half-life of only 3 days. IgD has a marked hinge region, which is afforded some protection by carbohydrates but which is still quite easily proteolytically cleaved. Most IgD would appear to be found together with IgM on the cell surface membranes of some lymphocytes, probably functioning much like IgM as an antigen receptor. It is assumed that IgD may serve as a second receptor, in addition to IgM, with equal specificity and can take on an immunoregulatory role in the activation and suppression of lymphocytes.

Relatively little is known about the functional significance of serum IgD. Specificity has been attributed to it as an autoantibody against thyreoglobulin or insulin and against cell nucleus antigens in autoaggressive illnesses.

IgE

Like IgG, the IgE molecule is made up of two H and two L-chains ($\varepsilon_2 L_2$). As in IgM, the H-chains have an additional constant domain, C_H4. It has a molecular weight of 190 000 Da and a relatively high carbohydrate content, like IgM and IgD, and is present at a low serum concentration, like IgD. Moreover, it has a very short half-life of 2 days in serum. Yet IgE remains fixed for a long time in the skin and after binding to specific IgE-Fc receptors on mast cells and basophilic granulocytes. When two molecules of membrane-bound IgE are bound by antigen or allergen and bridged, vasoactive and chemotactic mediator molecules are released from these cells, and anaphylactic and allergic reactions ensue (hay fever, exogen-mediated, extrinsic asthma; Prausnitz-Küstner skin reaction).

The main task of IgE is considered to be the protection of the mucous membranes, for instance after penetration of the IgA resistance barrier. Additional help provided by chemotactically attracted eosinophilic granulocytes and enhanced IgE synthesis as a reaction to parasitic pathogens constitutes a further and important defence mechanism. Circulating IgE cannot activate complement via the classical pathway, but it may activate it moderately via the alternative pathway.

The catabolism of immunoglobulins

Immunoglobulin turnover may be assessed using radioactively labelled immunoglobulin molecules on intravenous (i.v.) application. This shows the biological half-life of IgG to be around 18–23 days. Around 7% of intravascular IgG is catabolised daily, but only around 45% of the total amount of IgG is normally present in the circulation. This means that over half of all IgG antibodies must be present extravasally in interstitial fluid. Here they provide for local immune response to infection after penetration by an antigen.

It is assumed that approximately one-third of immunoglobulins are broken down in the liver and a further third in the intestines. During illness, IgG catabolism may be enhanced and the biological half-life shortened. Abnormal increases in IgG concentrations in the serum can inhibit B cell differentiation to plasma cells as well as IgG synthesis (negative feedback). A diminution of IgG, for instance as a result of plamapheresis, leads to an increased antibody synthesis (positive feedback).

IgM turnover, with a half-life of around 10 days, is a good deal faster than that of IgG. Something in the region of 80% of IgM is intravascular and available for acute response to infection.

Immunoglobulin preparations for medical use

The use of preparations containing antibodies for "serum therapy" was introduced by Emil von Behring and Shibasaburo Kitasato over 100 years ago [1] and found recognition through the award of the very first Nobel prize for physiology or medicine in 1901. These first "antitoxins" were heterologous serum preparations from hyperimmunised animals with antibody specificity against diphtheria and tetanus toxins. After initial and excellent medical success, particularly in diphtheria antisera, the side effects against the alien animal serum protein, known as serum sickness, became increasingly common. As a result, purer and therefore more compatible preparations were developed.

Early attempts were made at enzymatic treatment (Fig. 2) and purification, particularly with pepsin, trypsin and papain, but only the later introduction of the use of proteases in the 1930s gave rise to the "fermosera". Such preparations were at least equivalent to the purified heterologous immunoglobulins then available, and they caused far fewer anaphylactic reactions. However, this did not put an end to the risk of

"serum therapy"

"antitoxins"

fermosera

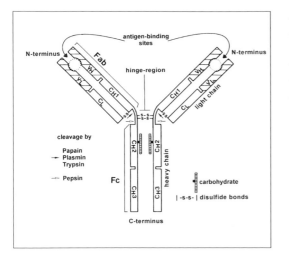

Figure 2 Important proteolytic cleavage sites of an immunoglobulin molecule

Two identical heavy-chains with four H-domains (three constant = C, one variable = V) and two identical light-chains with two L-domains (one constant = C, one variable = V) are combined by interchain disulfide bridges. Intradomain disulfide bridges are not shown.

serum sickness, which was not removed until the clinical introduction of homologous human immunoglobulin preparations [4]. In the meantime, a number of methods of concentrating and isolating immunoglobulins from serum or plasma were introduced. In most cases, alcohol or neutral salts were used for fractionated precipitation, later additions being polymers such as polyethylene glycol and hydroxyethyl starch and a number of adsorption substances and ion-exchange resins for chromatographic procedures.

The basic material for the production of common polyvalent homologous immunoglobulins either for intramuscular (i.m.) or i.v. application is a mixture of plasma from at least 1000 healthy and voluntary donors in order to guarantee the widest possible spectrum of antibody specificities. Special immunoglobulins, however, are gained from the plasma of specifically immunised donors or from the plasma of convalescents. For i.m. application of the smallest possible volumes of 0.2–1.0 ml per kg body weight, immunoglobulin is prepared as a 16% protein solution (w/v), whereby the preparation method should have increased the antiviral and antibacterial activity by at least 10-fold compared with the source plasma. The i.v. applications, however, normally take the form of 5%–10% immunoglobulin given at doses of 1–40 ml, with a maximum of 2 g per kg body weight.

Up to the 1960s immunoglobulin therapy was limited to i.m. use, and this situation was little altered by the introduction of homologous human **i.m. standard immunoglobulins** products, since these so-called i.m. standard immunoglobulins could commonly, if not generally, lead to serious side effects on i.v. application [5, 6]. The first compatible i.v. immunoglobulin was also a homologous "fermo-immunoglobulin" produced by pepsin treatment [7]. Here the Fc part of the antibody molecule was removed until virtually no more complement activation could be detected. [Side effects against the homologous protein are thought to be due to Fc-mediated reactions: activation of complement through aggregated or antigen-bound antibody molecules as well as stimulation of further physiological effector systems (Hagemann factor, kallikrein, kinins, prostaglandins, cytokines).

The great variety in the production procedures mentioned above generates differences in the resulting final products and becomes apparent in the physicochemical and functional profile of the i.v. immunoglobulins [8–10]. From a theoretical point of view, the doctor in attendance could choose a defined combination of properties within a certain range. The complexity of the real *in vivo* situation, which is often poorly understood, sometimes limits adequate therapy.

To some extent for historical reasons, some product properties are thought to be important criteria for tolerability (e.g. molecular size distribution, anticomplementary activity, content of isoagglutinins and prekallikrein activator), and these have thus been transformed into special requirements in the pharmacopoeiae. Considering the test results obtained today for most of the commercial products and the relatively low number of side reactions generally observed, these properties more likely represent parameters for the consistency of the production process.

Nowadays, i.v.-compatible immunoglobulin preparations are produced using a variety of the gentlest possible procedures which, on the one hand, lead to barely aggregated antibody molecules or, on the other hand, lead to molecules with structurally modified C_H2 domains and, therefore, altered Clq and Fc receptor binding properties. Following plasma fractionation by a cold ethanol method [11, 12] different specific processes are used for further purification and viral inactivation or removal (Table 2). The range of products can be divided into three groups on the basis of the three different methods used in their production:

(1) *Limited cleavage by proteases.* The main fragmentation product after pepsin treatment is the $F(ab')_2$ molecule. Treatment with small amounts of pepsin at pH 4 markedly lowers anticomplementary activity, and the antibody mostly remains intact as a 7S molecule. Limited cleavage by immobilised trypsin leads to a preparation containing some portions of Fab/Fc, Fab and Fc besides the unsplit IgG.

(2) *Chemical modification.* Irreversible chemical modification with β-propiolactone leads to a marked reduction of inherent complement binding [13], whereby β-propiolactone selectively modifies the amino acids lysine, cysteine and histidine [14]. Irreversible chemical modifica-

fermo immunoglobulins

methods used in production:

1. limited cleavage

2. chemical modifications

235

tion can also be achieved by reduction of the disulfide bridges with dithiothreitol and subsequent alkylation with iodoacetamide. S-sulfonation provides reversible chemical modification, either by means of sulfite and tetrathionate [15] or with sulfite and copper ions [16]. The interchain disulfide bridges in particular are cleaved and complement binding diminished. Repeated reduction and reoxidation enables the SO_3^- groups to be cleaved again *in vitro* and *in vivo*, and the disulfide bridges can be reconstituted.

3. specific precipitation, absorption and chromatography procedures

(3) *Special precipitation, absorption and chromatography procedures*. These comprise a series of individual procedures that may also be used in combination. In this context, particular mention should be made of the use of polymers (PEG = polyethylene glycol) for precipitation and stabilisation as well as the use of adsorbents like Aerosil, bentonite and calcium phosphate. Ion-exchange chromatography is used for polishing the IgG, especially for reduction of the IgA content. All these procedures aim to provide a gentle mode of production insofar as possible of non-cleaved, unaltered and functionally intact 7S immunoglobulins with almost normal IgG-subclass distribution and physiological half-life.

4. virus inactivation and removal

(4) *Virus inactivation and removal*. Single-process steps for the production of i.v. immunoglobulins (e.g. enzymatic cleavage, low pH, S-sulfonation and treatment with β-propiolactone) lead to a high level of viral safety because of viral inactivation. Furthermore, additional methods like pasteurisation (60 °C for 10 h), soluble detergent treatment for viral inactivation or nanofiltration for virus removal are introduced into production processes.

I.v. immunoglobulins are provided in freeze-dried as well as liquid formulations and contain different additives such as sugars, sugar alcohols, amino acids, human albumin and PEG in varying concentrations. The pH of the solutions is in the range 4.2–7.0.

Indications

From a historical perspective, important indications for the use of immunoglobulins are

important indications

- agamma- and hypogammaglobulinemia,
- deficiencies in certain subclasses of IgG sometimes combined with deficiency in IgA (e.g. IgA and IgG2),
- the prophylaxis and treatment of viral infections such as hepatitis A, measels and poliomyelitis and

- the neutralisation of bacterial toxins (e.g. enterotoxin of *Staphylococcus aureus*).

Later, autoimmune and systemic inflammatory diseases supplemented the spectrum of indications. Consensus panels initiated by the National Institutes of Health (NIH) in May 1990 and by the Australian Society for Blood Transfusion in July 1993 resulted in a nonofficial classification of diseases in which i.v. immunoglobulins were recommended for the therapy [17]. Their use is suggested as the initial therapy in category A and may be suggested in category B. Additional clinical data is necessary in category C to make recommendations.

Category A   **classification**
- immune thrombocytopenic purpura (ITP)
- Kawasaki syndrome

Category B
- Guillain Barre syndrome
- chronic inflammantory demyelinating polyneuropathy
- autoimmune hemolytic anemia
- autoimmune neutropenia
- acquired hemophilia A
- idiopathic thrombocytopenia purpura (ITP) in pregnancy
- myasthenia gravis

Category C (selection)
- systemic lupus erythematosus
- polymyositis and dermatomyositis
- rheumatoid arthritis
- insulin dependent diabetes mellitus
- systemic vasculitis
- antiphospholipid antibodies and recurrent abortions
- multiple sclerosis

Fc-mediated mechanisms (e.g. ITP: blockade of Fc receptors) and/or Fab-dependent reactions play or are thought to play an important role in the modulation of at least some of the autoimmune disorders listed above. The action of antiidiotypic antibodies representing a considerable portion of each polyclonal antibody preparation may be of causative importance for downregulation at the cellular level [18]. Still missing functional and quantitative characterisation of the specificities necessary, and therefore their nonstandardisable content in commercial products impedes a target-specific application. The availability of appropriate assays could be of some help in the future.

Dosage and administration

Originally, the use of immunoglobulin preparations in humans was limited to the prophylaxis and therapy of viral and bacterial infections. Additionally, substitution with immunoglobulins has proved possible in agamma- and hypogammaglobulinemic patients [19], larger amounts of immunoglobulin being administered. In severe infections with a broad spectrum of pathogens, the administration of larger amounts and volumes is also necessary. Finally, this development has led to high-dosage therapy with i.v. IgG, for instance in ITP, Kawasaki syndrome and other antibody-mediated autoimmune illnesses in which sometimes up to a maximum of 2 g/kg body weight may be administered per infusion. The general aim here is the immunoregulatory suppression of autoantibody synthesis.

The usual recommended average dose for i.v.-IgG replacement therapy in hypo- or agammaglobulinemic patients is 400 mg/kg per month [20]. The most suitable form of administration is an infusion with a catheter via the basilic, cephalic or medial antebrachial vein of the forearm. The dose may be adjusted individually since the half-life of immunoglobulins may vary from patient to patient (normal range 18–23 days).

For the therapy of ITP, a starting dose of 0.4 g/kg per day for two subsequent days or a single infusion of 0.8–1.0 g/kg is recommended. If the platelet count remains lower than $30 \times 10^9/l$ 2 days after starting therapy, i.v. IgG may be given additionally to complete a full dose of 2 g/kg [21].

Kawasaki disease is an acute illness of childhood characterised by inflammation of mucous membranes and, as a life-threatening complication, aneurysms caused by vasculitis. The recommended dose is 2 g/kg, which should be administered as a single infusion rather than giving the conventional dose of 0.4 mg/kg per day in multiple administrations.

Side effects of immunoglobulin therapy

Infusion-related adverse effects

Infusion of i.v. immunoglobulins may be considered safe and associated with relatively mild side effects in most cases. While 10 to 15% of all infusions with early i.v. IgG give rise to side effects, the figures have decreased to 2–6% with new products [22].

Mild side effects include back or lower abdominal pain, tachycardia, elevated blood pressure, muscle pain, headache, nausea, flushing, dizziness and chills. It is interesting to note that particularly aggammaglobulinemic patients have the most frequent adverse reactions. The reason for these reactions is most likely the formation of antigen-antibody (immune) complexes and complement activation when the exogenous antibodies interact with the antigen from possible infectious agents present in the patient. Thus, when i.v. IgG is administered during an active infection, the incidence of side effects is significantly higher. Adequate antibiotic treatment is therefore recommended prior to immunoglobulin infusion. However, these moderate inflammatory reactions ("phlogistic reactions") usually disappear when the infusion rate of the i.v. IgG is reduced or the infusion discontinued.

mild side effects

Sixty millilitres per hour is recommended as an initial infusion rate; the flow rate may be increased by 60 ml every 0.5 h, with a maximum of 240 ml/h. During subsequent infusions, flow rate increments should not exceed 30 ml every 30 min with a maximum of 180 ml/h. In some cases i.v. antiinflammatory treatment may be considered, either aspirin (5–10 mg) or methylprednisolone (1 mg/kg). The usefulness of antihistamines in these situations is unclear.

IgA deficiency

Severe anaphylactic reactions may occur in patients with IgA deficiency. Although a rare event, this could be life threatening and includes hypotension, respiratory or cutaneous reactions like urticarial skin rash. About 40% patients with an absolute IgA deficiency develop antibodies against IgA either of the IgG or IgE type. Binding of IgA-specific IgE in the recipient to the infused IgA-containing i.v. IgG results in activation of mast cells with degranulation and secretion of vasoactive agents such as histamine. Adverse events occur immediately after the start of infusions, and in such instances epinephrine (adrenaline) should be administered immediately.

It is advisable to select an i.v. immunoglobulin product with a very low concentration of IgA in order to minimise the reaction in these patients (see Table 2). Additionally, screening of patients for the presence of anti-IgA antibodies is recommended to lower the frequency of such adverse events.

Aseptic meningitis

As a complication of high-dose i.v.-IgG therapy (up to 2 g/kg) in patients with ITP or chronic neuropathy, severe headache, vomiting and nuchal rigidity may occur. This phenomenon, which is called acute aseptic meningitis, is a late event in immunoglobulin therapy; it occurs from 10 h up to 1 week after infusion. Analysis of the cerebrospinal fluid is negative for pathogens, although invasion of neutrophils is usually observed in patients suffering from aseptic meningitis.

The reason and the etiological agent responsible for this adverse event is unclear. One reason may be a contaminant present in the i.v. IgG, and this may induce the release of proinflammatory cytokines.

Viral safety of immunoglobulins

As early as the 1940s, the transmission of hepatitis viruses by blood components, especially by plasma, had been recognised as an inherent risk resulting from the practice of pooling plasma from a number of different donors, an occasional one of whom may be infected. Methods of plasma fractionation were developed which allowed the production of human serum albumin (HSA) and gammaglobulin preparations for intramuscular administration. Although the transmission of hepatitis by HSA did not represent a problem of practical relevance, an efficient virus inactivation procedure had been designed for safety considerations, making use of the marked thermal stability of this protein. It was also known that this special procedure of heating an aqueous solution of HSA at 60 °C for 10 h ("pasteurisation") in the presence of acetyltryptophan and sodium caprylate as stabilizers could not be directly applied to other more labile components of human plasma.

There was no reason at that time to develop a similar procedure for gammaglobulins, particularly because it was known that these proteins

HSA
hepatitis

could even be used to prevent infectious hepatitis in humans. Therefore, the presence of protective components in the antibody preparations was proposed. We know that today's immunoglobulins, which are purified from large plasma pools, contain a broad variety of specificities capable of neutralising infectious viruses. This fact is thought to be one of the reasons for the viral safety of human gammaglobulins.

Another contribution to safety originates from the process of plasma fractionation itself, since certain steps in the manufacturing process can bring about separation and inactivation of viruses. However, since the methods employed are different in detail, and the viruses concerned have distinct physicochemical properties, the virus-reducing capacity of the production procedure cannot be generalised and requires individual evaluation.

Moreover, and again originally conceived as a precautionary measure, manufacturers began introducing a separate virus inactivation method (e.g. a modified HSA pasteurisation) into the manufacturing procedure of immunoglobulins. This turned out to be reasonable, since reports have occasionally been published on the transmission of HCV (previously **HCV** non-A/non-B hepatitis virus) by certain preparations for intravenous application.

Apart from the presence of specific antibodies and the effect of the fractionation and inactivation process, the introduction of a serological check for parameters of infection, such as the absence of hepatitis B surface antigen (HBsAg), of alanine aminotransferase (ALT) and of antibodies to hepatitis C virus as well as to human immunodeficiency virus type 1 and 2 (HIV-1/2), is generally considered to constitute a further **HIV** improvement of virus safety of blood and blood-derived products. All single donations to the initial plasma pool are routinely subjected to such screening and are eliminated from fractionation in the case of positive test results. In addition, plasma for fractionation is quarantined and only released for further processing if the donor has been serologically checked again and found to be negative. This procedure helps to identify early infections still at levels below detection limit.

Despite the rationale underlying plasma screening, the implementation of anti-HCV testing for plasma used for fractionation in the United States caused an outbreak of hepatitis C following administration of a commercial i.v. IgG in early 1994. The basic manufacturing process for this product was lacking in an additional virus inactivation step. Investigations based on a sensitive polymerase chain reaction (PCR) assay re- **PCR** vealed that batches produced before introducing HCV antibody screening were HCV-RNA negative in contrast to almost all lots prepared from single donations without detectable antibodies of this specificity. Further

241

experiments suggested a process design appropriate to remove HCV in the presence of anti-HCV and of insufficient virus separation at significantly reduced levels of these antibodies. Consequently, the integration of an additional efficient validated step of virus reduction into the manufacturing process of all i.m. and i.v. immunoglobulins has been recommended by the U.S. and European authorities and, moreover, an HCV-PCR assay for all immunoglobulins without any convincing virus inactivation or removal step is now required.

From what we know today, HIV as well as hepatitis B virus (HBV) safety has certainly been achieved with the methods commonly used to prepare commercial immunoglobulins. A sensitive PCR technique established, for instance, to preselect HCV-RNA negative plasma donations for pooling may help to avoid future HCV transmissions by the final product.

Future interest in immunoglobulins

In the past few decades, the structure-to-function relationships of the antibody molecule have been revealed to a large extent. Nevertheless, even today, all regulatory functions on cells bearing Fc receptors and their involvement in stimulatory or suppressive immune processes are not comprehensively understood. The molecular basis for the clinical role of immunoglobulins in various forms of antibody-mediated autoaggression will require further elucidation to enable us to foresee and explain whether and under what premises immunoglobulins may be of clinical benefit to the individual patient. Certainly, further experimental and clinical investigations can help us to answer these questions.

Many believe that the future of immunoglobulin therapy may reside in and be challenged by the specificity inherent in monoclonal antibodies. Since their introduction some 20 years ago by Georges Köhler and Cesar Milstein [23] they have provided a greatly improved selectivity for antibody-based prevention and therapy. Surprisingly, the progress of monoclonal antibodies for clinical uses has proved to be slower than expected.

Antiallergic drugs and immunotherapy

Zdenek Pelikan

Antiallergic drugs represent a heterogeneous group, with particular agents expressing different biochemical and pharmacological properties and effects. The clinical use of particular antiallergic drugs in the treatment and control of allergic disorders in individual patients should be carefully considered and should depend on the results of diagnostic procedures. The management and treatment of allergic disorders should be a logical consequence of reliable diagnostic procedures.

Drugs listed in this chapter belong to classical, basic antiallergic drugs. Drugs having partial antiallergic effects such as β_2-sympathomimetics, immunosuppressive drugs, antileukotrienes and so on are listed and discussed in Chapters C4 and C8.

Disodium cromoglycate

Chemical structure

Disodium cromoglycate (cromolyn, DSCG), a disodium salt of 1,3-bis-(2-carboxychromone-5-yloxy)-2-hydroxypropane, has repeatedly been shown to be capable of preventing the activation and degranulation of animal and human mast cells and basophils as well as the semiselective secretion and release of various mediators and factors from these cells, both *in vitro* and *in vivo* [1–10].

Biochemical and pharmacological effects

The actions of DCSG are complex, and its clinical activity probably represents a combination of effects. Initial studies suggested two possible actions of DSCG on mast cells and basophils: inhibition of calcium transport and blocking of the antigen-induced opening of calcium gate in the

actions of DCSG

cellular membrane. Evidence has also been provided for a possible increase in membrane-associated cyclic adenosine monophosphate (cAMP) by DSCG, either directly or indirectly, through inhibition of phosphodiesterase, an enzyme involved in the breakdown of cAMP [5–10].

Inhibition of the IgE-mediated release of various mediators from mast cells and basophils and of the activation of other cell types by DSCG may be achieved by blocking the entry of calcium into the cell, which occurs through receptor-operated Ca^{2+} channels, a process that has also been shown to be a part of the signal transduction mechanism in other cell types [5]. It has further been shown that DSCG inhibits the IgE-mediated rise in intracellular calcium at concentrations that also inhibit histamine release [5].

Subsequent studies demonstrated that the inhibition of histamine release by DSCG involves the interaction of the drug and calcium ions (Ca^{2+}) with the participation of a membrane-bound protein [9]. In addition, a membrane-bound protein of 60 kDa, able to form SCG (cromolyn)-binding protein (CBP), has been isolated from RBL (rat basophilic leukemia) cells, and this protein revealed the properties characteristic of a calcium channel [8–10]. It can therefore be presumed that the site of action of DSCG is the calcium channel involved in signal transduction in cells, in this case mast cells and basophils.

However, DSCG cannot be considered to act solely through the calcium-signalling process; most probably other mechanisms are involved in the manifold effects of this drug. One of the other mechanisms proposed is protein phosphorylation, which is known to play an important role in the regulation of cell functions [5]. It has also been suggested that DSCG may reduce mediator release from mast cells by inhibiting the action of protein kinase C, an enzyme that requires calcium and phosphatidylserine for the full expression of its activity [9, 10]. Another factor which should be taken into account is the heterogeneity of mast cells and basophils. In this regard mast cells and basophils from different sources and locations may demonstrate variation in their susceptibility to the inhibitory effects of DSCG [7].

In humans, DSCG has demonstrated high and significant inhibitory effects on histamine release from bronchoalveolar lavage (BAL) mast cells, mast cells obtained by enzymatic degradation of human lung tissue fragments, conjunctival mast cells, nasal mucosal mast cells and basophils from the nasal washings or nasal secretions as well as basophils generally, whereas no significant inhibitory effects of this drug have been observed on mast cells from human skin. DSCG also inhibited isoprenaline ($IC_{50} = 10^{-7}$ M)-, gastrin ($IC_{50} = 10^{-8}$ M)- and forskolin ($IC_{50} = 10^{-7}$ M)-stimulated histamine secretion from isolated and har-

IC_{50} = concentration producing 50% inhibition

vested enterochromaffin-like cells (ELCs) of the rat gastric mucosa [5–10]. Moreover, low concentrations of DSCG (100 mM) are capable of completely suppressing the activating effects of chemoattractant peptides on human eosinophils, neutrophils and monocytes [5–10].

DSCG has been reported to reduce a number of complement reactions, e.g. C3b and immunoglobulin G (IgG) rosettes (Fcγ), on human eosinophils and to attenuate the enhanced capacity of these cells to kill *Schistosomula* of *Schistosoma mansoni* in response to *in vitro* stimulation with formyl-methionyl-leucyl-phenylalanine (fMLP). DSCG also inhibits [5–10]:

- the chemotaxis of human eosinophils induced by serum-opsonized zymosan ($IC_{50} = 1.5 \times 10^{-7}$ M; $EC_{50} = 1.0$ mM);
- tumor necrosis factor (TNFα) release from human lung and intestinal mast cells and from anti-IgE-stimulated rat peritoneal mast cells;
- IgE-dependent enzyme production and neutrophil chemotactic factor release from human alveolar macrophages; and
- serotonin release and chloride channel activity expressed by some cells.

DSCG also reduced the numbers of human eosinophils, mast cells and T-lymphocytes in the circulation as well as in tissue and macrophages in the human lung and significantly decreased the expression of adhesion molecules, especially ICAM-1, VCAM-1 and ELAM-1 in biopsies of the bronchial mucosa of patients with allergic bronchial asthma and on human nasal epithelial cells. DSCG inhibited the influx of neutrophils and the release of cytokines [TNFα and interleukin (IL-6)] into BAL fluid following allergen bronchial challenge [5–10].

DSCG has been reported to inhibit prostaglandin D_2 (PGD_2) and leukotriene C_4 (LTC_4) release from dispersed human lung cells [5–10]. Surprisingly, the drug has been shown to inhibit proliferative responses of cultured human T- and B-cells stimulated by mitogen together with rIL-2 and by allergen [9, 10]. DSCG may suppress the antibody-dependent cytotoxicity of human neutrophils and eosinophils, and the anti-IgG$_4$-induced degranulation of basophils. It increased both the survival time of human platelets from allergic patients *in vivo* and reduced IgE-dependent monoamine uptake in platelets from normal subjects *in vitro*. DSCG may inhibit IgE isotype switching and enhance IgG$_4$ production, whereas it has no direct effect on B-cells. DSCG was also shown to inhibit the switch recombination in IL-4-treated cells but had no effect on the induction of ε germline transcripts by IL-4 [9–10].

Clinical trials *in vivo*

Challenge studies

DSCG exhibits protective effects on different types of responses of various organs to challenge with (various) allergens, and in some cases to challenge with the nonspecific agents (= nonspecific hyperreactivity).

Bronchial challenges

In patients with allergic bronchial asthma, adults as well as children, DSCG in a daily dose of 4×2 inhalations (1 puff = 5 mg) has demonstrated significant protective effects on the immediate (IAR) and on the late asthmatic response (LAR) induced by bronchial challenge with allergen. However, DSCG did not significantly alter the delayed asthmatic response (DYAR) to allergen challenge [9–16].

No significant differences in the protective effects of DSCG on the asthmatic response have been observed between short- and long-term pretreatment [11–16].

In patients with allergic bronchial asthma, DSCG has been shown not only to reduce the number but also to decrease the activation/stimulation state of some cell types in the BAL fluid, such as mast cells, eosinophils and probably also neutrophils and platelets, and to reduce the activation of human alveolar macrophages. Finally, DSCG reduced the number of circulating leukocytes (especially eosinophils, neutrophils and basophils) during the immediate and the late asthmatic responses to allergen challenge, and it probably decreases the activation of circulating T-lymphocytes [9–16].

DSCG has been shown to inhibit asthmatic response, mostly of the immediate type that occurs after exercise in asthmatic subjects [9–10]. Moreover, DSCG has been found to significantly reduce bronchoconstriction due to nonspecific hyperreactivity mechanism(s), simulated by bronchial challenge with histamine, methacholine, cold air, distilled water and various chemical compounds [9, 10, 17].

Nasal challenges

In patients with nasal allergy (allergic rhinitis), both adults and children, the topical (intranasal) administration of DSCG in a daily dose of 4×2 puffs in each nostril (1 puff = 5 mg) significantly prevented both the immediate (INR) and the late nasal response (LNR) to nasal challenge with allergen. Similarly to the asthmatic response, DSCG did not significantly affect the delayed nasal response (DYNR) to allergen challenge [2, 3, 18–22].

The cytological changes in the nasal secretions – especially those in the numbers of eosinophils, neutrophils, basophils, mast cells and epithelial cells accompanying the nasal response following allergen challenge in patients with allergic rhinitis were significantly reduced by pretreatment with DSCG. DSCG also protected basophils, mast cells, eosinophils and neutrophils in the nasal secretions from degranulation and other intracellular changes that appear during nasal responses to allergen challenge such as INR, LNR and DYNR [2, 3, 18–22]. DSCG has been shown to downregulate some adhesion molecules, e.g. ICAM-1, expressed on human nasal epithelial cells. Intranasal DSCG also reduced the nasal response to challenge with histamine and methacholines [2, 3].

Conjunctival challenges

Cromolyn (DSCG), in a daily dose of 4×2 drops (1 drop = 1.6 mg DSCG), has also been found to prevent the immediate (ICR) and the late conjunctival response (LCR) to challenge with allergen [23].

Skin challenge

DSCG has not been found to significantly prevent any skin response to allergen challenge.

Oral challenge with foods

DSCG administered orally in a daily dose of 4×100–200 mg has been found to significantly prevent various organ responses to food ingestion challenge [2, 3, 5, 6, 9]. These responses to food ingestion challenge may be caused by so-called adverse reactions to foods, allergy being one of the most important mechanisms [2, 3, 23–26]. DSCG significantly prevented immediate and late types of asthmatic, nasal, paranasal sinus, middle ear, conjunctival, migraine, atopic eczema, urticarial and Quincke's edema responses to food ingestion challenge [2, 3, 23–29].

Therapeutic studies

Therapeutic studies have revealed and confirmed the clinical efficacy, highly significant protective effects, high safety, low side effect profile and manifold clinical effects, including the antiinflammatory profile, of this drug.

therapeutical studies

It can be concluded that DSCG, administered topically in a daily dose of four times, at least, is a very effective drug in the prophylaxis of allergic bronchial asthma, allergic rhinitis, allergic conjunctivitis and related disorders, especially in such cases in which the immediate and/or late types of allergic reaction play a predominant role. In these allergic dis-

effective drugs in prophylaxis

first-choice drug

orders, DSCG belongs to the first-choice therapeutic drugs, supplemented by β_2-sympathomimetics in the case of bronchial asthma and H_1-receptor antagonists in the case of allergic rhinitis and/or conjunctivitis. The oral formulation of DSCG is very effective in the prophylaxis of various clinical manifestations due to the food allergy.

Nedocromil sodium

Chemical structure

Nedocromil sodium (*NDS*), the disodium salt of a novel pyrano-quinoline dicarboxylic acid [9-ethyl-6,9-dihydro-4,6-dioxo-10-propyl-4H-pyranol (3,2-g) quinoline-2,8-dicarboxylic acid] has demonstrated a variety of antiallergic and antiinflammatory effects, especially in the respiratory tract, both in animal and in human studies [1–5, 7–9, 13–17, 21–23].

Biochemical and pharmacologic effects

In various experiments both *in vitro* and *in vivo*, NDS has been shown to inhibit the activation and various functions, such as release of mediators and/or other factors of various cell types, both in the animals and in humans, initiated by specific (antigenic) as well as by nonspecific stimuli. NDS has demonstrated inhibitory effects on human mast cells, basophils, eosinophils, neutrophils, macrophages, monocytes, epithelial cells in the airways and in the nose, platelets, T-lymphocyte, B-lymphocyte and sensory nerve cells [5, 7–9, 21, 22, 30, 31].

In human *in vitro* studies, NDS inhibited histamine release from the human "chopped lung" and showed a higher inhibitory activity on the IgE-mediated release of histamine from human mast cells from BAL ($IC_{50} = 0.5 \times 10^{-6}$ M) and from dispersed human lung fragments ($IC_{50} = 6 \times 10^{-6}$ M) than DSCG. However, mast cells from human BAL are protected by NDS to a higher degree than those from human dispersed parenchyma or chopped lung. In common with DSCG, tachyphylaxis to the inhibitory effects of NDS has only been observed with human lung parenchymal mast cells (dispersed lung), but not with the cells obtained by BAL [5, 7–9, 30]. NDS has also been shown to be capable of inhibiting the bronchoconstriction response to hyperosmolar challenge in humans, probably due to mediator release by activated mast cells and to the release of sensory neuropeptides [5–9, 30].

Like DSCG, NDS demonstrated significant inhibitory effects on IgE-dependent release of histamine and PGD_2 from human tonsillar mast cells, whereas mediator release from human intestinal mast cells was inhibited by NDS only to a slight degree. NDS also failed to inhibit IgE-dependent mediator release from animal and human skin mast cells *in vitro* as well as *in vivo*. NDS has been shown to inhibit substance P (SP)-induced histamine release and the release of $TNF\alpha$ from human lung mast cells [5, 8, 9, 30]. The variations in the inhibitory effects of NDS as well as DSCG on mast cells originating from various locations, even in one subject, animal or human, are related to the heterogeneity of the mast cells. In contrast to DSCG, the inhibitory and/or protective effects of NDS on human basophils have not yet been unequivocally confirmed. Nevertheless, some evidence has been provided for possible inhibitory effects of NDS on human basophils [5, 7–9].

NDS reduced the number of complement IgG rosettes on human eosinophils and attenuated the enhanced capacity of eosinophils to kill *Schistosomula* in response to fMLP and it can suppress the chemotaxis of human eosinophils induced by platelet activating factor (PAF) or LTB_4 ($EC_{50} = 1.0\ \mu M$ and $0.1\ \mu M$, respectively; $IC_{50} = 7.3 \times 10^{-9}$ M and 1.1×10^{-6} M, respectively). NDS inhibits the release of both preformed (granule-associated) eicosanoid mediators, such as eosinophil cationic protein (ECP) and newly generated eicosanoid mediators, such as leukotriene C_4 (LTC_4) from activated eosinophils. It also prevents a decrease in eosinophil density occurring in short-term culture. NDS, similarly to DSCG, has also been shown to inhibit activation, chemotaxis and mediator release from human neutrophils, and to inhibit the chemotactic response of human eosinophils to stimulation with PAF and LTB_4. NDS demonstrated inhibitory effects on the release of cytotoxic mediators from platelets of patients with aspirin-sensitive asthma, on the IgE-mediated activation of passively sensitized human blood platelets following exposure to *Schistosoma* antigen and on the generation of thromboxane B_2 (TXB_2) and intracellular messenger inositol triphosphate (IP_3), produced by thrombin-stimulated platelets [5, 8, 9, 30, 31].

Recently, NDS was reported to inhibit IL-4-induced IgE and IgG_4 production by human B-cells in atopic patients without affecting production of IgG_1, IgG_2, IgG_3, IgM or IgA. These NDS effects on the IL-4 stimulated B-cells are probably due to inhibition of the production of messenger RNA (mRNA) for the IgE antibody. In contrast, DSCG selectively inhibited IL-4-stimulated IgE production and IgA production by activated human B-cells even in the absence of T-cells. NDS inhibited the switch recombination in IL-4-treated cells and did not affect the induction of ϵ germ-line transcripts by IL-4 [5, 8, 9, 30, 31].

NDS has also been shown to possess inhibitory effects on various human cells from BAL fluid, such as mast cells stimulated *in vitro* with antibody to human IgE, activated eosinophils from asthmatic subjects and to prevent the decrease in density of eosinophils which occurs during the short-term culture.

In the cultured human bronchial epithelial cell model, NDS inhibited the release of TNFα, IL-8 and intracellular adhesion module-1 (ICAM-1) following exposure to ozone (50 ppb), the release of granulocyte-macrophage colony-stimulating factor (GM-CSF) and IL-8 caused by challenge with IL-1 and the expression of cell surface ICAM-1 induced by challenge of these cells with 1 mmol/L of histamine [5, 7–9, 30, 31].

An inhibitory effect of NDS on the production of IL-6 by human airway macrophages following challenge with specific antigen and/or with anti-IgE has been reported. NDS also inhibits lysosomal enzyme release from human alveolar macrophages and oxygen radical release from human monocytes following stimulation with anti-IgE [5, 8, 9, 30, 31].

Clinical trials *in vivo*

Challenge studies

Bronchial challenges
Inhaled NDS in a daily dose of THE 4×2 inhalations (1 puff = 2 mg) has significant protective effects on the IAR ($p < 0.01$ and $p < 0.001$) and on the LAR ($p < 0.001$) to bronchial challenge in adults as well as in children. Recently, an evidence also has been provided for the possible protective effects of NDS on the DYAR ($p \leq 0.05$). NDS is effective in prevention of the asthmatic response to exercise, which is mostly of an immediate type, as well as of the accompanying cellular changes in the blood [4–6, 9, 10, 13–17, 30].

Bronchoconstriction due to the nonspecific hyperreactivity mechanism(s), simulated by bronchial challenge with various agents, such as histamine, methacholine, cold air, bradykinin, metabisulphide, fog, hyperosmolar challenge and neurokinin A in patients with bronchial asthma, is also prevented significantly by inhaled NDS [4–6, 9, 10, 17, 30].

Nasal challenges
Topically (intranasally) administered NDS, in a daily dose of 4×2 puffs (1 puff = 4 mg) in each of the nostrils, significantly prevented both INR ($p < 0.01$) and LNR ($p < 0.001$), whereas DYNR was only partially prevented ($p = 0.05$). NDS significantly reduced the influx of eosinophils,

neutrophils, mast cells and basophils into nasal secretions, during INR, whereas it almost completely prevented the influx of neutrophils, eosinophils and basophils, and significantly decreased the epithelial and goblet cell count in nasal secretion during LNR [2, 3, 5, 6, 9, 10, 21, 22, 29, 32].

Intranasal NDS also reduced nonspecific hyperreactivity in the nose, a mechanism(s) simulated by nasal challenge with histamine and methacholine [2, 3, 5, 6, 9, 10, 29].

Conjunctival challenge

NDS applied intraconjunctivally in a daily dose of 4×2 drops (1 drop = 0.8 mg) provided significant protection against ICR as well as LCR to conjunctival challenge with allergen [5, 9].

Therapeutic studies

Therapeutic studies have confirmed the excellent clinical efficacy, tolerability and high degree of safety of NDS as well as its highly significant protective and therapeutic effects in patients with allergic bronchial asthma, allergic rhinitis and allergic conjunctivitis. The manifold clinical effects of this drug include both antiallergenic and antiinflammatory effects. Along with DSCG, NDS is the treatment of the first choice for bronchial asthma and in some cases of allergic rhinitis. NDS may be a useful drug in patients in whom DSCG fails to achieve full preventive effects and for whom corticosteroids are still not indicated.

excellent clinical efficacy tolerability and high degree of safety

first choice drug

Glucocorticosteroids

Chemical structure

The glucocorticosteroids (GCSs) are derived from hydrocortisone (cortisol), whose chemical structure is as follows: $11\beta,17\alpha,21$-trihydroxy-4-pregnene-3,20-dione [$C_{21}H_{30}O_5$], a compound consisting of four rings (three hexoses, one pentose), including 21 carbons [33–39].

Biochemical and pharmacological effects

The GCSs possess a variety of very potent antiinflammatory activities and effects on various cell types, biochemical and immunological processes and mechanisms, at various levels and stages [33–39] (see Chapter C9).

The classical GCS responses have been attributed to the cascade of cellular events initiated by GCS binding to specific GCS receptors. These receptors appear widely in the cytoplasm of almost all mammalian and also human cells, such as lymphocytes, neutrophils, monocytes and eosinophils. However, the existence of such GCS-specific receptors on human mast cells and basophils has not yet been confirmed [33–39].

The manifold biochemical and pharmacological effects of GCSs are described and discussed in detail in a number of reviews [33–39]. The GCSs exhibit the following effects:

1) they increase and potentiate the action of cAMP, whereas they decrease and inhibit the action of cyclic guanosine monophosphate (cGMP);
2) they inhibit the synthesis of various metabolites of arachidonic acid (AA) such as prostaglandins, leukotrienes and thromboxanes;
3) they inhibit the synthesis and release of vasoactive kinins;
4) they influence the cellular transport of calcium by an effect on Ca^{2+} channels, resulting in some cell types in an increased accumulation of calcium, and in other cell types in a decreased entry of Ca^{2+};
5) they decrease histamine synthesis and histamine concentration in tissue;
6) they prevent the reaccumulation of histamine in the tissues and regulate gene expression and transcription in a variety of cells, among others in human pulmonary and bronchial epithelial cells and peripheral blood mononuclear cells;
7) they influence several biochemical processes, such as regulation of carbohydrate, lipid and protein metabolism, water and electrolyte exchanges, and glucose metabolism. They also facilitate the release of fatty acids from neutral lipids, and cause urine retention by stimulating the reabsorption of sodium at the renal distal tubules;
8) they may have some inhibitory effects on complement activation, such as a decrease in C3 and B-factor secretion and an increase in secretion of alternative pathway factor H;
9) they decrease vascular permeability and increase the resistance of capillary walls;
10) they suppress *in vivo* the production and serum levels of immunoglobulins, particularly of IgG and IgA;

11) they inhibit the proliferation of eosinophils *in vitro*, and decrease the total number of circulating eosinophils, inhibiting their accumulation in the tissue, probably through inhibition of PAF and IL-1, and inhibit the release of mediators from eosinophils;

12) they decrease the chemotaxis of neutrophils, both directly and through the suppression of LTB_4 production, the accumulation of neutrophils in the tissue, and they inhibit production and release of some cellular products of neutrophils, such as superoxide, selected peptides and plasminogen activator;

13) they decrease the numbers of circulating basophils, eosinophils, monocytes and T-lymphocytes, especially of the helper/inducer (CD4) subset, but not of the cytotoxic/suppressor (CD8) subset, whereas they increase the number of circulating neutrophils by increasing their release from bone marrow and delaying their migration from the intravascular space;

14) they inhibit the adherence of neutrophils to vascular endothelium;

15) they inhibit the proliferation and activation of T-lymphocytes as well as the synthesis and production of some of their cytokines, such as mRNA for IL-2 and interferon γ (IFNγ);

16) they inhibit the activation of monocytes and macrophages, their recruitment to the site of inflammatory processes as well as the synthesis and release of some of their products, such as AA metabolites (TXB_2, LTB_4), plasminogen activator, collagenase elastase, IL-1 and TNFα;

17) they inhibit the prolongation of eosinophil survival *in vitro* as well as *in vivo*, by both a direct effect on the eosinophils and by diminishing the levels of the relevant cytokines (e.g. IL-3, IL-5, GM-CSF);

18) they inhibit the production and release of some chemotactic factors and cytokines, whereas they antagonize the effects of other chemotactic factors and cytokines. GCSs inhibit the production and also the partial effects of IL-1, IL-2, IL-3, IL-6, IL-8, IFNγ, GM-CSF and TNFα in human epithelial cells, whereas they increase the number of receptors for IL-1 and IL-6 and enhance the production of acute-phase reactants and immunoglobulins induced by IL-1 and IL-6 in human mononuclear phagocytes. GCSs also inhibit *in vitro* production of monocyte chemotactic and activating factor (MCAF) by human monocytes;

19) they stimulate the growth and reduce the synthesis of collagen due to a decrease in the level of RNA for the collagen types I and II;

20) they may also have direct inhibitory effects, at the level of gene transcription, on the expression of adhesion molecules, such as ICAM-1 and E-selectin, which are expressed on human monocytes and bronchial epithelial cells;

21) they decrease the transcription of genes coding for some receptors, e.g. neurokinin 1 receptor (NK1), whereas they increase the expression of β2-adrenoreceptors, and they are potent inducers of decoy IL-1 receptors.

Despite these manifold antiinflammatory effects of GCSs on various cell types, direct inhibitory effects on the mast cells and basophils, especially in humans, have not yet been unequivocally confirmed. In human studies *in vivo*, topical GCSs reduced the numbers of epithelial and mucosal mast cells after allergen challenge in the nose and in the BAL fluid, but had no inhibitory effects on the release of their mediators [33–39].

Clinical trials *in vivo*

Challenge studies

Bronchial challenge
The GCSs demonstrated significant protective effects on the antigen-induced LAR and DYAR, whereas they do not significantly affect IAR. No significant differences in these protective effects have been observed between the oral forms, such as prednisone, prednisolone, hydrocortisone, dexamethasone (daily dose of 2×5 mg to 2×10 mg) and the inhaled forms, such as beclomethasone, budesonide, fluticasone, triamcinolone (daily dose 4×100–200 mcg) [4, 11–16, 33–39].

GCSs have been shown to reduce the number and functions of various types of cells, such as bronchoalveolar mast cells, eosinophils, T-lymphocytes ($CD4^+/CD25^+$), goblet cells, epithelial cells, macrophages, monocytes, neutrophils and fibroblasts, and they may suppress the airway microvascular leakage induced by several mediators. GCSs have been reported to reduce bronchial nonspecific hyperreactivity, including bronchial responsiveness to challenge with histamine, methacholine, cold air and various chemical compounds [33–39]. It has been suggested that GCSs decrease the asthmatic response due to the exercise [4, 11–16, 33–39].

Nasal challenge
Topically (intranasally) administered glucocorticosteroids, in a daily dose of 4×50–100 mcg in each of the nostrils, have significantly prevented both the LNR and DYNR, whereas they did not affect INR. GCSs were shown to reduce the counts of some types of cells, such as eosinophils, neutrophils, epithelial cells and basophils, in nasal secretions (NS) accompanying LNR and those accompanying the DYNR, such as neu-

trophils, epithelial cells and lymphocytes, whereas they did not significantly influence the cell counts in the nasal secretions accompanying the INR [2, 3, 18–22, 29, 33, 36–39].

GCSs have also been reported to reduce the concentration or to inhibit the appearance of some of the mediators, factors or chemical compounds in the nasal lavage fluid or nasal secretions during the LNR, such as histamine, ECP, TAME-esterase activity (N-α-tosyl-L-arginine methyl esther), kinins, albumin, MBP (major basic protein), eosinophil-derived neurotoxin or during the INR, such as histamine, TAME-esterase activity and kinins to a very slight degree. However, GCSs do not affect the increased concentrations of LTB_4 in the nasal lavage fluid during the INR or LNR. Topically administered GCSs (beclomethasone dipropionate, budesonide, fluticasone) do not inhibit the nasal response to challenge with histamine or methacholine (bromide, chloride) [2, 3, 29, 33, 36–39].

Conjunctival challenge

There is a dearth of data concerning the possible effects of GCSs on the conjunctival responses induced by an allergen as well as by the nonspecific hyperreactivity agent. Recently, some protective effects of GCSs in some forms of allergic conjunctivitis have been reported [33, 36–39].

Skin challenge

GCSs such as prednisone and prednisolone, administered orally or topically, significantly inhibit the antigen-induced late skin response, whereas they do not affect the antigen-induced immediate skin response. They also inhibit the release of some of the skin mast cell mediators – the influx of basophils and eosinophils accompanying late skin response – but they do not affect the number of skin mast cells [33, 36–39].

Therapeutic studies

Therapeutic studies with GCSs have revealed manifold antiinflammatory and therapeutic effects, clinical efficacy and safety of these drugs, though with some differences among particular drugs.

Studies have been shown GCSs in topical formulations to be very effective drugs in the prophylaxis of cases of allergic bronchial asthma, allergic rhinitis, allergic conjunctivitis, atopic eczema and related disorders, in which a delayed-type allergic reaction plays a predominant role and/or where the late type of allergic reaction cannot be sufficiently controlled by DSCG or NDS. Systemic GCSs are indicated in cases of ana-

effective in prophylaxis

phylactic reaction or other allergic, life-threatening disorders and allergic disorders with insufficient response to the nonsteroidal treatment.

H-receptor antagonists

Histamine, 2-(4-imidazolyl)ethylamine or 5-aminoethylimidazole, is formed by decarboxylation of the amino acid histidine by the pyridoxal phosphate-dependent enzyme L-histidine decarboxylase in the Golgi apparatus of mast cells and basophils [8, 40–42].

The majority of the histamine is synthesized and stored in a preformed form in the cytoplasmic granules of the mast cells and basophils (~4–10 pg/human mast cell and 1 pg/human basophil) in close association with the anionic side chains of proteglycans comprising the granule matrix (see also Chapters A7 and A9). There is evidence for the possible synthesis of histamine by other cell types and tissues, also in humans, such as monocytes, endothelial cells, central nervous system and platelets [8, 40–44].

Histamine has a variety of biological effects and activities which have been extensively described in a number of excellent reviews [43–46]. These biological effects are mediated through the activation of specific surface receptors, called H-receptors. Histamine receptors have two basic functions: they recognize the specific molecular structures of the agonist by a process of high-affinity binding, and after having been bound by this agonist, they initiate a cascade of biological reactions, resulting in particular biochemical responses. Histamine is the major messenger for all three external H-receptor types [40–42, 44].

Three types of histamine receptors have been identified, H_1-, H_2- and H_3-receptors. Histamine receptors are distributed widely in various mammalian tissues, in animals as well as in humans [40–42].

In general, four basic signal transduction processes by which the receptors operate have been defined through biochemical analysis. These processes include (1) receptor-operated ion channels; (2) receptor-controlled guanine nucleotide-binding proteins (G proteins); (3) intrinsic protein kinase activity; (4) transcription factors directly regulating gene expression [40–42, 44].

H_1-receptors

The molecular size of the H_1-receptor protein in the human cerebral cortex is 160 kDa. Different states of receptor glycosylation may, however, contribute to heterogeneity of H_1-receptor-binding properties [8, 40–42].

In humans, H_1-receptors have been identified and localized on the following cell surfaces (membranes): (1) central nervous system: brain tissue cells, cerebellum, cerebral cortex; (2) vascular system: human umbilical endothelial cells, vascular endothelial cells; (3) respiratory system: airway smooth muscle cells, lung tissue and bronchial epithelium including mucus-secreting glands; (4) platelets, lymphocytes, monocytes and fibroblasts [40–42].

cells and organs with H_1-receptors

Interestingly, H_1- and H_3-receptors have not yet been demonstrated on the cellular membranes of either human mast cells or human basophils. Some evidence has been provided for a possible existence of H_2-receptors on the membrane of the human circulating basophil [40–42].

Biochemical characterization of H_1-receptors

Signal transduction by H_1-receptors probably occurs through the hydrolysis of inositol phospholipids bound to the membrane of the target cell. Stimulation of the H_1-receptor, by histamine among others, leads in most tissue types to its interaction with the phospholipase C system, resulting in the hydrolysis of membrane-related inositol phospholipids. The phospholipase C system acts as one of the first messengers of the H_1-receptor. Hydrolysis of membrane-bound inositol phospholipids results in the formation of inositol-1,4,5-triphosphate (IP_3) and 1,2-diacyl-glycerol (DAG), both of them acting as second messengers [40–42, 44].

stimulation of the H1-receptors

IP_3, which is released into the cytosol of the target cell, mobilizes the calcium ions (Ca^{2+}) from intracellular stores, whereas DAG, which is retained within the cellular membrane structure, may activate protein kinase C. The activation of phospholipase C is probably regulated by G proteins. DAG is an important factor in the transduction of signals to calcium-mobilizing receptors, and it is also the main physiological activator of protein kinase C. DAG increases protein kinase C affinity for Ca^{2+}, which results in the activation of this enzyme without any significant rise in the cytosolic Ca^{2+} concentration [40–42, 44].

Two different calcium-mobilization pathways, leading to biphasic responses, have been proposed. IP_3 is responsible for the release of Ca^{2+} from the intracellular stores, and this mobilization of calcium ions may cause a primary transient peak response, which occurs even in the absence of extracellular calcium, whereas secondary sustained intracellular Ca^{2+} elevation may be due to the influx of extracellular Ca^{2+} into the target cell [40–42, 44].

consequences of elevation of Ca^{2+} concentration

Histamine-induced elevation of the intracellular Ca^{2+} concentration has important consequences: (1) the rise in intracellular Ca^{2+} levels can further stimulate the activity of phospholipase C; (2) elevation of intracellular Ca^{2+} also stimulates the activities of other enzymes; (3) H$_1$-receptor-mediated production of cGMP has been demonstrated; (4) H$_1$-receptor-mediated, endothelium-dependent relaxation in vascular tissue is probably related to the production of nitric oxide [40–42, 44].

Histamine is also a very potent stimulant of the elevation of cAMP and its accumulation in various tissues [40–42].

The most important clinical effects of of H$_1$-receptor stimulation can be summarized as follows:

chemical effects

1) upper airways: nasal pruritus and sneezing due to the stimulation of H$_1$-receptors on sensory nerves; mucosal edema due to the stimulation of H$_1$-receptors in the nasal mucosa; hypersecretion due both to H$_1$-receptor stimulation and vagal reflex pathways causing muscarinic-induced mucous gland discharge;

2) lower airways: bronchial smooth muscle contraction, both via direct effects on smooth muscle cells and through stimulation of vagal afferent nerve fibers; pulmonary vasoconstriction; increased capillary permeability and serous fluid secretions; increase in airway epithelial permeability; induction of prostaglandin and thromboxane production;

3) cardiovascular system: peripheral vasodilation; increased vasal and capillary permeability; positive chronotropy; vasoconstriction of coronary arteries;

4) gastrointestinal system: spasmodic contraction of the gall bladder;

5) skin: sensory nerve-induced pruritus and flare responses through the release of neuropeptides, especially substance P, which enhances these responses both directly by causing vasodilatation and edema, and indirectly by degranulating the cutaneous mast cells (this mechanism exists in animals only);

6) central nervous system: neurotransmission and neuromodulation;

7) endothelial cells: contraction of these cells and stimulation of synthesis of a variety of factors, such as prostacyclin, EDRF (endothelium-derived relaxing factor) and PAF;

8) some circulating cell types: inhibition of neutrophil and eosinophil chemotaxis; stimulation of the release of AA metabolites from platelets [8, 40–42].

H$_1$-receptor antagonists

These compounds, classically termed antihistamines, form a large heterogeneous group which can be divided by various criteria such as: (1) time sequence of their absorption, distribution and action in tissues; (2) antihistamines of the first, second and third generation, the latter also called nonsedating antihistamines; (3) chemical families; (4) clusters of their clinical effects; (5) affinity for particular tissue types; (6) side effects (e.g. sedation versus no sedation) [2, 3, 8, 41, 43–45].

criteria for division

The basic H$_1$-receptor antagonists can be divided into seven groups, six chemical "families" and one "miscellaneous" group:

1) *ethylendiamines*, e.g. mepyramine, pyrilamine, clemizole, tripelennamine;
2) *ethanolamines*, e.g. doxylamine, clemastine, bromdiphenhydramine;
3) *akylamines*, e.g. chlorpheniramine, triprolidine, dimethindene;
4) *phenothiazines*, e.g. promethazine, oxatomide, trimeprazine;
5) *piperazines*, e.g. hydroxyzine, cyclizine, cinnarizine, meclizine, buclizine;
6) *piperidines*, e.g. azatadine, thenalidine, phenindamine, piprinhydrinate;
7) *miscellaneous*, such as mebhydroline, mequitazine, cabastine, levocabastine, ketotifen, astemizole, temelastine, mianserine, epinastine, terfenadine, fexofenadine, loratadine, cetirizine, azelastine, acrivastine, ebastine [2, 3, 41, 43–45].

H$_1$-receptor antagonists groups

Biochemical and pharmacological effects

At low concentrations H$_1$-receptor antagonists are pharmacological antagonists of histamine at H$_1$-receptor sites and act by binding to the H$_1$-receptors, which results in blocking of the H$_1$-response. This binding is readily reversible for most of the H$_1$-receptor antagonists. The relative number of the receptors occupied by histamine and the relative number of receptors occupied by the H$_1$-antagonists depend on the relative concentrations of histamine and on the distance of the H$_1$-receptor antagonist to the receptor site. The mode of receptor interaction with the H$_1$-receptor antagonists, especially of the newer generations, seems to be more complex than the simple competitive binding, and is probably noncompetitive. The absence of all three H-receptor types on the surface of human mast cells and of H$_1$- and H$_3$-receptors on the surface of human basophils would exclude the direct effects of H-receptor antagonists, es-

antagonists of histamine

pecially H_1-receptor antagonists, on these cell types through H-(H_1-)receptor-mediated mechanism(s) [8, 41, 43, 44].

Two hypotheses have been postulated to try to explain suggested inhibitory effects of H_1-receptor antagonists on mediator release from mast cells [8, 41, 43].

first hypothesis

The first hypothesis concerns the proposed stabilizing effects of the H_1-receptor antagonists on the cellular membrane of mast cells. Since H_1-receptor antagonists are lipophilic compounds, they are taken up into the cell membranes. Low concentrations of these drugs may stabilize the cell membrane, whereas higher concentrations may lead to cytologic effects. The stabilized cellular membrane may then be less permeable to transmembrane ion traffic, thereby reducing sodium influx. The consequent release of calcium ions (Ca^{2+}) from their intracellular sites may be reduced.

second hypothesis

The second hypothesis concerns the suggested effects of these drugs on several stages of the process of calcium mobilization. The activation of mast cells involves a complex network of various biochemical processes which include both the mobilization of intracellular calcium (Ca^{2+}) and the opening of specific calcium channels in the cellular membrane to permit the influx of extracellular calcium ions. The increase in cytosolic calcium concentrations results in the activation of several intracellular factors, including calmodulin. Calmodulin is capable not only of binding calcium but also of modulating the catalytic activity of a variety of enzymes, such as protein kinase, adenylate cyclase, guanylate cyclase, phospholipase, adenosine triphosphatase, phosphodiesterase, myosin light-chain kinase, diglyceride kinase and lipase. By corollary, these enzymes may then be involved in the progression of or in the negative feedback on the secretory and/or degranulation responses of the mast cells.

proposed effects

H_1-receptor antagonists have been proposed (1) to prevent the increase in intracellular calcium concentration due to the increased influx of extracellular calcium into the mast cells; (2) to displace calcium from the lipid monolayers at the same concentrations as those that probably inhibit the histamine release (this suggested capacity may probably be related to their cationic amphiphilic properties); (3) to prevent binding of calcium to the membrane calcium channels and also in this way to inhibit the influx of calcium (these effects may probably be due to the inhibition of calmodulin by these drugs); (4) to activate adenylate cyclase, leading to increased intracellular levels of cAMP, and ultimately result in the prevention of mobilization of intracellular calcium [8, 41, 43, 44].

However, the validity of such hypotheses for the H_1-receptor antagonists is very limited, since these drugs are not capable of inhibiting antigen-related mediator release from the activated human mast cells and basophils *in vivo*.

Clinical trials *in vivo*

H_1-receptor antagonists represent a large group that includes a high number of compounds, some of them belonging to the first drugs used in the treatment of allergic disorders. To date numerous studies of these drugs have been conducted and published. Inclusion of these studies would exceed the scope of this chapter; moreover, they are excellently reviewed elsewhere [43–46].

Challenge studies

Bronchial challenges

Results reported in the literature concerning the possible protective effects of H_1-receptor antagonists on the antigen-induced asthmatic response, mostly of the immediate/early type, in patients with bronchial asthma vary widely [13–16, 44].

In a number of bronchial challenge studies with various inhaled allergens, carried out according to different designs, we failed to observe inhibitory effects of any of the H_1-receptor antagonists, including those of the second and the third generation (promethazine, clemastine, methydroline, cinnarizium, ketotifen, astemizole, terfenadine, azelastine, cetirizine, acrivastine, claritine, hydroxyzine, azatadine) on either AR or LAR [13–16, 37]. These drugs did not even affect DYAR to allergen challenge [16]. The existence of inhibitory effects of H_1-receptor antagonists on antigen-induced IAR and LAR is therefore questionable [37, 44]. According to our preliminary results, none of the H_1-receptor antagonists studied (ketotifen, cinnarizine, hydroxyzine, astemizole, cetirizine, loratadine) affected histamine- or methacholine-induced bronchospasm.

Thus the clinical effects of H_1-receptor antagonists on bronchoconstriction in patients with bronchial asthma appear to vary markedly. Relief of some symptoms of bronchial asthma is mild, and the clinical importance of these effects is limited. Therefore, these drugs do not rank among the first-choice treatments for allergic bronchial asthma; they may be useful as additional or supplementary therapy.

Nasal challenges

H_1-receptor antagonists, such as orally administered terfenadine, diphenhydramide, clemastine, ketotifen, cetirizine, loratadine, as well as topically administered azatadine, azelastine and levocabastine, have been reported to reduce or to inhibit some of the nasal symptoms accompanying the immediate nasal response to allergen challenge (INR), especially sneezing, hypersecretion and itching, to various degrees [2, 3, 21, 22]. However, most of these drugs are not able to reduce or to significantly inhibit nasal obstruction associated with INR, LNR or DYNR nasal response to allergen challenge [2, 22].

Some investigators have reported the lack of significant inhibitory effects of some of these drugs, such as cetirizine, terfenadine, azelastine, loratadine, levocabastine, astemizole and acrivastine on the antigen-induced influx of eosinophils into nasal secretions which accompanies INR. In contrast, other investigators have reported significant reduction of the influx of eosinophils and of other kinds of cells into nasal secretions accompanying antigen-induced INR after pretreatment with some of the H_1-receptor antagonists. Cetirizine, loratadine, clemastine and azelastine have been reported to reduce the influx of eosinophils into the nasal secretions, whereas cinnarizine, loratadine and clemastine may decrease the counts of eosinophils, neutrophils and basophils in the nasal secretions [21, 22, 29, 43–45].

H_1-receptor antagonists can also inhibit to different degrees the antigen-induced release of various mediators into the nasal secretions or nasal lavage fluid associated with the INR. Terfenadine has been reported to inhibit the release of histamine, kinins, TAME-esterase, albumin and prostaglandin D_2, whereas it was ineffective in inhibiting of leukotriene C_4 and prostaglandin D_2 release. Cetirizine has been shown to inhibit the release of TAME-esterase, albumin and leukotriene C_4, whereas it did not affect the release of histamine and prostaglandin D_2. Loratadine demonstrated inhibitory effects on the release of prostaglandin D_2, albumin and histamine, whereas it did not inhibit the release of TAME-esterase, prostaglandin D_2, leukotriene C_4 or histamine. Azatadine has been shown to inhibit release of histamine, kinins and TAME-esterase, whereas azelastine, ketotifen and diphenhydramine did not inhibit the release of histamine. Clemastine did not affect the release of albumin [43-45].

None of the drugs studied (cetirizine, loratadine, terfenadine, cinnarizine, clemastine, acrivastine, astemizole, levocabastine, ketotifen, chlorphenamine, promethazine, mebhydroline, azelastine) was able to significantly prevent LNR. However, some of these drugs reduced the influx of some kinds of cells into nasal secretions during LNR [21, 22, 29, 37]. Nasal response to the challenge with histamine was reduced or prevented by cetirizine, loratadine and azelastine, and also partly by cinnarizine and clemastine. Histamine-induced nasal response has not been affected by astemizole, acrivastine, azatadine, levocabastine and terfenadine [43–45].

These results suggest that none of the above-mentioned H_1-receptor antagonists has been able to fully inhibit the antigen-induced nasal response, especially the accompanying nasal obstruction and antigen-induced release of the whole complex of mediators as well as associated cellular changes in the nasal secretions. These results may also indicate that the H_1-receptor antagonists affect not only H_1-receptors but probably also muscarinic (M_1, M_3) receptors and through them subsequently mediated sneezing, hypersecretion and itching [21, 22, 43–45].

H_1-receptor antagonists should therefore be considered to be the treatment of choice in cases of allergic rhinitis, especially in mild cases, but not as an exclusive and definitive therapy. In severe cases of this disorder, they may be used to supplement the treatment with cromolyn and corticosteroids [2, 3].

Skin challenge

Clemastine has been shown to inhibit the antigen-induced skin responses, especially flare, but not wheal. Terfenadine inhibited histamine-induced skin responses, whereas it did not affect antigen-induced skin response or histamine release in patients with urticaria. Cetirizine has been reported to inhibit antigen-induced cutaneous response (wheal and flare reactions), whereas other data failed to confirm an inhibitory effect on antigen-induced release of histamine and PGD_2 within 6 h following the challenge. However, this drug does inhibit histamine-induced skin wheal.

Loratadine demonstrated inhibitory effects on antigen-induced skin response, although to a lesser degree than cetirizine, and also inhibited histamine-induced skin response. Ebastine also inhibited histamine-induced skin response, whereas astemizole is only partial effective in suppressing the skin response to injected histamine [43–45].

Conjunctival challenge

Levocabastine, administered topically, has been shown to inhibit antigen-induced conjunctival response of the immediate type but did not affect the late conjunctival response. Cetirizine, administered orally seems to be able to reduce the antigen-induced immediate conjunctival response [43–45].

Therapeutic studies

Extensive results of clinical studies are discussed in several review papers and books. From these, it appears that various H_1-receptor antagonists, especially those of the second and the third generation, have shown very good therapeutic properties and clinical effectiveness, especially in patients with allergic disorders of the upper airways, urticaria, anaphy-

very good therapeutic properties and clinical effectiveness

laxis and atopic dermatitis, whereas they did not substantially affect the symptoms of bronchial asthma, food allergy or gastrointestinal allergy.

Allergic disorders, especially of the upper airways and skin, with mild symptoms, can be effectively controlled by H_1-receptor antagonists. In allergic disorders with more severe symptoms, and a complicated clinical picture or nonimmediate types of reactions (late and/or delayed), H_1-antagonists should be used as a supplementary therapeutic measure only.

H_2-receptors, H_3-receptors and their antagonists

Antagonists of H_2- and H_3-receptors are currently not considered to be relevant drugs for the treatment of allergic responses. However, the H_2-receptor antagonists having been shown to potentiate the effects of H_1-receptor antagonists, came to be used in the treatment of anaphylactic reactions, upon simultaneous intravenous administration. The interested reader is referred to other reviews for information [46].

Anticholinergic (parasympatholytic, antimuscarinic) drugs

According to the classical hypothesis, neural control of the airways is determined by the balance between the cholinergic and the adrenergic nervous systems as well as by the NANC (nonadrenergic, noncholinergic) nervous system. Neuropeptides in the respiratory tract represent neurotransmitters of the NANC system [47].

cholinergic nervous system

The cholinergic (parasympathetic) nervous system in the respiratory tract is considered to be "excitatory" in nature, and it plays an important role in maintaining bronchial muscle tone and in mediating acute bronchoconstriction. The cholinergic nervous system acts through vagal afferent fibers in and around the airway lumen, which travel to the central nervous system and then terminate in the efferent fibers innervating the airway smooth muscles. Vagal stimulation induces diffuse constriction of the airways over their whole length. This effect may be antagonized by atropine and potentiated by acetylcholine-esterase inhibitors, indicating that the effect is mediated by acetylcholine acting on muscarinic

muscarinic receptors

receptors. The muscarinic receptors are present at a high density in the airways. However, their concentration is highest in the large airways. In the human lung, three muscarinic receptor subtypes have been identified (M_1, M_2, M_3), However, five different muscarinic receptor subtypes are thought to exist. The muscarinic receptors of human airway smooth muscles are mainly of the M_3-subtype, whereas the human alveolar wall contains only the M_1-subtype [47].

The adrenergic (sympathetic) nervous system in the respiratory tract is considered to be an "inhibitory" system, since stimulation of the β-receptors results in relaxation of the bronchial smooth muscles and dilatation of the airways. The terminal segments of the adrenergic system in human airways are formed by the α- and β-adrenergic receptors that are involved in regulation of smooth muscle tone [47]. **adrenergic nervous system**

The β-receptors can be divided into $β_1$- and $β_2$-receptors, the ratio of which in the human lung is 1:3. $β_2$-Receptor stimulation results in relaxation of bronchial smooth muscles, inhibition of antigen-induced mast cell mediator release, release of surfactants, fluid and protein exchange, ion transport and decrease in cholinergic neurotransmission [47]. α-Adrenergic receptors also exist in two subtypes, $α_1$- and $α_2$-receptors. Their exact role in the airways is, however, not yet fully understood. **β-receptors**

α-receptors

The NANC system consists of the nonadrenergic inhibitory system pathways and noncholinergic excitatory system pathways. The nonadrenergic inhibitory system appears to be the predominant neural bronchodilatory system in the human lung. Potential neurotransmitters of this system in humans include vasoactive intestinal peptide, peptide histidine methionine, and probably also nitric oxide. The noncholinergic excitatory system in human lung induces a bronchoconstriction, which is not inhibited by atropine but is blocked by antagonists of substance P. Potential neurotransmitters of this system include substance P, neurokinin A, neurokinin B and calcitonin gene-related peptide. The possible participation of the noncholinergic excitatory system in the mechanism of asthma has been proposed by Barnes, formulating the so-called axon-reflex hypothesis [47] (see also Chapter C4).

Innervation of the nasal mucosa includes the classical nervous systems, the sensory nervous system and the autonomic nervous system, consisting of the sympathetic (adrenergic) system containing noradrenaline as neurotransmitter and of the parasympathetic (cholinergic) system with acetylcholine as neurotransmitter. The nasal mucosa also contains other neurogenic processes, such as "the third nervous system", which is comparable to NANC in the lower respiratory airways, various neuropeptides playing a role as neurotransmitters, e.g. substance P, neurokinin A, neuropeptide Y, vasoactive intestinal peptide, calcitonin gene-related peptide and bombesin/gastrin-releasing peptide. **nasal mucosa**

The basic types of neuroreceptor, cholinergic (muscarinic) as well as adrenergic, have also been demonstrated in the human nasal mucosa.

subtypes M₁, M₃

Muscarinic receptors of subtypes M_1 and M_3 have been detected in the submucosal glands and M_1-receptors in the wall of the blood vessels in the human nasal mucosa, but only to a slight degree.

Adrenergic receptors of the α-class (α_1 and α_2) as well as of the β-class (β_1 and β_2) have also been demonstrated in the human nasal mucosa. In general, in the nasal mucosa, α-receptor stimulation is mostly excitatory, whereas β-receptor stimulation is usually inhibitory [47].

Anticholinergic agents

tertiary ammonium compounds

guaternary ammonium compounds

varia

These agents can be divided into three groups: (1) tertiary ammonium compounds, such as classical atropine and its congeners, e.g. scopolamine, hyoscine, hyosciamine sulphate (Egacene), oxyphencyclimine hydrochloride (Daricon), and others; (2) the guaternary ammonium compounds, such as ipratropium bromide (N-isopropyl-nortropine-tropic acid ester methyl bromide) (Atrovent), oxitropium bromide (Oxivent), oxyphenonium bromide (Antrenyl), butylscopolamine hydrobromide (Buscopan), propantheline bromide (Pro-Banthine) and glycopyrrolate (Robinul), and (3) varia, such as thiazinamium hydrochloride (= derivative of phenothiazine) (Multergan) [47].

Pharmacological effects of anticholinergic drugs

effects of atrophine

Atropine, together with other anticholinergic drugs, causes relaxation of smooth muscles in the airways, gastrointestinal tract, biliary tract, peripheral vasculature, urinary bladder, ureter and iris. In contrast, atropine inhibits the relaxation of the urinary sphincter. Atropine at low doses causes a slight bradycardia, whereas it causes a tachycardia at higher doses.

Atropine reduces the rate of apocrine and salivary secretions, inhibits mucociliary clearance in the airways, and because it crosses the blood-brain barrier, it can cause a mild central stimulation, excitement and restlessness. However, ipratropium bromide and other members of this group, such as oxyphenonium and oxitropium, being only very poorly absorbed and crossing the blood-brain barrier to a negligible degree, do not cause central nervous system stimulation. Atropine and the other anticholinergic drugs block the responses of ciliary muscles and the ocular sphincter muscle, resulting in cycloplegia, mydriasis and an increase in intraocular pressure. These drugs are able to inhibit salivary secretion, whereas gastric secretion is decreased only after larger doses. Atropine inhibits the function of the salivary and sweat glands, dries out the mucosal membranes and the skin, and may increase body temperature. These drugs inhibit nasal secretions, itching and sneezing, but not nasal obstruction [47].

The study thus shows that anticholinergic drugs are effective in allergic disorders in which cholinergic mechanism(s) may participate in the development of symptoms. They are usually used as supplementary drugs in the treatment of bronchial asthma and allergic rhinitis, where the non-specific hyperreactivity component participates in the patient's complaints. Sometimes these drugs are useful in cases of cholinergic, cold-induced and/or idiopathic urticaria and/or skin itching.

Immunotherapy

Immunotherapy with inhalant allergens is one of the oldest therapies for allergic diseases. However, immunotherapy remains controversial. From its early use as a general therapy applied to many patients suffering from a variety of allergic disorders, immunotherapy has evolved into a very specific therapy administered to a limited number of highly selected patients with a limited spectrum of allergen sensitivities in whom allergen avoidance is not possible and/or the patient exhibits poor response to drug treatment [48–53].

Despite various theories and hypotheses concerning the mode of action and rationale for immunotherapy, the exact mechanism(s) is poorly understood and largely unknown. The limited role of immunotherapy in the clinical practice has various explanations, including

1) IgE antibodies are no longer considered to play an exclusive role in allergic disorders – other classes of immoglobulins, e.g. IgG, IgA, IgM, are also now known to be involved; **explanations for limited role of immunotherapy**

2) the existence and role of the so-called blocking antibodies, the IgG subclasses, has not yet been unequivocally confirmed;

3) various side effects of immunotherapy from local reactions to fatal events have already been reported;

4) the effectiveness of immunotherapy cannot be guaranteed and varies greatly. In any event, it would not be expected to be higher than 50%;

5) requirements for the quality of the allergenic extracts, skill of the attending staff, general and specific emergency facilities have become more stringent;

6) the duration of immunotherapy, usually 2–4 years, possesses a problem for some patients;

7) the availability of a number of highly effective antiallergic drugs with few or no side effects are available, such as cromolyn, nedocromil, glucocorticosteroids, β_2 sympathomimetics and H_1-receptor antagonists of the second and the third generations;

8) immunotherapy must be administered under supervision by allergologists or specially trained physicians in specialized departments with possible emergency treatment and reanimation facilities regarding point 3) [48–53].

Immunotherapy appears to be a reliable treatment for patients with upper airway and/or ocular allergies, such as allergic rhinitis and allergic conjunctivitis, but it is less suitable for allergic bronchial asthma, urticaria or atopic eczema (dermatitis) [48–53].

basic requirements

The basic requirements for immunotherapy can be summarized as follows: (1) the allergic disorder must be due to an immediate, IgE-mediated hypersensitivity; (2) the complete avoidance of allergen(s) is almost impossible; (3) the patient should not suffer from anaphylactic reactions, other serious, e.g. metabolic disorders, or use contraindicated drugs or treatments, and should not be pregnant [48–53].

Immunotherapy should also be used in combination with pharmacotherapy, and the patient should carry an emergency set comprising a potent H_1- and probably also H_2-receptor antagonist and ready-to-use adrenaline (e.g. Epipen autoinjector).

Venom (wasp, bee) immunotherapy represents a very special field. This therapy should meet even stronger criteria than those for immunotherapy with inhalant allergens [48–53].

The other modifications of immunotherapy described in the literature, such as immunotherapy with food extracts, molds, bacteria, skin-end-point titration (Rinkel's method), skin neutralization, as well as sublingual and oral administration of the allergenic extracts, for which the scientific value and/or efficiency have not yet been confirmed, should be considered unproven and dangerous methods, and are therefore not recommended for use in the practice [48–53].

Antiasthma drugs

Peter J. Barnes

Introduction

Currently available therapy for asthma is highly effective in the majority of patients. Asthma therapy is traditionally divided into bronchodilator therapy, which gives immediate relief of symptoms mainly by relaxation of airway smooth muscle, and antiinflammatory therapy, which suppresses chronic inflammation in asthmatic airways and results in long-term control of asthma. Some drugs may have both actions and may be difficult to classify. Bronchodilators include β_2-agonists, theophylline and anticholinergics, whereas antiinflammatory drugs are best exemplified by corticosteroids. Cromones are used as asthma controllers, although their antiinflammatory effect is minimal.

β_2-Agonists

Inhaled β_2-agonists are the bronchodilator treatment of choice, as they are the most effective bronchodilators and have minimal side effects when used correctly [1].

Mode of action

β-Agonists produce bronchodilatation by directly stimulating β_2-receptors in airway smooth muscle, which leads to relaxation [2] (Table 1). This can be demonstrated *in vitro* by the relaxant effect of isoprenaline on human bronchi and lung strips (indicating an effect on peripheral airways) and *in vivo* by a rapid decrease in airway resistance. β-Receptors have been demonstrated in airway smooth muscle by direct receptor-binding techniques, and autoradiographic studies indicate that β-receptors are localised to smooth muscle of all airways from trachea to terminal bron-

bronchodilatation

β-receptors

Table 1 Effects of β-agonists on airways

- Relaxation of airway smooth muscle (proximal + distal airways)
- Inhibition of mast cell mediator release
- Inhibition of plasma exudation and airway edema
- Increased mucociliary clearance
- Increased mucus secretion
- No effect on chronic inflammation

chioles [2]. The molecular mechanisms by which β-agonists induce relaxation of airway smooth muscle have been extensively investigated.

adenylyl cyclase   Activation of adenylyl cyclase increases intracellular cyclic adenosine 3,5 monophosphate (cAMP), leading to activation of a protein kinase A which phosphorylates several target proteins within the cell, leading to relaxation (Fig. 1). These processes include lowering of intracellular calcium ion (Ca^{2+}) concentration by active removal of Ca^{2+} from the cell and into intracellular stores; an inhibitory effect on phosphoinositide hy-

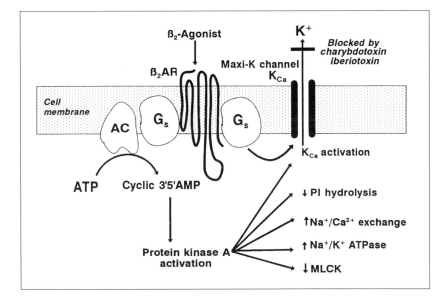

Figure 1 Molecular mechanism of action of β₂-agonists on airway smooth muscle cells

Activation of β₂-receptros (β₂AR) results in activation of adenylyl cyclase (AC) and increase in cyclic AMP. β₂-receptors may also be directly coupled to large conductance Ca^{2+} activated K^+ channels (K_{Ca}).

drolysis; direct inhibition of myosin light-chain kinase; and opening of a large conductance calcium-activated potassium channel (K_{Ca}) which repolarises the smooth muscle cell and may stimulate the sequestration of Ca^{2+} into intracellular stores [3]. Recently it has become apparent that β-agonists may be directly coupled to K_{Ca} and that relaxation of airway smooth muscle may occur independently of an increase in cAMP. β-Agonists act as functional antagonists and reverse bronchoconstriction irrespective of the contractile agent. This is an important property, since many bronchoconstrictor mechanisms (neural and mediators) are likely to be contributory in asthma.

β-Agonists may have additional effects on airways, and β-receptors are localised to several different airway cells. β-Agonists have potent effects in preventing mediator release from isolated human lung mast cells (via $β_2$-receptors). β-Agonists may also reduce and prevent microvascular leakage and thus the development of bronchial mucosal edema after exposure to mediators such as histamine. β-Agonists increase mucus secretion from submucosal glands and ion transport across airway epithelium; these effects may enhance mucociliary clearance, and therefore reverse the defect in clearance found in asthma. β-Agonists appear to selectively stimulate mucous rather than serous cells, which may result in a more viscous mucus secretion. β-Agonists reduce neurotransmission in human airway cholinergic nerves by an action at pre-junctional $β_2$-receptors to inhibit acetylcholine release. This may contribute to their bronchodilator effect by reducing cholinergic reflex bronchoconstriction. In animal studies $β_2$-receptors on sensory nerves inhibit the release of bronchoconstrictor and inflammatory peptides such as substance P.

additional effects of β-agonists

Although these additional effects of β-agonists may be relevant to the prophylactic use of these drugs against various challenges, their rapid bronchodilator action can probably be attributed to a direct effect on airway smooth muscle.

Antiinflammatory effects?

Whether $β_2$-agonists have antiinflammatory effects in asthma has become an important issue, particularly with their increasing use and the introduction of long-acting inhaled $β_2$-agonists. The inhibitory effects of β-agonists on mast cell mediator release and microvascular leakage are clearly antiinflammatory, suggesting that β-agonists may modify acute inflammation. However β-agonists do not appear to have a significant inhibitory effect on the chronic inflammation of asthmatic airways, which is controlled by corticosteroids. This has now been confirmed by biopsy studies in patients with asthma who are taking regular β-agonists, which demonstrate no significant reduction in the number or activation in inflammatory cells in the airways, in contrast to resolution of the inflammation which occurs with inhaled steroids. This is likely to be related to the fact that β-agonists do not have an important inhibitory effect on macrophages, eosinophils or lymphocytes.

Current use

inhalation

Inhaled β$_2$-agonists are the most widely used and effective bronchodilators in the treatment of asthma. When inhaled from metered-dose aerosols, they are convenient, easy to use, rapid in onset and without significant side effects. In addition to an acute bronchodilator effect, they are effective in protecting against various challenges, such as exercise, cold air and allergen. They are the bronchodilators of choice in treating acute severe asthma, when the nebulised route of administration is as effective as intravenous use. The inhaled route of administration is preferable to the oral route because side effects are less, and also because it may be more effective. β-Agonists should not be used on a regular basis in the treatment of mild asthma, but should be used "as required" by symptoms, since increased usage then is an indicator for the need for more antiinflammatory therapy. Oral β-agonists are indicated as an additional bronchodilator. Slow-release preparations (such as slow-release salbutamol and bambuterol) may be indicated in nocturnal asthma, but are less useful than inhaled β-agonists because of an increased risk of side effects.

oral application

Side effects

Unwanted effects are dose-related and are due to stimulation of extrapulmonary β-receptors (Table 2). Side effects are not common with inhaled therapy, but more common with oral or intravenous administration. Muscle tremor is due to stimulation of β$_2$-receptors in skeletal muscle, and is the commonest side effect. It may be more troublesome with elderly patients. Tachycardia and palpitations are due to reflex cardiac stimulation secondary to peripheral vasodilatation, from direct stimulation of atrial β$_2$-receptors (human heart is unusual in having a relatively high proportion of β$_2$-receptors), and possibly also from stimulation of myocardial β$_1$-receptors as the doses of β$_2$-agonist are increased. These side effects tend to disappear with continued use of the drug, reflecting

muscle tremor

tachycardia, palpitation

Table 2 Side effects of β-agonists

- Muscle tremor (direct effect on skeletal muscle β_2-receptors)
- Tachycardia (direct effect on atrial β_2-receptors, reflex effect from increased peripheral vasodilatation via β_2-receptors)
- Hypokalaemia (direct effect on skeletal muscle uptake of K^+ via β_2-receptors)
- Restlessness
- Hypoxaemia (increased V/Q mismatch due to pulmonary vasodilatation)
- Worsening of asthma control? (controversial)

the development of tolerance. Metabolic effects (increase in free fatty acid, insulin, glucose, pyruvate and lactate) are usually seen only after large systemic doses. Hypokalaemia is a potentially more serious side effect. This is due to β_2-receptor stimulation of potassium entry into skeletal muscle, which may be secondary to a rise in insulin secretion. Hypokalaemia might be serious in the presence of hypoxia, as in acute asthma, when there may be a predisposition to cardiac dysrrhythmias. In practice, significant arrhythmias after nebulised β_2-agonist have not been reported in acute asthma, however. β-Agonists may increase ventilation-perfusion (V/Q) mismatching by causing pulmonary vasodilatation in blood vessels previously constricted by hypoxia, resulting in the shunting of blood to poorly ventilated areas and a fall in arterial oxygen tension. Although in practice the effect of β-agonists on PA_{O2} is usually very small (<5 mmHg fall), occasionally in severe chronic airways obstruction it is large; it may be prevented by giving additional inspired oxygen.

metabolic effects

Tolerance

Continuous treatment with an agonist often leads to tolerance (subsensitivity, desensitisation), which may be due to downregulation of the receptor. For this reason there have been many studies of bronchial β-receptor function after prolonged therapy with β-agonists [4]. Tolerance of non-airway β-receptor responses, such as tremor and cardiovascular and metabolic responses, is readily induced in normal and asthmatic subjects. Tolerance of human airway smooth muscle to β-agonists *in vitro* has been demonstrated, although the concentration of agonist necessary is high and the degree of desensitisation is variable. Animal studies suggest that airway smooth muscle β-receptors may be more resistant to desensitisation that β-receptors elsewhere due to a high receptor reserve. In normal subjects bronchodilator tolerance has been demonstrated in some studies after high-dose inhaled salbutamol, but not in others. In asthmatic patients tolerance to the bronchodilator effects of β-agonists has not usually been found. However, tolerance develops to the bronchoprotective effects of β_2-agonists, and this is more marked with indirect constrictors such as adenosine, allergen and exercise (that activate mast cells) than with direct constrictors such as histamine and methacholine. The reason for the relative resistance of airway smooth muscle β-receptors to desensitisation remains uncertain, but perhaps reflects the fact that, in asthmatic airways, β-receptors may always be downregulated as a result of the chronic inflammatory process. The high level of β_2-receptor gene expression in airway smooth muscle compared with peripheral lung may also contribute to the resistance to tolerance, since there is likely to be a high rate of β-receptor synthesis. Tolerance to the bronchodilator effects of the long-acting β_2-agonist formoterol has been reported.

Experimental studies have shown that corticosteroids prevent the development of tolerance in airway smooth muscle, and prevent and reverse the fall in pulmonary β-receptor density. However, recent studies suggest that inhaled steroids do not prevent the development of tolerance to the bronchoprotective effect of inhaled β_2-agonists.

Concerns about β-agonists

asthma deaths

fenoterol

Because of a possible relationship between adrenergic drug therapy and the rise in asthma deaths in several countries during the early 1960s, doubts have been cast on the safety of β-agonists. A causal relationship between β-agonist use and mortality has never been established, although in retrospective studies this would not be possible. A particular β_2-agonist, fenoterol, has been linked to the recent rise in asthma deaths in New Zealand since significantly more of the fatal cases were prescribed fenoterol than were case-matched control patients. This association was strengthened by two subsequent studies, and since fenoterol has not been available the asthma mortality has fallen dramatically. An epidemiological study based in Saskatchewan, Canada, examined the links between drugs prescribed for asthma and death or near death from asthma attacks, based on computerised records of prescriptions. There was a marked increase in the risk of death with high doses of all inhaled β-agonists. The risk was greater with fenoterol, but when the dose was adjusted to the equivalent dose for salbutamol, there was no significant difference in the risk for these two drugs. The link between high β-agonist usage and increased asthma mortality does not prove a causal association, since patients with more severe and poorly controlled asthma, and who are therefore more likely to have an increased risk of fatal attacks, are more likely to be using higher doses of β-agonist inhalers and less likely to be using effective antiinflammatory treatment. Indeed in the patients who used regular inhaled steroids, there was a significant reduction in risk of death.

Regular use of inhaled β-agonists may increase asthma morbidity. In a study carried out in New Zealand, the regular use of fenoterol was associated with poorer control and a small increase in airway hyperresponsiveness compared with patients using fenoterol "on demand" for symptom control over a 6-month period. However, this was not found in a studies with salbutamol. There is some evidence that regular inhaled salbutamol may increase exercise-induced asthma. One possible mechanism is that β-agonists may inhibit the antiinflammatory action of glucocorticoids.

While it is unlikely that normally recommended doses of β_2-agonists worsen asthma, it is possible that this could occur with larger doses. Furthermore, some patients may be particularly susceptible if they have polymorphic forms of the β_2-receptor (Arg16 → Gly) that more rapidly downregulate [5]. Short-acting inhaled β_2-agonists should only be used "on demand" for symptom control, and if they are required frequently (more than three times weekly), then an inhaled antiinflammatory drug is needed. There is an association between increased risk of death from asthma and the use of high doses of inhaled β-agonists; while this may reflect severity, it is also possible that high-dose β-agonists have a deleterious effect on asthma. High concentrations of β-agonists interfere with the antiinflammatory action of steroids. Patients on high doses of β-agonists (>1 canister per month) should receive effective antiinflammatory treatments and attempts should be made to reduce the daily dose of inhaled β-agonist.

Long-acting inhaled β_2-agonists

The long-acting inhaled β_2-agonists salmeterol and formoterol have been a major advance in asthma therapy. Both drugs have a bronchodilator action of >12 h and also protect against bronchoconstriction for a similar period [6]. They are particularly useful in treating nocturnal asthma. Both improve asthma control (when given twice daily) compared with regular treatment with short-acting β_2-agonists four times daily. Both

salmeterol, formoterol

nocturnal asthma

drugs are well tolerated. Tolerance to the bronchodilator effect of formoterol and the bronchoprotective effects of formoterol and salmeterol have been demonstrated, but this is not a loss of protection, does not appear to be progressive and is of doubtful clinical significance. While both drugs have a similar duration of effect in clinical studies, there are some differences. Formoterol has a more rapid onset of action and is a fuller agonist than salmeterol. This might confer a theoretical advantage in more severe asthma, whereas it may also make it more likely to induce tolerance. Studies comparing the clinical efficacy of both drugs in mild and severe asthmatic patients are now needed.

Recent studies suggest that inhaled long-acting β_2-agonists might be introduced earlier in therapy. In asthmatic patients not controlled on either 400 or 800 µg inhaled steroids, addition of salmeterol gives better control of asthma than increasing the dose of inhaled steroid. This has also been found with formoterol, which also reduces the frequency of asthma attacks. This suggests than long-acting inhaled β_2-agonists may be added to low-dose inhaled steroids if asthma is not controlled, as an alternative (and perhaps in preference) to increasing the dose of inhaled steroids.

At present it is recommended that long-acting inhaled β_2-agonists should only be used In patients who are also prescribed inhaled steroids. In the future, long-acting inhaled β_2-agonists may be used in fixed combination inhalers (formoterol + budesonide, salmeterol + fluticasone) in order to improve compliance and reduce the risk of patients using these drugs as sole long-term treatment.

Theophylline

methylxanthine Methylxanthines such as theophylline, which are related to caffeine, have been used in the treatment of asthma since 1930. Indeed, theophylline is still the most widely used antiasthma therapy worldwide because it is inexpensive. Theophylline became more useful with the availability of rapid plasma assays and the introduction of reliable slow-release preparations [7]. However, the frequency of side effects and the relative low efficacy of theophylline have recently led to reduced usage, since β-agonists are far more effective as bronchodilators, and inhaled steroids have a greater antiinflammatory effect. In patients with severe asthma it still remains a very useful drug, however. There is increasing evidence that theophylline has an antiinflammatory or immunomodulatory effect [8].

Table 3 Mode of action of theophylline?

- Phosphodiesterase inhibition
- Adenosine receptor antagonism
- Increased adrenaline secretion
- Prostaglandin inhibition
- Inhibition of calcium entry/release
- Inhibition of phosphoinositide hydrolysis

Mode of action

The mechanism of action of theophylline is still uncertain (Table 3). It is likely that the bronchodilator effect of theophylline is due to inhibition of phosphodiesterases (PDEs), which break down cAMP in the cell, thereby leading to an increase in intracellular cAMP concentrations (Fig. 2). Theophylline is a nonselective PDE inhibitor, but the degree of inhibition is fairly small at concentrations of theophylline which are within the "therapeutic range". Furthermore, inhibition of PDE should lead to synergistic interaction with β-agonists, but this has not been convincingly demonstrated *in vivo*. Several isoenzyme families of PDEs have

inhibition of phosphodiesterases

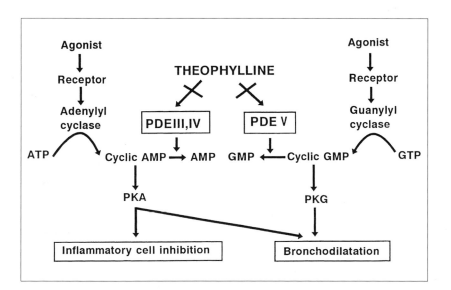

Figure 2 Theophylline inhibits PDEs resulting in an increase in cAMP and cGMP

now been recognised, and some are more important in smooth muscle relaxation. Theophylline is also an adenosine receptor antagonist at therapeutic concentrations, suggesting that this could be the basis for its

bronchodilator effects

enprofylline

bronchodilator effects. Inhaled adenosine causes bronchoconstriction in asthmatic subjects when given by inhalation, by releasing histamine from airway mast cells, which is prevented by therapeutic concentrations of theophylline. However, a related xanthine derivative enprofylline, which is more potent than theophylline as a bronchodilator, has no significant inhibitory effect on adenosine receptors at therapeutic concentrations, suggesting that adenosine antagonism is an unlikely explanation for the bronchodilator effect of theophylline. However, adenosine antagonism may account for some of the side effects of theophylline, such as central nervous system stimulation, cardiac arrhythmias and diuresis.

It is possible that any beneficial effect in asthma is related to its action on other cells (such as platelets, T-lymphocytes or macrophages) or on airway microvascular leak and edema in addition to airway smooth muscle relaxation. It is possible that theophylline acts as an immunomodulator and has effects on T-lymphocyte function *in vitro*. A placebo-controlled theophylline withdrawal study indicates that theophylline appears to have an immunomodulatory effect and decreases the number of activated T-cells in the airways probably by blocking their trafficking from the circulation. Theophylline inhibits the late response to allergen challenge more effectively than the early response and inhibits the influx of eosinophils into the airways.

Clinical use

aminophylline

In patients with acute asthma, intravenous aminophylline is less effective than nebulised β-agonists, and should therefore be reserved for those patients who fail to respond to β-agonists. Theophylline should not be added routinely to nebulised β-agonists since it does not increase the bronchodilator response and may only increase their side effects.

theophylline

Theophylline has little or no effect on bronchomotor tone in normal airways, but reverses bronchoconstriction in asthmatic patients, although it is less effective than inhaled β-agonists and is more likely to have unwanted effects. Indeed, any role of theophylline in the management of asthma has been questioned. There is good evidence that theophylline and β-agonists have additive effects, even if true synergy is not seen, and there is evidence that theophylline may provide an additional bronchodilator effect even when maximally effective doses of β-agonist have been given. This means that, if adequate bronchodilatation is not achieved by a β-agonist alone, theophylline may be added to the maintenance therapy with benefit. Theophylline may be useful in some patients with nocturnal asthma, since slow-release preparations are able to provide therapeutic concentrations overnight and are more effective than slow-release β-agonists. Although theophylline is less effective than a β-agonist and corticosteroids, there are a minority of asthmatic patients who appear to derive unexpected benefit, and even patients on oral steroids may show a deterioration in lung function when theophylline is withdrawn.

Theophylline is readily and reliably absorbed from the gastrointestinal tract, but there are many factors that affect plasma clearance, and therefore plasma concentration, which make the drug relatively difficult to use (Table 4).

Side effects

Unwanted effects of theophylline are usually related to plasma concentration and tend to occur when plasma levels exceed 20 mg/l. However, some patients develop side effects even at low plasma concentrations. To some extent side effects may be reduced by gradually increasing the dose until therapeutic concentrations are achieved.

The commonest side effects are headache, nausea and vomiting, abdominal discomfort and restlessness (Table 5). There may also be increased acid secretion and diuresis. At high concentrations convulsions

commonest side effects

Table 4 Factors affecting theophylline clearance

- Increased clearance

  Enzyme induction (rifampicin, phenobarbitone, ethanol)
  Smoking (tobacco, marijuana)
  High-protein, low-carbohydrate diet
  Barbecued meat
  Childhood

- Decreased clearance

  Enzyme inhibition (cimetidine, erythromycin, ciprofloxacin, allopurinol)
  Congestive heart failure
  Liver disease
  Pneumonia
  Viral infection and vaccination
  High-carbohydrate diet
  Old age

and cardiac arrhythmias may occur. Some of the side effects (central stimulation, gastric secretion, diuresis and arrhythmias) may be due to adenosine receptor antagonism and may therefore be avoided by drugs such as enprofylline, which has no significant adenosine antagonism at bronchodilator doses.

Table 5 Side effects of theophylline

- Nausea and vomiting
- Gastrointestinal disturbance
- Headache
- Restlessness
- Gastroesophageal reflux
- Diuresis
- Cardiac arrythmias
- Epileptic seizures
- Behavioural disturbance in children (controversial)

Future use

Theophylline use is declining, partly because of the problems with side effects, but mainly because more effective therapy with inhaled steroids has been introduced. Oral theophylline is still a very useful treatment in some patients with difficult asthma and appears to have effects beyond those provided by steroids. Rapid release theophylline preparations are cheap and are the only affordable antiasthma medication in some developing countries. There is increasing evidence that theophylline has some antiasthma effect at doses that are lower than those needed for bronchodilatation and plasma levels of 5–10 mg/l are recommended, instead of the previously recommended 10–20 mg/l. A recent study has demonstrated that addition of low-dose theophylline gives better control of asthma than doubling the dose of inhaled steroids in patients not controlled on a dose of 800 µg daily, so it may be a less-expensive alternative to the addition of a long-acting β_2-agonist.

Anticholinergics

Atropine, a related naturally occurring compound, was also introduced for treating asthma but because this compound caused side effects, particularly drying of secretions, less-soluble quaternary compounds, such as atropine methylnitrate and ipratropium bromide, were introduced. These compounds are topically active and are not significantly absorbed from the respiratory tract or from the gastrointestinal tract.

atropine methyl-nitrate, ipratro-pium bromide

Mode of action

Anticholinergics are specific antagonists of muscarinic receptors and, in therapeutic use, have no other significant pharmacological effects. The bronchodilator effect of anticholinergics is likely to be through blockade of M_3-receptors on airway smooth muscle, but additional blocking effects on M_1 receptors in parasympathetic ganglia may also contribute. In animals and humans there is a small degree of resting bronchomotor tone which is probably due to tonic vagal nerve impulses which release acetylcholine in the vicinity of airway smooth muscle, since it can be blocked by anticholinergic drugs. Cholinergic pathways may play an important role in regulating acute bronchomotor responses in animals, and there are a wide variety of mechanical, chemical and immunological stimuli which are capable of eliciting reflex bronchoconstriction via vagal pathways. However, while these drugs may afford protection against acute challenge by sulphur dioxide, inert dusts, cold air and emotional factors, they are less effective against antigen challenge, exercise and fog. This is not surprising, as anticholinergic drugs will only inhibit reflex cholinergic bronchoconstriction and could have no significant blocking effect on the direct effects of inflammatory mediators such as histamine and leukotrienes on bronchial smooth muscle. Furthermore, cholinergic antagonists probably have little or no effect on mast cells, microvascular leak or the chronic inflammatory response.

M_3-receptor blockade

cholinergic pathways

Clinical use

In asthmatic subjects anticholinergic drugs are less effective as bronchodilators than β-agonists and offer less efficient protection against various bronchial challenges. They may be more effective in older patients with asthma in whom there is an element of fixed airway obstruction.

acute severe asthma

Nebulised anticholinergic drugs are effective in acute severe asthma, although they are less effective than β-agonists in this situation. Nevertheless, in the acute and chronic treatment of asthma, anticholinergic drugs may have an additive effect with β-agonists and should therefore be considered when control of asthma is not adequate with β-agonists, particularly if there are problems with theophylline, or inhaled β-agonists give troublesome tremor in elderly patients. The time course of bronchodilatation with anticholinergic drugs is slower than with β-agonists, reaching a peak only 1 h after inhalation, but persists for over 6 h.

COPD

In chronic obstructive pulmonary disease (COPD) anticholinergic drugs may be as effective as, or even superior to β-agonists. Their relatively greater effect in chronic obstructive airways disease than in asthma may be explained by an inhibitory effect on vagal tone which, while not necessarily being increased in COPD, may be the only reversible element of airway obstruction, which is exaggerated by geometric factors in a narrowed airway. Anticholinergics may inhibit mucus hypersecretion in chronic bronchitis.

Side effects

glaucoma

bronchoconstriction

Inhaled anticholinergic drugs are usually well tolerated, and there is no evidence for any decline in responsiveness with continued use. Systemic side effects after ipratropium bromide are very uncommon because there is virtually no systemic absorption. Because cholinergic agonists stimulate mucus secretion there have been several studies of mucus secretion with anticholinergic drugs as there has been concern that they may reduce secretion and lead to more viscous mucus. However, this has not been observed even with high doses of ipratropium bromide. Nebulised ipratropium bromide may precipitate glaucoma in elderly patients due to a direct effect of the nebulised drug on the eye. This may be prevented by nebulisation with a mouthpiece rather than a face mask. There are several reports of paradoxical bronchoconstriction with ipratropium bromide, particularly when given by nebuliser. This is largely explained by the hypotonicity of the nebuliser solution and by antibacterial additives, such as benzalkonium chloride and EDTA. Nebuliser solutions free of these problems are less likely to cause bronchoconstriction. Occasionally, bronchoconstriction may occur with ipratropium bromide given by metered dose inhaler (MDI). It is possible that this is due to blockade of prejunctional M_2-receptors on airway cholinergic nerves which normally inhibit acetylcholine release.

Corticosteroids

Corticosteroids were introduced for the treatment of asthma shortly after their discovery in the 1950s and remain the most effective therapy available for asthma. However, side effects and fear of adverse effects have limited their use, and there has therefore been considerable research into discovering new or related agents which retain the beneficial action on airways without unwanted effects. The introduction of inhaled steroids has revolutionised the treatment of chronic asthma [9]. Now that asthma is viewed as a chronic inflammatory disease, inhaled steroids may even be considered as first-line therapy in patients with chronic asthma.

Mode of action

Corticosteroids enter target cells and bind to cytosolic glucocorticoid receptors (GRs). There is only one type of GR and no evidence for different subtypes which might mediate different aspects of steroid action [10]. The steroid-receptor complex is transported to the nucleus, where it binds to specific sequences on the upstream regulatory element of certain target genes, resulting in increased or decreased transcription of the gene, which leads to increased or decreased protein synthesis. GRs may also interact directly with protein transcription factors in the cytoplasm and thereby influence the synthesis of certain proteins independently of an interaction with DNA in the cell nucleus [10]. The direct repression of transcription factors, such as AP-1 and NF-κB, is likely to account for many of the antiinflammatory effects of steroids in asthma.

glucocorticoid receptors

The mechanisms of action of corticosteroids in asthma are still poorly understood, but are most likely to be related to their antiinflammatory properties. There is compelling evidence that asthma and airway, hyperresponsiveness are due to an inflammatory process in the airways and there are several components of this inflammatory response which might be inhibited by steroids (Fig. 3). Several studies of bronchial biopsies in asthma have demonstrated a reduction in the number and activation of inflammatory cells in the epithelium and submucosa after regular inhaled steroids, together with a healing of the damaged epithelium. Indeed, in mild asthmatics the inflammation may be completely resolved after inhaled steroids. Steroids potently inhibit the formation of cytokines, such as interleukin (IL)-1, IL-2, IL-3, IL-4, IL-5, IL-13, granulocyte macro-

steroids

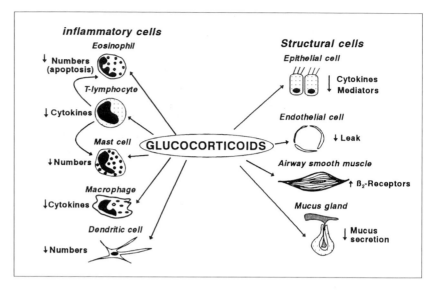

Figure 3 Glucocorticoids have inhibitory effects on many inflammatory and structural cells that are activated in asthma

phage colony-stimulating factor (GM-CSF) by lymphocytes and macrophages. Indeed this may be the most important action of steroids in suppressing asthmatic inflammation, since cytokines may play a very critical role in the maintenance of the chronic eosinophilic inflammation. Steroids prevent and reverse the increase in vascular permeability due to inflammatory mediators in animal studies and may therefore lead to resolution of airway edema. Steroids also have a direct inhibitory effect on mucus glycoprotein secretion from airway submucosal glands, as well as indirect inhibitory effects by downregulation of inflammatory stimuli.

Steroids have no direct effect on contractile responses of airway smooth muscle, and improvement in lung function is presumably due to an effect on the chronic airway inflammation and airway hyperresponsiveness. After a single dose, inhaled steroids have no effect on the early response to allergen (reflecting their lack of effect on mast cell mediator release), but inhibit the late response (which may be due to an effect on macrophages and eosinophils) and also inhibit the increase in airway hyperresponsiveness. Inhaled steroids also reduce airway hyperresponsiveness, but this effect may take several weeks or months and presumably reflects the slow healing of the damaged inflamed airway.

It is important to recognise that steroids suppress inflammation in the airways but do not cure the underlying disease. When steroids are withdrawn there is a recurrence of the same degree of airway hyperresponsiveness, although in patients with mild asthma it may take several months to return. Steroids increase β-adrenergic responsiveness, but whether this is relevant to their effect in asthma is uncertain. Steroids potentiate the effects of β-agonists on bronchial smooth muscle and prevent and reverse β-receptor tachyphylaxis in airways *in vitro* and *in vivo*. At a molecular level steroids increase the gene transcription of β-receptors in human lung, and systemic glucocorticoids prevent downregulation of β_2-receptors in animal lungs. Unfortunately, inhaled steroids do not appear to prevent the development of tolerance to inhaled β_2-agonists in human airways.

airway hyperresponsiveness

Current use

Hydrocortisone is given intravenously in acute asthma. While the value of corticosteroids in acute severe asthma has been questioned, others have found that they speed the resolution of attacks. There is no apparent advantage in giving very high doses of intravenous steroids (such as methylprednisolone 1 g). Intravenous steroids are indicated in acute asthma if lung function is <30% predicted normal and in whom there is no significant improvement with nebulised β-agonists. Intravenous therapy is usually given until a satisfactory response is obtained and then oral prednisolone may be substituted. Oral prednisolone (40–60 mg) has an effect similar to intravenous hydrocortisone and is easier to administer. Inhaled steroids have no proven effect in acute asthma, but trials with nebulised steroids are underway.

hydrocortisone

Inhaled steroids are now recommended as first-line therapy for all but the mildest of asthmatic patients [9]. Inhaled steroids should be started in any patient who needs to use a β-agonist inhaler for symptom control more than three times a week. Oral steroids are reserved for patients who cannot be controlled on other therapy, the dose being titrated to the lowest which provides acceptable control of symptoms. For any patient taking regular oral steroids objective evidence of steroid responsiveness should be obtained before maintenance therapy is instituted.

inhaled steroids

Short courses of oral steroids (such as 30 mg prednisolone daily for 1–2 weeks) are indicated for exacerbations of asthma, and the dose may be tailed off over 1 week once the exacerbation is resolved (although the taIL-off period is not strictly necessary, patients find it reassuring). Nebulised steroids (budesonide 8 mg twice daily) may have a steroid-sparing effect in more severe asthmatic patients who are on maintenance oral steroids.

oral steroids

dosage of steroids

For most patients, inhaled steroids should be used twice daily, which improves compliance, once control of asthma has been achieved (which may require four-times daily dosing initially). If a dose of more than 800 µg daily is used, a spacer device should be used as this reduces the risk of orpharyngeal side effects. Inhaled steroids may be used in children in the same way as adults, and at doses of 400 µg daily or less there is no evidence of growth suppression.

pharmacokinetics

The pharmacokinetics of inhaled steroids is important in relation to systemic effects [11]. The fraction of steroid which is inhaled into the lungs acts locally on the airway mucosa and may be absorbed from the airway and alveolar surface and therefore reach the systemic circulation. The fraction of inhaled steroid which is deposited in the oropharynx is swallowed and absorbed from the gut. The absorbed fraction may be metabolised in the liver before reaching the systemic circulation. Budesonide and fluticasone have a greater first-pass metabolism than BDP and is therefore less likely to produce systemic effects at high inhaled doses. The use of a large-volume spacer chamber reduces oropharyngeal deposition and therefore reduces systemic absorption of steroids. Similarly, rinsing the mouth and discarding the rinse has a similar effect, and this procedure should be used with high-dose dry powder steroid inhalers, since spacer chambers cannot be used with these devices.

Some patients, usually with severe asthma, apparently fail to respond to corticosteroids. "Steroid-resistant" asthma is likely to be due to an increase in binding of the glucocorticoid receptor to the transcription factor AP-1, due to increased activation of AP-1.

COPD patients

COPD patients occasionally respond to steroids, and these patients are likely to be undiagnosed asthmatics. Steroids have no objective short-term benefit on airway function in patients with true chronic bronchitis, although they may often produce subjective benefit because of their euphoric effect. It is not yet certain whether the use of steroids delays the progressive fall in lung function seen in patients with COPD, and large-scale clinical trials to answer this important question are now underway.

Side effects

inhibition of ACTH and cortisol secretion

Steroids inhibit adrenocorticotrophic hormone (ACTH) and cortisol secretion by a negative feedback effect on the pituitary gland. Hypothalamo-pituitary-adrenal (HPA) axis suppression is dependent on dose, and usually only occurs when a dose of prednisolone greater than 7.5–10 mg daily is used. Significant suppression after short courses of steroid therapy is not usually a problem, but prolonged suppression may occur after several months or years. Steroid doses after prolonged oral therapy must therefore be reduced slowly. Symptoms of "steroid withdrawal syndrome" include lassitude, musculoskeletal pains and occasionally fever. HPA suppression with inhaled steroids is seen only when the daily inhaled dose exceeds 2000 µg daily.

Side effects of long-term corticosteroid therapy are well described and include fluid retention, increased appetite, weight gain, osteoporosis, capillary fragility, hypertension, peptic ulceration, diabetes, cataracts and psychosis. Their frequency tends to increase with age. Very occasionally adverse reactions (such as anaphylaxis) to intravenous hydrocortisone have been described, particularly in aspirin-sensitive asthmatics.

The incidence of systemic side effects after inhaled steroids is an important consideration. Systemic absorption occurs not only from the gastrointestinal tract, but also from the lung, so that all inhaled steroids currently available have some systemic absorption. Initial studies suggested that adrenal suppression only occurred when inhaled doses of over 1500–2000 µg daily were used. More sensitive measurements of systemic effects include indices of bone metabolism, such as serum osteocalcin and urinary pyridinium cross-links, and in children knemometry, which may be increased with inhaled doses as low as 800 µg in some patients. The clinical relevance of these measurements is not yet clear, however. Nevertheless, it is important to reduce the likelihood of systemic effects by using the lowest dose of inhaled steroid needed to control the asthma, by the use of a large volume spacer to reduce oropharyngeal deposition (and therefore the fraction absorbed from the gastrointestinal tract).

systemic side effects

Several systemic effects of inhaled steroids have been described (Table 6) and include dermal thinning and skin capillary fragility, which is relatively common in elderly patients after high-dose inhaled steroids. Other side effects such as cataract formation and osteoporosis are reported, but often in patients who are also receiving courses of oral steroids. There has been particular concern about the use of inhaled steroids in children because of growth suppression. Most studies have been reassuring in that doses of 400 µg or less have not been associated with impaired growth, and there may even be a growth spurt as asthma is better controlled. A meta-analysis of over 20 studies with inhaled BDP showed no effect on growth or overall height of children.

Inhaled steroids may have local side effects due to the deposition of inhaled steroid in the oropharynx. The most common problem is hoarseness and weakness of the voice (dysphonia) which is due to laryngeal deposition. It may occur in up to 40% of patients and is noticed particularly by patients who need to use their voices during their work (lecturers, teachers and singers). It may be due to atrophy of the vocal cords.

local side effects

Table 6 Side effects of inhaled steroids

Local side effects
- Hoarseness (dysphonia)
- Oropharyngeal candidiasis
- Throat irritation and cough (due to additives)

Systemic side effects
- Adrenal suppression
- Easy bruising
- Skin thinning
- Increased bone metabolism, osteoporosis
- Cataracts
- Stunted growth in children
- Behavioural disturbances?
- Glaucoma

Throat irritation and coughing after inhalation are common with MDIs and appear to be due to the additives, since these problems are not usually seen if the patients switch to the dry powder inhalers. Oropharyngeal candidiasis may occur in 5% of patients. The incidence of local side effects may be related to the local concentrations of steroid deposited and may be reduced by the use of large-volume spacers, which markedly reduce oropharyngeal deposition. Local side effects are also less likely when inhaled steroids are used twice daily rather than four times daily. There is no evidence for atrophy of the lining of the airway, or of an increase in lung infections (including tuberculosis) after inhaled steroids.

Future potential

There has been a dramatic increase in the use of inhaled steroids in asthma treatment. This is due to the recognition that asthma is an inflammatory condition and to the introduction of treatment guidelines that emphasise the early use of inhaled steroids. There is also increasing recognition that at the dose of inhaled steroids needed to control asthma in most patients there are no systemic effects. At present it is estimated that in the United Kingdom approximately half of the adult asthmatic population are prescribed inhaled steroids, and the proportion is rising. While this is commendable, there is also evidence that some patients are being overtreated in general practice. This may lead to a backlash against the use of inhaled steroids if persistent high doses of inhaled steroids lead to systemic side effects such as osteoporosis. The step-down of treatment has not been sufficiently stressed, and it is important to educate general practitioners (GPs) and patients to maintain patients on the minimum dose of inhaled steroid required to control asthma optimally. In other countries, in Europe and the United States only a small proportion of patients with asthma are being treated with inhaled steroids, but the numbers are rapidly rising. It is now recommended that patients should be started on relatively high doses of inhaled steroids in order to establish control of asthma in all patients, then to reduce the dose once control is achieved after 3 months or so [12].

Children with asthma are often treated with cromoglycate before inhaled steroids are tried, but there is an increasing tendency to use inhaled steroids as first-line antiinflammatory therapy in children, as they are more effective than cromoglycate and work in every patient. The dose of inhaled steroid equivalent in effect to cromoglycate is 100–200 µg BDP/budesonide daily, at which dose there is no risk of systemic effects. The use of inhaled steroids in the treatment of childhood asthma will increase as these low doses are shown to be safe.

treatment of children

Early treatment with inhaled steroids in both adults and children gives a greater improvement in lung function than if treatment with inhaled steroids is delayed (and other treatments such as bronchodilators are used). This may reflect the fact that steroids are able to modify the underlying inflammatory process and prevent any structural changes (fibrosis, smooth muscle hyperplasia etc.) in the airway as a result of chronic inflammation. It is not yet certain how early inhaled steroids should be introduced. There is evidence for inflammation in the airways, even when patients have episodic asthma, but at present it is recommended that inhaled steroids be introduced when there are chronic symptoms (e.g. use of an inhaled β_2-agonist on a daily basis).

early treatment in adults and children

Cromones

Cromones include sodium cromoglycate and nedocromil sodium. Cromoglycate is a derivative of khellin, an Egyptian herbal remedy which was found to protect against allergen challenge without bronchodilator effect. Nedocromil sodium is structurally related and has very similar clinical effects, although there is some evidence that it is more potent.

sodium cromoglycate and nedocromil sodium

Mode of action

Initial investigations indicated that cromoglycate inhibited the release of mediators by allergen in passively sensitised human and animal lung, and inhibited passive cutaneous anaphylaxis in rat, although it was without effect in guinea pig. This activity was attributed to stabilisation of the mast cell membrane, and thus cromoglycate was classified as a mast cell stabiliser. However, cromoglycate has a rather low potency in stabilising human lung mast cells, and other drugs which are more potent in this respect have little or no effect in clinical asthma. This has raised doubts about mast cell stabilisation as the mode of action of cromoglycate.

inhibition of bronchoconstriction

Cromoglycate and nedocromil potently inhibit bronchoconstriction induced by sulphur dioxide, metabisulphite and bradykinin, which are believed to act through activation of sensory nerves in the airways. In dogs, cromones suppress firing of unmyelinated C-fibre nerve endings, thereby reinforcing the view that they might be acting to suppress sensory nerve activation and thus neurogenic inflammation. Cromones have variable inhibitory actions on other inflammatory cells which may participate in allergic inflammation, including macrophages and eosinophils. *In vivo* cromoglycate is capable of blocking the early response to allergen (which may be mediated by mast cells) but also the late response and airway hyperresponsiveness, which are more likely to be mediated by macrophage and eosinophil interactions. There is also evidence that long-term treatment with cromones reduces airway hyperresponsiveness.

The molecular mechanism of action of cromones is not understood, but recent evidence suggests that they may block a particular type of chloride channel that may be expressed in sensory nerves, mast cells and other inflammatory cells. It remains to be explained why cromones are only effective in allergic inflammation.

Current use

prophylaxis

Cromoglycate is a prophylactic treatment and needs to be given regularly. Cromoglycate protects against various indirect bronchoconstrictor stimuli, such as exercise and fog. It is only effective in mild asthma, but does not appear to be effective in all patients and there seems no sure way of predicting which patients are likely to respond. Cromoglycate is often the antiinflammatory drug of first choice in children because it has almost no side effects. In adults, steroids by inhalation are preferred as they are effective in all patients, although adults with mild asthma (even when it is nonallergic in type) do respond to cromoglycate. Cromoglycate must be given four times daily to provide good protection, which makes it less useful than inhaled steroids which may be given twice daily. It may also be taken prior to exercise in children with exercise-induced asthma that is not blocked by an inhaled β-agonist. In clinical practice nedocromil has a very similar efficacy to cromoglycate and is therefore indicated in patients with mild asthma.

Side effects

Cromoglycate is one of the safest drugs available, and side effects are extremely rare. The dry powder inhaler may cause throat irritation, coughing and, occasionally, wheezing, but this is usually prevented by prior administration of a β-agonist inhaler. Very rarely a transient rash and urticaria are seen, and a few cases of pulmonary eosinophilia have been reported, all of which are due to hypersensitivity. Side effects with nedocromil are not usually a problem, although some patients have noticed a sensation of flushing after using the inhaler. Many patients find the bitter taste unpleasant, but a menthol-flavoured version is now available which seems to overcome this problem.

safe drugs

Other treatments

Antileukotrienes

Recently, leukotriene receptor antagonists (e.g. zafirlukast, pranlukast, montelukast) and 5'-lipoxygenase inhibitors (e.g. zileuton) have been introduced as antiasthma therapies [13]. These treatments have been shown to reduce asthma symptoms and the need for rescue inhaled β_2-agonists, and to improve lung function in patients with mild to moderate asthma. They are less effective than inhaled steroids, although some patients show a good response. Their great advantage is that they are active orally and do not appear to have any class-related side effects. It is likely that they will be a useful additional medication and may be a useful add-on treatment to low-dose inhaled steroids in patients who still have symptoms. It is likely that they will be particularly effective in patients who have aspirin-sensitive asthma.

useful additional medication

aspirin-sensitive asthma

Ketotifen

Ketotifen is described as a prophylactic antiasthma compound. Its predominant effect is H_1-receptor antagonism, and it is this antihistaminic effect which accounts for its sedative effect. Ketotifen has little effect in clinical asthma, either in acute challenge, on airway hyperresponsiveness or on clinical symptoms. A long-term placebo control trial of oral ketotifen in children with mild asthma showed no significant clinical benefit. It is claimed that ketotifen has disease-modifying effects if started early in asthma in children and may even prevent the development of asthma in atopic children. More carefully controlled studies are needed to assess the validity of these claims.

Immunosuppressive and steroid-sparing therapy

Immunosuppressive therapy has been considered in asthma when other treatments have been unsuccessful or to reduce the dose of oral steroids required [14]. They are therefore only indicated in a very small proportion of asthmatic patients at present.

asthmatic patients
methotrexate

Low-dose methotrexate (15 mg weekly) has a steroid-sparing effect in asthma and may be indicated when oral steroids are contraindicated because of unacceptable side effects (e.g. in postmenopausal women when osteoporosis is a problem). Some patients show better responses than others, but whether a patient will have a useful steroid-sparing effect is unpredictable. In some studies no useful beneficial effect is reported. Side effects of methotrexate are relatively common and include nausea (reduced if methotrexate is given as a weekly injection), blood dyscrasias and hepatic damage. Careful monitoring of such patients (monthly blood counts and liver enzymes) is essential. Methotrexate has been found to be disappointing in most people's clinical experience.

gold

Gold has long been used in the treatment of chronic arthritis. There is anecdotal evidence that it may also be useful in asthma, and it has been used in Japan for many years. A controlled trial of an oral gold preparation (Auranofin) demonstrated some steroid-sparing effect in chronic asthmatic patients maintained on oral steroid. Side effects such as skin rashes and nephropathy are a limiting factor.

cyclosporin A

Cyclosporin A is active against $CD4^+$ lymphocytes and might therefore be useful in asthma, in which these cells are implicated. A trial of low-dose oral cyclosporin A, in patients with steroid-dependent asthma, indicates that it can improve control of symptoms in patients with severe asthma on oral steroids, but other trials have been unimpressive. Its use is likely to be limited by side effects, such as nephrotoxicity and hypertension, which are common. In clinical practice it is very disappointing as a steroid-sparing agent.

Intravenous immunoglobulin has been reported to have steroid-sparing effects in steroid-dependent asthma, when high does were used (2 g/kg), although in a controlled trial in children at lower doses it was ineffective.

intravenous immunoglobulin

Immunotherapeutic properties of immunoaugmenting agents

James E. Talmadge

Introduction

The use of immunostimulants to treat human disease has its origins in the experimental use of mixed bacterial toxins to treat cancer by William B. Coley early in the century. These early studies have spawned the clinical approval and use of such microbially derived substances as BCG (bladder cancer, USA), Krestin, Picibanil and Lentinan (gastric and other cancers, Japan) and Biostim and Broncho-Vaxom (recurrent infections, Europe). While these crude drugs induce immunopharmacologic activities, they pose considerable regulatory problems due to impurity, lot-to-lot variability, unreliability and side effects. Similarly, traditional herbal medicines (Japan and the Orient) also provide a source of active substances for immunotherapy. Further, the purification, characterization and synthetic production of the active moieties from these products provides a source of drug candidates for development. However, current clinical emphasis is on the use of recombinant proteins (cytokines), although the utility of these drugs is somewhat limited due to their focused bioactivity and pharmacologic deficiencies, such as limited pharmacokinetics. Thus there remains a potentially important role for classical biological response modifiers (BRMs) due to their oral bioavailability and ability to induce multiple cytokines for optimal immunoaugmentation and hematopoietic restoration and as adjuvants for use with more traditional therapeutics including antibiotics, chemotherapy and/or radiotherapy.

immunostimulants

BCG

cytokines

BRMs

Recombinant proteins

Therapeutic proteins have emerged as a new and important class of drugs for the treatment of cancer, immunodepression, myeloid dysplasia and infectious disease. However, their development has been slowed by our limited understanding of their pharmacology and mechanism of action. To

surrogate

colony stimulating
factor

optimal immuno-
modulating dose

facilitate the development of these immunoregulatory proteins, additional information is needed on their pharmacology [1, 2]. One approach to the development of these proteins is to identify a clinical hypothesis based on a therapeutic surrogate identified during preclinical studies of a drug's immunopharmacology [3, 4]. A surrogate for clinical efficacy may be a phenotypic, biochemical, enzymatic, functional (immunologic, molecular or hematologic) or quality-of-life measurement which is believed to be associated with therapeutic activity. Phase I clinical trials can then be designed to identify the optimal immunomodulatory dose (OID) and treatment schedule for protein administration which maximizes the augmentation of the surrogate end point(s). Subsequent phase II/III trials can then be established to determine if the changes in the surrogate

Table 1 Approved biotechnology drugs

Product type	Abbreviated indication
erythropoietin	anemia associated with chronic renal failure anemia in HIV-infected patients anemia associated with cancer chemotherapy
CSF-G	febrile neutropenia associated with chemotherapy treatment of marrow transplants treatment of severe chronic neutropenia (chemotherapy) peripheral blood progenitor cell transplants
CSF-GM	neutropenia associated with transplants acceleration of myeloid recovery following autologous bone marrow transplantation reduce immunosuppression in AML peripheral blood progenitor cell transplants allogeneic bone marrow transplantation from HLA-matched related donors
IFNα 2a	treatment of hairy cell leukemia treatment of AIDS-related Kaposi's sarcoma treatment of Philadelphia chromosome-positive CML
IFNα 2b	treatment of hairy cell leukemia treatment of AIDS-related Kaposi's sarcoma treatment of patients with non-A, non-B/C hepatitis treatment of patients with chronic hepatitis B systemic recurrence of malignant melanoma
IFNγ	chronic granulomatous disease rheumatoid arthritis
IFN alfacon-1	chronic hepatitis C
IFNβ	multiple sclerosis
IL-2	Renal cell carcinoma

levels correlate with therapeutic activity. Table 1 lists the immunologically and hematologically active cytokines which are approved for general use in the United States.

In contrast to strategies based on the identification of surrogates for therapeutic efficacy, many protocols for recombinant proteins have been identified based on practices developed for conventional drugs and may not be advantageous for the development of proteins. This is because of the pharmacologic attributes of proteins which require selective or targeted delivery to the desired site (i.e. the bone marrow, spleen or tumor) [5]. To administer proteins optimally as drugs and assure their targeting is the primary challenge for their development. One additional difficulty in the development of a recombinant protein is that in many instances there is little relationship between the dose administered and the biologic effect. Indeed, in some instances there is a nonlinear dose relationship that has been described as bell-shaped [6]. This dose-response relationship, or lack thereof, may be due to the nonlinear manner in which the drug is dispersed in the body; a poor ability to enter into a saturatable receptor-mediated transport process; chemical instability; sequence of administration with other agents or an incorrect time of administration; and or due to an inappropriate location and response of the target cells. Further, a "bell-shaped" dose-response curve may be associated with the tachyphylaxis of receptor expression or a signal transduction mechanism whereby the cells become refractory to subsequent receptor-mediated augmentation. Because the regulation of immune reactivity can lead to physiologically unwanted events, it is important that the administration of recombinant proteins be optimal to ensure the desired biological activity.

dose response curve

bell-shaped curve

surrogate

Interferon-α (IFNα)

The initial, nonrandomized, clinical studies with IFNα suggested that it had therapeutic activity for malignant melanoma, osteosarcoma and various lymphomas [7]. However, subsequent randomized trials with IFNα demonstrated significant therapeutic activity only against less common tumor histiotypes including hairy cell and chronic myelogenous leukemia (CML) [7–9] and a few types of lymphoma [9], including low-grade non-Hodgkin's lymphoma [10] and cutaneous T-cell lymphoma [11]. Subsequently, the list of responding indications was expanded to include renal cell carcinoma [12, 13], acquired immunodeficiency syndrome (AIDS) and Kaposi's sarcoma [14], genital warts, hepatitis and bladder papillomatosis.

interferon

It has taken almost three decades to translate the concept of IFNα as an antiviral to its routine utility in clinical oncology and infectious diseases. Despite extensive study, the development of IFNα is still in its early stages, and such basic parameters as optimal dose and therapeutic schedule remain to be determined [8, 9]. The mechanism of activity is also controversial, since IFNα has been shown to have dose-dependent antitumor activities *in vitro*, yet to be active at low doses for hairy cell leukemia [8, 9]. Immunomodulation as the mechanism of therapeutic activity with IFNα is perhaps best supported by its action against hairy cell leukemia. Treatment with IFNα in this disease is associated with a 90–95% response rate; however, this is not fully achieved until the patients have been on the protocol for a year, and it appears that low doses of IFNα are as active as higher doses [15].

hairy cell leukemia

Initial dose-finding studies, determined that a dose of 12×10^6 U/M^2 of human recombinant (r-IFNα) was not tolerable in patients with hairy cell leukemia [9]. Subsequently it was demonstrated that a dose of 2×10^6 U/M^2 was both well tolerated and effective when administered three times per week. Later [16] it was demonstrated that highly purified natural IFNα at a dose of 2×10^6 U/M^{2,}, administered for 28 days, was well tolerated in most patients. However, it retained some toxicity, including myelosuppression as well as neurotoxicity and cardiotoxicity. In these studies, a lower dose of 2×10^5 U/M^2 was also administered for 28 days and was found to be better tolerated and to also induce improvements in peripheral neutrophil and platelet counts as rapidly as the standard dose. In this trial substantial clinical improvement, primarily in terms of increased platelet and neutrophil counts, was also observed within the first 4 to 8 weeks of treatment. This resulted in an improved quality of life, a depression in cardiac and neurologic toxicity, flulike syndrome, myelosuppression, the need for platelet transfusions and a reduced incidence of bacterial infections. It appears that once improvements are obtained at 2×10^5 U/M^2, and patients become tolerant to the acute toxicity associated with IFNα, the dose can be increased to 2×10^6 U/M^2 to obtain the greater antileukemia effect of the higher dose. Further, it appears that significant improvements in thrombocytopenia and neutropenia can be rapidly induced in the majority of patients when low and minimally toxic doses of IFNα are used. However, there is also a therapeutic dose-response effect, whereby higher doses of IFNα will induce a quantitatively greater antileukemic response than that observed with low doses of IFNα.

toxicity

IFNγ

Preclinical studies have suggested that r-IFNγ has significant therapeutic activity in animal models of experimental and spontaneous metastasis which occurs with a reproducible bell-shaped dose-response curve [6]. Studies of immune response in normal animals have revealed the same bell-shaped dose-response curve for the augmentation of macrophage tumoricidal activity [6, 17]. Thus, optimal therapeutic activity is observed with the same dose and protocol of r-IFNγ but with significantly less therapeutic activity at lower and higher doses. A significant correlation between macrophage augmentation and therapeutic efficacy has been reported [17], suggesting that immunological augmentation provides an indirect mechanism for the therapeutic effect of r-IFNγ and supports the hypothesis that treatment with the maximum tolerated dose (MTD) of r-IFNγ may not be optimal in an adjuvant setting.

chronic granulous disease

The preclinical hypothesis of a bell-shaped dose-response curve for r-IFNγ has been confirmed in numerous clinical studies of the immunoregulatory effects of r-IFNγ which defined an OID [18, 19]. In general, the OID for r-IFNγ has been found to be between 0.1 and 0.3 mg/M^2 following intravenous (i.v.) or intramuscular injection. In contrast, the MTD for r-IFNγ may range from 3 to 10 mg/M^2 depending upon the source of the r-IFNγ and/or the clinical center. The identification of an OID for r-IFNγ in patients with minimal tumor burden has resulted in the development of clinical trials to test the hypothesis that the immunological enhancement induced by r-IFNγ will result in prolongation of the disease-free period and overall survival of patients in an adjuvant setting [19]. However, r-IFNγ was found, on an empirical basis, to have therapeutic activity in chronic granulomatous disease (CGD) [20] and it was for this indication that the U.S. Federal Drug Administration (FDA) approved r-IFNγ. The studies in CGD suggested that the mechanism of therapeutic activity for IFNγ is associated with enhanced phagocytic oxidase activity and increased superoxide production by neutrophils. However, more recent data suggests that the majority of CGD patients obtain clinical benefit by prolonging IFNγ therapy, and the mechanism of action may not be due to enhanced neutrophils oxidase activity but rather to the correction of a respiratory burst deficiency in a subset of monocytes [21]. In addition to its licensing for CGD, IFNγ has also been approved for the treatment of rheumatoid arthritis in Germany.

arthritis

Interleukin-2 (IL-2)

IL-2 is a T-cell proliferative cytokine, as well as a potent natural killer (NK) cell augmenting agent, and can activate lymphokine activated killer (LAK) cells. These are cells which have been cultured with IL-2 *in vitro* for 72 h or longer and have markedly increased, nonspecific cellular cytotoxicity. As such, IL-2 is important to all facets of T-cell and NK-cell augmentation and proliferation. IL-2 has been approved for use as a single agent for the treatment of renal cell carcinoma, although it is also administered in conjunction with LAK or T-cell infiltrating lymphocytes (TILs) in adoptive cellular therapy protocols. TIL cells are T-cells obtained from a tumor which are expanded *in vitro* with lower levels of IL-2 then that used with LAK cells and in the presence of tumor antigen(s). The overall goal is to expand a population of tumor-specific cytotoxic T-cells. However, it has been questioned whether the adoptive transfer of LAK cells is necessary or adds to the clinical efficacy of r-IL-2. Indeed, there has been little indication of an improved therapeutic effect of r-IL-2 plus LAK cells versus IL-2 alone [22, 23]. When the clinical trials with IL-2 are rigorously examined, neither strategy has impressive (as opposed to significant) therapeutic activity [22, 23]. The overall response rate with r-IL-2 is 7–14% and is associated with considerable toxicity [24]; however, it should be remarked that these responses are durable. In one of the first clinical studies [25], partial responses were observed in 4 out of 31 patients. Interestingly, these partial responders did not correspond to the patients with increased LAK- or NK-cell activity. The antitumor effect of both TIL and LAK cells could be due either to a direct effect or secondary to the generation of other cytokine mediators as suggested by the observation that r-IL-2-stimulated lymphocytes produce IFNγ and tumor necrosis factor (TNF) as well as other cytokines and that the therapeutic activity of r-IL-2 may be synergistic with these cytokines [25].

Many of the intravenous IL-2 infusion clinical trials with or without LAK cells in metastatic renal cell carcinoma have used an MTD of IL-2. A study by the laboratory of Fefer et al. [26] compared maintenance IL-2 therapy at the MTD of 6×10^6 U/M^2/day to 2×10^6 U/M^2/day. They found that it was possible to maintain the patients for a median of 4 days at 6×10^6 U/M^2/day, but in the presence of severe hypertension and capillary leak syndrome. In the lower-dose protocol none of the patients experienced severe hypertension or capillary leak syndrome, and the median duration of maintenance IL-2 therapy was 9 days. Further, in the lower-dose protocol there was a total response rate of 41%, which contrasted with the higher-dose protocol (with a shorter duration of ad-

natural killer cell

tumor infiltrating cells

maximum tolerated dose

LAK

ministration), which had a 22% response rate. These investigators suggest that there may be an improved therapeutic activity associated with a longer-maintenance protocol at lower doses.

A recent study which examined the transcriptional regulation of cytokine messenger RNA (mRNA) levels in the peripheral blood leukocytes (PBL) of cancer patients suggested that (1) doses of r-IL-2 as low as 3×10^4 U/day could augment T-cell function, and (2) higher doses of r-IL-2 $> 1 \times 10^5$ U/day increase not only T-cell but also macrophage function [27]. The latter was measured since TNF levels and the upregulation of TNF at the higher dose of IL-2 combined with the T-cell production of IFNγ which occurs at the lower dose of IL-2 may be responsible for the toxicity of IL-2 [28]. Recently, renal cell cancer patients were randomized to receive a high-dose regimen (FDA-approved dose), or one using one-tenth of the dose (72 000 IU/kg/8 h) administered by the same schedule (days 1–5 and 15–19, which was repeated every 4–6 weeks). An interim report of this trial [29] reported similar response rates in the two groups of approximately 7% complete responses (CR) and 8% partial responses (PR) in the low-dose group, versus 3% CR and 17% PR in the high-dose group. However, the toxicity of the low-dose regimen was substantially less than that of the high-dose regimen.

Recently, chronic IL-2 administration at low doses ($\sim 200\,000$ IU/M^2/day) has been found to increase CD4$^+$ cell number and the CD4:CD8 ratio in AIDS patients [29, 30]. The goal of one of these studies [30] was to give asymptomatic immunodeficiency virus-positive (HIV$^+$) individuals IL-2 without promoting viral replication, using an approach patterned after that described by Ritz et al. [31], who reported that low doses of IL-2 could be given to cancer patients for periods up to 3 months with minimal toxicity. The results indicate that extremely low IL-2 doses are nontoxic and effective in stimulating immune reactivity.

AIDS
renal cell
carcinoma

Natural BRMs

The use of BRMs (Table 2) to treat human disease has its origins in the use of bacterial toxins to treat cancer by William B. Coley [32]. These early studies resulted in the use of microbially derived substances such as BCG or Picibanil, carbohydrates from plants or fungi, such as Krestin, and Lentinan, and other products such as Biostim and Broncho-Vaxom (Table 2). However, there is considerable lot-to-lot variation in the amount and purity of these compounds. In addition, due to their particulate nature, intravenous injection can result in pulmonary thrombosis

Table 2 Licensed BRMs

Agent	Chemical nature	Action	Clinical use
Microbial-derived			
BCG (USA and Eur)	live mycobacteria	macrophage activator	bladder cancer
Picibanil (OK432) (Jap)	extract *Streptococcus pyogenes*	macrophage activator	gastric/other cancers
Krestin (PSK) (Jap)	fungal polysaccharide	macrophage activator	gastric/other cancers
Lentinan (Jap)	fungal polysaccharide	macrophage activator	gastric/other cancers
Biostim (Eur)	extract *Klebsiella pneumoniae.*	macrophage activator	chronic or recurrent infections
Thymus-derived			
Thymostimulin (Eur)	thymic peptide extract	T-cell stimulant	cancer and infection
T-activin (Russia)	thymic peptide extract	T-cell stimulant	cancer and infection
Thym-uvocal (FRG)	thymic peptide extract		cancer and infection
Chemically defined			
Romurtide (Jap)	18 lys MDP	macrophage stimulant	bone marrow recovery
Thymopentin TP-5 (Italy and FRG)	pentapeptide	T-cell stimulant	Rheumatoid arthritis infection and cancer
Levamisole (US)	phenylimidothiazole	T-cell stimulant	cancer
Bestatin (Jap)	dipeptide	macrophage and T-cell stimulant	AML
Isoprinosine (Eur)	inosine:salt complex	T-cell stimulant	infection

BCG

bladder cancer

thymosine

bestatin

and respiratory distress as well as the potential development of focal or multifocal granulomatous disease following either dermal administration, scarification or intravenous administration.

The most commonly used microorganism for cancer therapy trials in the USA is BCG, which has been used systemically for metastatic disease or adjuvant therapy, intralesionally (especially for cutaneous metastatic malignant melanoma), topically for superficial bladder cancer and in combination with other immune modulators, tumor vaccines, and chemotherapy. Its greatest proven efficacy has been when given intravesically or both intravesically and intradermally to treat superficial bladder cancer in the setting of residual disease and in the adjuvant setting [33]. A well-controlled, randomized study has shown a prolonged disease-free interval and time to progressive disease in patients treated with intradermal and intravesical BCG as compared with controls [34] and is one of several currently accepted treatment modalities for patients with superficial bladder cancer, especially post-fulguration. The mechanism by which BCG mediates its antitumor response is not known, but granulomatous inflammation is induced in the bladder by BCG treatment [35], and elevated IL-2 levels are detectable in the urine of treated patients [36], suggesting that an augmented local immune response may be important.

Chemically defined BRMs

The use of nonspecific immunostimulants has also been extensively studied (Table 2). The microbially derived agents have in common widespread effects on the immune system and side effects akin to infection (e.g. fever, malaise, myalgia etc.). The administration of these agents can enhance nonspecific resistance to microbial or neoplastic challenge when administered prior to challenge (immunoprophylactic) but rarely when administered following challenge (immunotherapeutic). This is an important distinction in that the primary objective for the oncologist is the treatment of preexistent metastatic disease. Following a long history of experimental use in many different cancers and diseases, levamisole became the first chemically defined, orally active immunostimulant to be licensed (USA) for clinical use [37, 38]. It was approved for the treatment of Duke's C colon cancer in combination with 5-fluorouracil. This agent promotes T-lymphocyte, macrophage and neutrophil function. It stimulates T-cell function *in vivo*, particularly in immunodeficient individuals, presumably through the action of its sulfur moiety. It is relatively nontoxic (flulike symptoms, gastrointestinal upset, metallic taste, skin rash and antibuse reaction), but can produce an agranulocytosis particularly in human lymphocyte antigen (HLA) B-27$^+$ patients with rheumatoid arthritis, where its use has been discontinued. It is currently being considered for use in other cancers, with an emphasis on gastrointestinal disease.

levamisole

One of the largest and best-studied classes of synthetic agents are the muramyl dipeptides (MDP). The first to be licensed, Romurtide (Japan), is employed to induce bone marrow recovery following cancer chemotherapy [39]. Its mechanism of action is the activation of macrophages to secrete colony stimulating factors (CSFs), IL-1 and TNF, resulting in the stimulation of marrow precursors to produce increased numbers, progenitor and mature granulocytes and monocytes. Therefore, the period of granulocytopenia and the risk of secondary infections

muramyl dipeptides

are reduced, allowing more frequent and/or intense chemotherapy. Murabutide, an orally active form of MDP which does not induce fevers, is currently in clinical trials in cancer and infection in France. Muramyl tripeptide phosphatidylethanolamine (MTP-PE) encapsulated in liposome is also in clinical trials for cancer (USA and Europe). The MDPs are also potent adjuvants alone and with oil and are under consideration for use with HIV vaccines employing various synthetic peptide epitopes.

MDP was discovered based on the isolation of the minimally active substitute for intact BCG in Freund's adjuvant [40]. Unfortunately, as with many of the polypeptides due to their low molecular weight, MDP has a short serum half-life and requires high doses given frequently to be active. In addition, agents such as MDP are strongly pyrogenic, presumably due, in part, to their ability to induce IL-1. MDP has been incorporated into multilamellar vesicles (MLVs) for higher stability and to facilitate monocytic phagocytosis of the MLV. In order to further stabilize the incorporation of MDP into MLV, lipophilic analogs of MDP such as MTP-PE have been developed. Clinical trials using MTP-PE in liposomes are currently ongoing for osteosarcoma [41, 42] but it is too early to know what the therapeutic efficacy of this agent will be.

ANLL

GVHD

Bestatin (ubenimex) is a potent inhibitor of aminopeptidase N and aminopeptidase B [43], which was isolated from a culture filtrate of *Streptomyces olivoreticuli* during the search for specific inhibitors of enzymes present on the membrane of eukaryotic cells [44]. Inhibitors of aminopeptidase activity are associated with macrophage activation and differentiation. Bestatin has shown significant therapeutic effects in several clinical trials [45]. In a multiinstitutional study, 101 patients with acute nonlymphocytic leukemia (ANLL) were randomized to receive Bestatin or control [46]. Patients received 30 mg of Bestatin orally after completion of induction and consolidation therapy, and concomitant with maintenance chemotherapy. Remission duration was prolonged in the Bestatin group, although this difference did not reach statistical significance. However, overall survival was prolonged in the Bestatin group. Recently, a confirmatory phase III trial in ANLL was reported which extended the observation to a significant prolongation of remission [47]. In a recent multicenter study, Bestatin was administered to acute leukemia and chronic myelogenous leukemia patients who did not develop any graft versus host disease (GVHD) within 30 days following bone marrow transplantation (BMT) [48]. Bestatin-treated acute leukemia patients had an increased incidence of chronic low-grade GVHD compared with the control arm and a lower rate.

Combination chemotherapy and immunotherapy

Because the cytokines have unique mechanisms of action, they are ideal candidates for combination therapy with chemotherapeutic agents. However, increased knowledge and consideration of the potential interactions between these two classes of drugs is necessary for optimal clinical use. The use of high-dose chemotherapy (HDT) and stem-cell rescue provides the ultimate in cytoreductive therapy and posttransplant immunotherapy. As shown later in this chapter, stem-cell transplantation provides one of the few statistically supported demonstrations of therapeutic efficacy by T-cell augmentation (comparison of allogeneic to autologous transplantation). Thus, strategies to upregulate T-cell function postautologous stem-cell transplantation is one focus for cytokine therapy post-transplantation. This is important, as the return of immunologic function in transplanted patients is slow and is accompanied by depressed numbers of CD-4$^+$ T-cells, a low CD-4/CD-8 T-cell ratio, and depressed cellular responses [49] .

peripheral blood stem cell transplantation

The role of T-cells in controlling neoplastic disease has been demonstrated in allotransplanted patients and described as a graft versus tumor (GVT) reaction. A significantly higher risk of relapse is associated with the use of T-cell depleted bone marrow cells or the clinical use of cyclosporin A (CSA) to prevent GVHD [49–52]. It has been postulated that T-lymphocyte depletion increases leukemia relapse by removing the cells responsible for the GVT effect [50–53]. Similar relapse rates are observed in recipients of non-T-cell depleted transplants receiving CSA, suggesting that it inhibits the same GVT-cells that are removed by T-cell depletion. Clearly, GVHD can also have unfavorable effects on transplant-related mortality. In first remission, the decreased relapse rate with acute and/or chronic GVHD is more than offset by the increased risk of death from other causes. Consequently, patients with GVHD have a lower risk of treatment failure, but an increased risk of morbidity due to GVHD.

bone marrow transplantation

Thus, one approach to improving survival of cancer patients has been to use immunotherapy following HDT and stem-cell transplant to induce an autologous GVT response. Based on this strategy, studies using r-IL-2 alone following BMT, have shown an increase in NK-cell phenotype and function [54–57]. In one such study [56] with 18 evaluable patients, three responses were observed. In another study, r-IL-2 was infused following both autologous and allogeneic transplants for a median of 85 days at a dose of 2×10^5 units/M^2/day [57]. Toxicity was minimal, and the treatment could be undertaken in the outpatient setting via a Hick-

tumor necrosis factor

man catheter. In this study no patient developed any signs of GVHD, hypertension or pulmonary capillary leak syndrome. The treatment did not affect the absolute neutrophil count or hemoglobin level, although eosinophilia was observed. Despite the administration of this low dose of r-IL-2, significant immunological changes were noted with a 5- to 40-fold increase in NK cell number. In addition, there was a significant augmentation of *ex vivo* cytotoxicity against K-562 and colon tumor targets. In a similar study, it was shown that following continuous infusion of r-IL-2 in patients receiving autologous BMT (AuBMT), the CD-3⁺ and CD-16⁺ cells secrete increased levels of IFNγ and TNF, leveled following *in vitro* culture and that there was a significant increase in serum levels of IFNγ but not TNF following the administration of r-IL-2 [57].

Similar posttransplantation strategies with r-IFNα have been undertaken with the observation of a reduced risk of relapse and an increase in myelosuppression [58, 59]. The Seattle Group [59] reported an early study of the prophylactic use of r-IFNα following allogeneic (Ao) BMT, and that adjuvant treatment with IFNα had no effect on the probability or severity of cytomegalovirus (CMV) infections or GVHD in acute lymphocytic leukemia (ALL) patients who were in remission at the time of transplantation. However, in this large study, there was a significant reduction in the probability of relapse in the r-IFNα recipients ($P = 0.004$) as compared with transplant patients who did not receive r-IFNα, although survival rates did not differ between the r-IFNα recipients and control patients. It was suggested that the administration of r-IFNα following transplantation reduced the risks of relapse but did not affect CMV infection, perhaps because r-IFNα was not initiated until a median of 18 days following transplantation and was not administered chronically. Recently, Ratanatharathorn et al. [60] extended the approach of the induction of a GVT reaction to a combination study which utilized both CSA-induced GVHD and IFNα augmentation of this effect in autologous transplant patients. Twenty-two patients were enrolled of which 17 were considered evaluable. Thirteen of the patients who received r-Hu-IFNα2a developed GVHD regardless of whether they received CSA, whereas only 2 of the 4 patients who received CSA alone developed detectable GVHD. Patients receiving 1×10^6 U/day of r-Hu-IFNα2a concomitant with CSA showed a trend towards increased severity of clinical GVHD as compared with patients receiving CSA alone ($P = 0.06$). They concluded that IFNα administration can be safely started on day 0 of AuBMT and can induce autologous GVHD as a single agent with the potential to improve therapy.

In similar studies Kennedy et al. [61] treated women with advanced breast cancer with therapy of CSA for 28 days in combination with

0.025 mg/m^2 of subcutaneous IFNγ every other day on days 7–28 after high-dose chemotherapy and AuBMT. They observed that autologous GVHD developed in 56% of the patients, an incidence comparable with that previously observed with CSA alone. The severity of GVHD was greater with CSA plus IFNγ than with CSA alone, as 16 patients required corticosteroid therapy for dermatologic GVHD. Note that strategies to induce an autologous GVT, while conceptually interesting, have not matured to allow a discussion of efficiency.

BRMs

Conclusion

In the last 20 years, nonspecific immunostimulation has progressed from the initial trials with crude microbial mixtures and extracts to more sophisticated uses with a large collection of targeted immunopharmacologically active compounds (only a few of which are discussed here) having diverse actions on the immune system. A body of immunopharmacologic knowledge has evolved which shows substantial divergence from conventional pharmacology, particularly in terms of the relationship of dosing schedules to immunopharmacodynamics. This knowledge is important in evaluating agents and predicting appropriate use. While much remains to be learned and new compounds to be extracted and/or cloned, the future of immunotherapy seems bright. A number of the cytokines have been approved, as well as numerous supplemental indications [62], in the United States, Europe and Asia. However, it is apparent that the combinations of cytokines and BRMs will have optimal activity when used as adjuvants with more traditional therapeutic modalities.

Immunostimulants as anti-infectives

K. Noel Masihi

Introduction

Infectious diseases continue to impact human health and development. The global pandemic of acquired immunodeficiency syndrome (AIDS) infects over 1 million people a year, and communicable diseases are among the most frequent infectious conditions worldwide. The current public awareness of microbial infections has been heightened by recent episodes of bacterial food poisoning, diphtheria from areas in political turmoil, the rapid spread of cholera in South America and highly publicized reports of bovine spongiform encephalitis-related Creutzfeld-Jakob disease.

Infections which caused ravages in the 19th century, such as tuberculosis, are once again resurging with vehemence. Newly emerging pathogens capable of causing human diseases such as Ebola haemorrhagic fever, for which there is no cure or vaccine, continue to surface. Antibiotic-resistant nosocomial (hospital-related) infections remain significant. Some infections are now so resistant to drug therapy that they are virtually untreatable. Multidrug resistance and infections with opportunistic pathogens in immunocompromised patients will predictably persist as problems well into the next millenium. Many experts are openly concerned about a postantibiotic era. The World Health Organization has estimated that there are at least 17 million infection-related deaths every year and that up to half the approximately 5.7 billion people on earth are at risk of many endemic diseases. It is disconcerting that there are still a vast number of diseases afflicting humans and domestic mammals for which no vaccines or specific chemotherapy will be available in the near future. The struggle to control infectious diseases, far from being over, has acquired new poignancy. Novel concepts acting as adjunct to established therapies are urgently needed.

antibiotic resistance

Immunostimulants

definition of
immunostimulants

The immune system can be manipulated by vaccination or immunomodulation. Immunostimulants are agents that are capable of modulating the immune response towards protection against microbial pathogens or tumors. This can occur by augmentation of the antiinfectious or antitumor immunity by immune system cells including lymphocyte subsets, macrophages and natural killer cells. Other mechanisms can involve induction or restoration of immune effector functions. Synonymous terms for immunostimulants include biological response modifiers, immunoaugmentors or immunorestoratives. Microbial products, drugs of natural and synthetic origin, and proteins derived from the immune system represent some of the immunostimulants that are currently in use [1–5] (Table 1).

Table 1 Classification of immunostimulants

Type of immunostimulant	Representatives
Whole microbes	attenuated strains, whole heat-killed bacteria
Microbial products	bacterial homogenates, isolated fractions
Compounds of natural origin	calf thymic hormones, plant fractions
Synthetic compounds	isoprinosine, muramyl peptides
Compounds of endogenous origin	interferons, interleukins, colony-stimulating factors

Microbial Immunostimulants

Whole microbes

Viable *Mycobacteria*, in particular the attenuated vaccine strain of bacillus Calmette-Guérin (BCG), and heat-killed or formalin-inactivated *Propionibacterium* (*Corynebacterium*) *parvum* have been employed as nonspecific first-generation microbial immunomodulators for enhancing resistance against neoplasms and several experimental infections. Currently, preparations containing formalinized *Corynebacterium* sp. are licensed in Europe for stimulation of the body's own host defence.

Whole cell microbial immunomodulators showed limited anecdotal efficacy in early empirical studies which could not be reliably reproduced in randomized clinical trials. The general consensus among clinical investigators has been that immunomodulatory treatments with whole bacteria need elucidation of underlying mechanisms and development of more specific immunotherapeutic agents.

Bacterial lysates

Bacterial extracts are widely used as immunostimulants to prevent recurrent infections of the respiratory tract. There exists a large body of primary literature on placebo-controlled and double-blind clinical trials which have been conducted with these agents. Several preparations containing bacterial lysates are licensed for use in Europe (Table 2).

The current concept of the mucosal immune system postulates that activated lymphocytes from the gut are capable of conferring protective immunity by disseminating into the intestinal tract and other mucosal tissues located in respiratory and urogenital organs. Stimulation of the gut-associated lymphoid tissue can thus lead to the induction of a generalized response in the whole mucosal-associated lymphoid tissue.

mucosal immunity

Patients, most often children, with recurrent episodes of infections of the respiratory tract and of the ear, nose and throat have been treated with oral bacterial lysates. In most cases, the frequency and the severity of infections was reduced and both the physician and the patient considered the treatment to be beneficial. In some patients, increases in the levels of immunoglobulin A (IgA) in saliva, bronchoalveolar lavage and/or serum have been observed. Functional tests on alveolar macrophages have shown increases in motility and in the production of superoxide anion,

Table 2 Composition of typical bacterial lysate preparations used for treatment of respiratory infections

Example 1 (Broncho-Munal)	Example 2 (Luivac)
Haemophilus influenzae	*Streptococcus pneumoniae*
Diplococcus pneumoniae	*Streptococcus pyogenes*
Klebsiella pneumoniae	*Streptococcus mitis*
Klebsiella ozaenae	*Staphylococcus aureus*
Staphylococcus aureus	*Haemophilus influenzae*
Streptococcus pyogenes	*Klebsiella pneumoniae*
Streptococcus viridans	*Branhamella catarrhalis*
Neisseria catarrhalis	

and chemiluminescence. It is of interest that many studies have reported a decrease in antibiotic consumption in bacterial lysate-treated patients.

Preparations containing extracts or heat-killed organisms of *Escherichia coli* alone or mixed with other bacteria mentioned in Table 2 are being used for the treatment of recurrent urinary tract infections. The number of recurrences, consumption of antibiotics, the incidence of bacteriuria and dysuria were reported to be significantly reduced after such treatment, and urinary and vaginal IgG and IgA levels were increased in treated patients.

Bacterial components

Preparations containing bacterial components are also licensed in Europe, mainly for recurrent respiratory tract infections. A glycoprotein preparation, Biostim/RU41740, extracted from *Klebsiella pneumoniae*, has been shown to decrease the number, duration and complications of respiratory infections in children and elderly patients and to reduce the duration of antibiotic therapy. Another preparation, Ribomunyl, contains ribosomes isolated from *Klebsiella pneumoniae*, *Streptococcus pneumoniae*, *S. pyogenes*, *Haemophilus influenzae* and proteoglycan from *K. pneumoniae*. It has been shown to improve bronchopulmonary infections in children and adults.

Immunostimulants of natural origin

Thymic hormones

thymus

The thymus is a double-lobed lymphoid gland and the key organ for the development of immunocompetent T-lymphocytes. Specialised thymic cells secrete hormonelike substances which play a pivotal role in the intrathymic maturation of precursor T-lymphocytes. The thymus, however, shows an early age-dependent involution with a concurrent decrease in T-cell immunity. This has prompted intense interest in restoring declining thymic functions.

Preparations containing bovine thymus extracts are currently licensed in Europe for adjunct therapy of immune defects arising during infectious diseases, and are indicated for generally weakened host defence occurring in viral diseases and recurrent bacterial infections.

Recurrent herpes simplex, herpes zoster and human papilloma virus infections are sometimes difficult to control by traditional antiviral therapy. Therapy with thymus extracts administered by either oral or parenteral routes has been shown to reduce the frequency and intensity of recurrences of herpes labialis infections. Contrary to antiviral drugs, the effect of thymic-derived preparations appears to be long-lasting even after discontinuation of treatment.

The main concern in use of crude mixtures from bovine thymus extracts has been the possibility of eliciting allergic responses to bovine proteins, which have been observed in some cases.

Immunostimulants of synthetic origin

Isoprinosine

Isoprinosine (Inosiplex) is a complex of the *p*-acetamidobenzoate salt of *N,N*-dimethylamino-2-propanol: inosine in a 3:1 molar ratio (Fig. 1). It is a white cystalline powder soluble in water. The inosine portion of isoprinosine is metabolically labile and half-life in rhesus monkeys is 3 min after intravenous and 50 min after oral administration. Isoprinosine has been shown to augment production of cytokines such as interleukin (IL)-1 and -2 and interferon (IFN)-γ. It enhances proliferation of lymphocytes in response to mitogenic or antigenic stimuli, increases active T-cell rosettes and induces T-cell surface markers on prothymocytes.

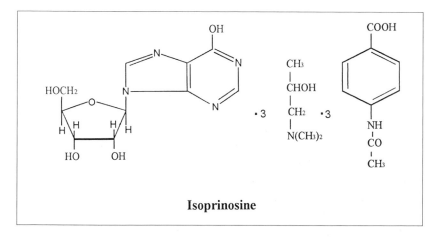

Isoprinosine

Figure 1 Chemical structure of Isoprinosine

313

Isoprinosine can augment the production of interferon and was developed as an antiviral agent. It has been found to be useful in the treatment of several viral diseases such as herpes simplex, herpes zoster, influenza and rhinovirus infections. Isoprinosine increases survival in subacute sclerosing panencephalitis, although it does not inhibit the replication of measles virus. Multicenter double-blind clinical trials of isoprinosine in asymptomatic human immunodeficiency virus (HIV)-positive patients with more than 400 CD4$^+$ counts have shown significant delay in the progression of HIV infection to AIDS.

Isoprinosine is currently licensed in Europe for treatment of herpes simplex infections, subacute sclerosing panencephalitis, acute viral encephalitis caused by herpes simplex, Epstein-Barr and measles viruses and for treatment of these viral infections in immunosuppressed patients.

Isoprinosine has been reported to have minor central nervous system (CNS) depressant but no neuromuscular, sedative or antipyretic activities in pharmacologic studies in animals. In humans, isoprinosine may cause transient nausea and an increase in uric acid in serum and urine at high doses.

Splenopentin

Splenopentin is a pentapeptide corresponding to the amino acid sequence 32–36 (Arg-Lys-Glu-Val-Tyr) of the splenic hormone splenin (Fig. 2). The difference between splenopentin and thymopentin, a synthetic thymic peptide preparation, is in the substitution of Glu for Asp. Splenopentin induces the differentiation of T-cell precursors, T helper and suppressor cells, and increases dose-dependently the number of bone marrow colonies.

Diacetylsplenopentin is a pentapeptide of splenin modified by two-fold acetylation. Diacetylsplenopentin is currently licensed in Europe for use in patients with HIV infection with manifest immunodeficiency and, in combination with the antiretroviral zidovudine, in patients with AIDS.

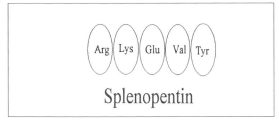

Figure 2 Amino acid sequence of Splenopentin

The main limitation with smaller peptides is that they generally have short half-lives. This necessitates frequent injections of relatively large amounts of the peptide preparation.

Immunostimulants of endogenous origin

Cytokines are intimately involved in antimicrobial immune responses by modulating the expression of major histocompatibility (MHC) complex and various adhesion molecules regulating the activity of effector cells. Certain cytokines stimulate the production of other cytokines in synergistic or antagonistic networks. Local and systemic effects of cytokines produced by infiltrating cells appear to play an important role in control of infections. Recent advances in the monoclonal antibody and recombinant DNA technologies have led to availability of large quantities of cytokines with immunomodulatory activities.

Interferons

Interferons can confer resistance to cells against diverse viruses and were first described in 1957. Interferons play an important role in host defence against infectious pathogens and in the regulation of immune responses.

There is a vast body of literature on the activity of IFNα as an antiviral agent. Natural IFNα obtained from human serum and leukocytes is currently licensed for the treatment of a rare form of cancer, hairy cell leukemia. Recombinant IFNα-2a is licensed for treatment of chronic active hepatitis B and for hepatitis C virus infections. However, only a small subset of patients with hepatitis B and around 40% of cases with hepatitis C are responsive to interferon therapy. IFNα is also approved for treating condyloma acuminata caused by human papilloma virus and for Kaposi's sarcoma in patients with HIV infection. **IFNα**

IFNβ obtained from human FS-4 fibroblast cell lines is licensed for use in severe uncontrolled virus-mediated diseases occurring in cases of viral encephalitis, herpes zoster and varicella in immunosuppressed patients. A further indication is viral infection of the inner ear with loss of hearing. Recently, IFβ has been licensed for treatment of multiple sclerosis. **IFNβ**

IFNγ is a potent macrophage-activating factor produced by both CD4$^+$ and CD8$^+$ T-cells and can induce class I and class II MHC products. Patients with chronic granulomatous disease are unable to gener- **IFNγ** ate oxidative respiratory burst. As a consequence, they develop recurring catalase-positive bacterial infections such as *Staphylococcus aureus*, *Pseudomonas cepacia*, and *Chromobacterium violaceum*. Multicenter clinical trials have shown that sustained administration of IFNγ to chronic granulomatous disease patients markedly reduces the relative risk of serious infection. IFNγ is licensed as a therapeutic adjunct for use in patients with chronic (septic) granulomatosis for the reduction of the frequency of serious infections.

The major side effects of all interferon therapies include flulike syndromes, fever, myalgia, headache and fatigue. Hypotension, granulocytopenia and thrombocytopenia can also occur. Deleterious effects on the CNS, particularly at high doses, have been observed.

Colony-stimulating factors

CSFs

The colony-stimulating factors (CSFs) are intimately involved in the production and differentiation of stem cells in the bone marrow to phagocytic cells. CSFs are classified into four major types, namely IL-3, macrophage CSF (M-CSF), granulocyte CSF (G-CSF) and granulocyte-macrophage CSF (GM-CSF).

GM-CSF produced by recombinant technology from *E. coli* 12 has been licensed for the reduction of risk of infection by diminishing the severity of neutropenia in patients treated with usual doses of myelotoxic chemotherapy.

Emerging therapies

Experimental immunostimulants of natural and synthetic origin

A number of immunostimulants of natural and synthetic origin are currently being investigated in clinical trials. While many of these immunostimulants have been studied in patients with cancer, vast amounts of preclinical data from animal experiments and some results from human clinical trials in various infectious disease models have been published [1–5].

Thymic peptide analogs and thymomimetics

Crude bovine thymic extracts have been used to isolate and identify hormones responsible for physiological functions of the thymus gland. Thymic extracts have yielded peptide mixtures such as thymosin fraction 5 and purified peptide preparations such as thymopoietin, thymic humoral factor, thymulin and thymosin (Fig. 3). Partial peptide sequences such as thymopentin have been synthesised. These preparations can induce T-lymphocyte surface markers on prothymocytes and can modulate

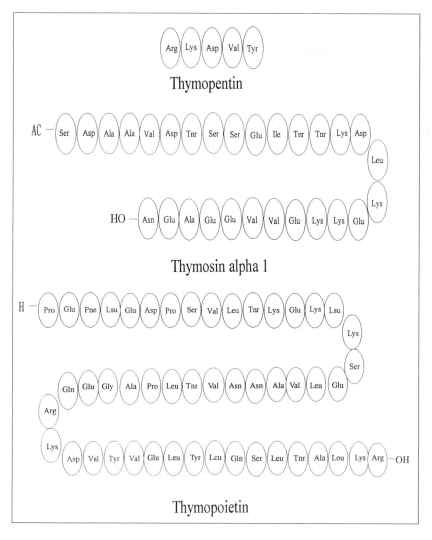

Figure 3 Amino acid sequence of thymic peptides

thymopentin

T-cell proliferation, as well as helper, suppressor, cytotoxic and cytokine functions.

Thymopentin is a synthetic pentapeptide (Arg-Lys-Asp-Val-Tyr) representing the active biologic site of 49 amino acid thymic hormone thymopoietin. At present thymopentin is licensed in Europe for treatment of primary immundeficiencies characterised by reduced T-cell numbers or showing limited T-lymphocyte function, as occurs in DiGeorge and Louis-Bar syndromes.

The significant degree of immunologic dysfunction in HIV infection has generated interest in possible immune stimulation and reconstitution. Thymopentin was evaluated in a double-blind, randomized, placebo-controlled trial in zidovudine (AZT)-treated asymptomatic HIV-infected subjects with 200–500 CD4 cells/mm^3 at entry. Thymopentin treatment reduced the relatively high progression rates to AIDS or death in AZT-experienced placebo-treated subjects [6]. In another randomized

thymosin α_1

nonblinded study, combination therapy with *thymosin α_1*, IFNα and AZT in patients with CD4$^+$ lymphocytes ranging from 200 to 500/mm^3 was well tolerated after 12 months and was associated with a substantial increase in the number and function of CD4$^+$ T-cells [7].

A survey of 11 clinical studies shows that thymopentin treatment reduces the incidence of recurrent respiratory tract infections. Thymopentin treatment resulted in a statistically significant decrease in infective recurrences. The need for symptomatic and antibiotic drugs was also reduced. The clinical effect appears to be long-lasting, i.e. up to 3–4 months after discontinuation of treatment.

thymosin fraction

Chronic hepatitis B is a severe and frequently progressive disease. The safety and efficacy of *thymosin fraction* 5 and thymosin α_1 were assessed in a prospective, placebo-controlled trial in patients with chronic hepatitis B. All patients had histological and biochemical evidence of active liver disease for at least 6 months before treatment and were positive for serum hepatitis B virus DNA and hepatitis B surface antigen (HBsAg). By the end of 1 year, serum aminotransferase levels had improved significantly, and more than half of the treated patients cleared hepatitis B virus DNA from serum.

MIMP

Methyl inosine monophosphate (MIMP) is a recently dveloped thymomimetic immunomodulator capable of inducing the expression of T-lymphocyte differentiation markers and IL-2 receptors in human prothymocytes. MIMP has been shown to enhance mitogen-induced proliferation of lymphocytes, augment IgM plaque-forming cells, induce delayed-type hypersensitivity and normalise an impaired response to IL-2. Depressed phytohaemagglutinin responses of lymphocytes suppressed by an HIV-derived peptide, IFNα, prostaglandin PGE$_2$ or lymphocytes from pre-AIDS (ARC) patients could be progressively restored by MIMP. Moreover, the mean survival time in mice infected with Friend leukaemia virus, employed as a murine model of AIDS, could be significantly increased by MIMP [8].

Another new synthetic thymic-derived immunomodulator, *pidotimod* [(*R*)-3-(*S*)-(5-oxo-2-pyrrolidinyl)-carbonyl)-thiazolidine-4-carboxylic acid], has been shown to significantly increase survival time after challenge with low doses of mengovirus, herpes simplex virus and influenza virus in animal models. A number of multicenter clinical trials with pidotimod in children have shown a decrease in the number of episodes of recurrent respiratory infections, less antibiotic consumption and reduced periods of absence from kindergarten or school [9].

pidotimol

The main drawback with most of these smaller purified peptides is the fact that they have short half-lives and necessitate frequent injections of relatively large amounts.

Muramyl peptides

N-acetyl-muramyl-L-alanyl-D-isoglutamine (MDP) is a small glycopeptide which represents the minimal structure essential for mycobacterial adjuvanticity. Synthetic MDP and its analogs (Fig. 4) possess pleiotropic properties including the ability to enhance nonspecific resistance against diverse microbial infections.

MDP

MDP-Lys(L18), a muramyl peptide analog, is a potent inducer of a variety of cytokines such as IL-1, IL-6, CSFs, tumor necrosis factor (TNF), and IFNγ in mice and humans. MDP-Lys(L18) is licensed in Japan under the trademark Romurtide, and has been shown to be effective for restoration of decreased neutrophils and platelets in cancer patients. The incidence of infectious diseases in the MDP-Lys(L18)-treated group was lower than in the control groups during the clinical trials [10]. A placebo-controlled double-blind clinical trial of glucosaminyl analog, GMDP, for immunotherapy of septic complications arising after abdominal surgery has also been reported. Prophylactic administration of GMDP and postoperative treatment of patients who acquired infections resulted in decreased frequency of septic complications and reduced mortality.

MDP-Lys(L18)

MDP and analogs such as threonyl MDP and MTP-PE, alone or in combination with other agents, have been shown to be capable of conferring resistance against experimental infections by influenza, herpes simplex, Sendai, Semliki-Forest, vaccinia and murine hepatitis viruses. MDP was found to exhibit an inhibitory activity against HIV infection in CD4$^+$ H9 lymphocytes and U937 monocytoid cells [11]. Monocyte-de-

MTP-PE

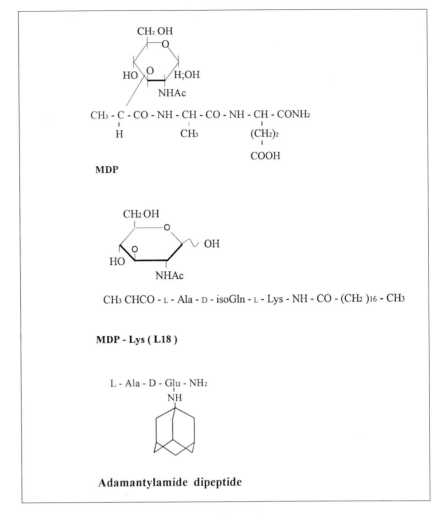

Figure 4 Chemical structures of muramyl peptides

rived macrophages infected with HIV *in vitro* and treated with a liposo-mal formulation of lipophilic MTP-PE were shown to a have an in-hibitory effect on HIV production. Interestingly an MDP analog, **MDP(thr)-GDP**, has shown a complete lack of cellular transcription fac-tor nuclear factor-κB (NF-κB) activation which is known to play a key role in HIV infection. Recombinant HIV envelope protein administered with MTP-PE has been shown to generate cytotoxic T-lymphocytes in mice and induced specific binding antibodies and lymphoproliferative re-sponses in human volunteers.

In an innovative approach, a novel hybrid entity combining pertinent components of both an antiviral and an immunomodulator in a single synthetic compound have been synthesized. *Adamantylamide dipeptide* consists of an antiviral 1 amino-amantadine moiety linked to the essential L-alanine-D-isoglutamine portion of immunomodulator MDP. Amantadine is a primary symmetric amine with an interesting tricyclic structure that has been extensively employed in humans since 1966 for the prophylaxis and chemotherapy of influenza and Parkinson's disease. Adamantylamide dipeptide showed significant activity against influenza virus in cell cultures, and preclinical animal studies have demonstrated that the homotypic immunity induced by influenza subunit vaccines can be broadened to the desirable heterologous immune response [12].

adamantylamide dipeptide

Glucans

Lentinan is a chemically well defined 1-3-β-D-glucan with 1-6-β-D-glucopyranoside branches and is isolated from an edible Japanese mushroom. It is licensed as an adjunct for antitumor therapy in Japan. Experimental studies have demonstrated that lentinan can confer protection against influenza virus and *Listeria monocytogenes* and prevent relapse of *Mycobacterium tuberculosis* [13]. Sulfated polysaccharides, such as *curdlan sulfate*, have been shown to exert inhibitory activity on HIV replication. Curdlan sulfate may exert an inhibitory effect on HIV infection by delaying the events that precede and/or include reverse transcription and by interfering with the membrane fusion process [14]. Curdlan sulfate is currently being investigated in clinical trials in several countries.

lentinan

curdlan sulfate

Yeast glucan has been shown to enhance resistance against herpes simplex and murine hepatitis viruses, and prolong survival against parasitic infections by *Plasmodium berghei* and *Leishmania donovani*. It also exerts antifungal activity against *Candida*, *Cryptococcus* and *Sporotichum*. Glucans have been shown to induce nonspecific resistance against *K. pneumoniae* infection and to protect patients from sepsis, bacteraemia and peritonitis resulting from *E. coli*, *Stapylococcus aureus* and *Pseudomonas aeruginosa* infections. The safety and efficacy of poLy-β-1-6-glucotriosyl-β-1-3-glucopyranose (PGG) glucan in surgical patients at high risk for postoperative infection who underwent major thoracic or abdominal surgery has recently been reported. Patients who received PGG-glucan had significantly fewer infectious complications, decreased intravenous antibiotic requirement and a shorter intensive care unit length of stay [15].

PGG-glucan

Cytokines as experimental immunostimulants

The last decade has seen the emergence of cytokines as promising therapeutic agents in infectious diseases. There are burgeoning reports in the literature on the protective effects of diverse cytokines in a variety of infectious diseases in animals and humans [3, 5, 16].

IFNγ

IFNγ

There is growing evidence from a number of studies that IFNγ plays a central role in protection against diverse intracellular infections. Mice immunosuppressed with cyclosporin A can be protected against fatal infection by *Listeria monocytogenes* when treated with IFN, and administration of IFNγ can enhance resistance to *Francisella tularensis*. IFNγ is essential for the resolution of parasitic infections by *Toxoplasma gondii*, *Pneumocystis carinii* and against *Plasmodium berghei* infection in rodents. Human neutrophils treated with IFNγ significantly augmented the killing of asexual blood forms of *Plasmodium falciparum*. IFNγ also plays an important role in the control of pneumonia caused by *Chlamydia trachomatis* and represents a crucial component in the host defence against against *Rikettsia conorii*.

CSFs

M-CSF

M-CSF can enhance the production of other cytokines such as interferons and TNF. Murine macrophages treated with M-CSF became resistant to vesicular stomatitis virus infection and reduced the amount of HSV-1 virus produced in cultures. Resident peritoneal macrophages treated with M-CSF exhibited enhanced phagocytosis and killing of *L. monocytogenes*. Treatment with M-CSF of human monocytes and murine

G-CSF

macrophages induces killing of *Candida albicans*. G-CSF induced resistance in neutropenic animals to infections by *Pseudomonas aeruginosa*, *Staphylococcus aureus*, *Serratia marcescens*, or *C. albicans*. Pretreatment and presence of GM-CSF during culture of U937 human monocytic cells provided protection against HIV infection. A synergisitc activity of

GM-CSF

GM-CSF with AZT could be observed in HIV-infected cells, and the toxic effect of AZT on human myeloid progenitor cells could be ameliorated. Human monocytes treated *in vitro* with recombinant human GM-CSF were capable of inducing antifungal activity against *C. albicans*. Recombinant murine GM-CSF administered to mice could confer protection against *listerial* infections and enhanced clearance of *Salmonella typhimurium*. Macrophages activated by GM-CSF exhibit enhanced capacity to kill *Leishmania donovani*, *L. tropica* and *Trypanosoma cruzi*.

Interleukins

Treatment with recombinant murine IL-1α significantly enhanced resistance of mice to *Listeria monocytogenes*. Mice rendered granulocytopenic by cyclophosphamide, infected with *Pseudomonas aeruginosa* and given gentamicin showed increased survival when IL-1β was administered before infection. Recombinant human IL-1α given before *P. aeruginosa* infection also enhanced survival of neutropenic mice. Recombinant human IL-1α administered simultaneously and after infection with *K. pneumoniae* conferred maximal protection. The growth of *C. albicans* in mice immunosuppressed with either cyclophosphamide or irradiation was significantly reduced when recombinant human IL-1α was administered before, given simultaneously or within 6 h after infection. Prophylactic treatment with recombinant human IL-1β enhanced resistance of normal and cyclophosphamide-treated mice to systemic infection with *C. albicans*.

IL-1α

IL-1β

    IL-12, also known as natural killer cell-stimulating factor, is a heterodimeric cytokine produced by monocytes and B-cells. It has multiple effects on T and natural killer cells and is a potent inducer of Th1 cytokine IFNγ. Treatment with IL-12 prolonged survival of SCID mice infected with *Toxoplasma gondii*. Treatment with murine IL-12 during the first week of infection with *Leishmania major* cured a majority of the normally susceptible BALB/c mice and provided durable resistance against reinfection. IL-12 may prevent Th2 responses that are deleterious in certain infections and promote protective IFNγ-based Th1 responses.

IL-12

TNF

TNF has been shown to possess protective effects against a variety of pathogens. Recombinant human TNFα exhibited a distinct antiviral activity on various cell cultures infected with encephalomyocarditis virus and against vesicular stomatitis virus. Administration of TNF has been shown to confer protection against bacterial infections by *K. pneumoniae*, *Streptococcus pneumoniae*, *Legionella*, disseminated *Mycobacterium*

TNF

avium, salmonellosis and *Listeria monocytogenes* infections in mice. *In vivo* injection of recombinant TNF in parasitic infections has been shown to inhibit experimental infections with *Plasmodium* species, cutaneous leishmaniasis, *Trypanosoma cruzi* and *Toxoplasma gondii* infections in mice.

An excessive production of TNF with subsequent dysregulation of physiologic responses can, however, occur in cases of severe infection. The evidence for a pathophysiological involvement of TNF in a variety of disease states including AIDS, sepsis and malaria has steadily accumulated during the last decade. An immunopathological role has been ascribed to TNF also in other states such as inflammatory joint disease, allograft rejection and cachexia. Downregulation of TNF in these conditions should have a potential for therapy. This has provided the rationale for development of potential therapeutic strategies based on interrrupting the production of inflammatory TNF.

Dichotomy of cytokine application

The examples cited above amply demonstrate that cytokines have the potential for enhancing resistance against diverse pathogens. IL-2, IL-12, TNF and interferons may be useful in potentiating host antimicrobial defense via stimulation of the host effector cells. Other cytokines such as IL-1, IL-3 and haematopoietic growth factors alone and in combination are considered to be beneficial in treatment of infections associated with neutropenia, neonatal septicaemia or in prevention of infections accompanying aplastic anaemia, chemotherapy, immunodeficiency or burn injury.

IL-2

Host response to exogenously administered cytokines can, however, be dichotomous. Cytokines are often described as double-edged swords and have been attributed both beneficial and harmful effects. IL-2 acts as a potent growth factor for clonal expansion of T-lymphocytes, plays a pivotal role in T-cell-mediated immune responses, and has been shown to confer protection in several infectious disease models. Application of IL-2 in immunodeficiency states has been an obvious choice. Several studies with IL-2 therapy in AIDS patients showed that, although certain immunological parameters were improved, the results in terms of survival were poor. Paradoxically, a higher incidence of bacterial infections has been observed in AIDS patients receiving IL-2. *In vitro* investigations showed that IL-2 increased the production of HIV by naturally infected mononuclear cells from seropositive donors [17] and enhanced the translocation of bacteria from intestines to other organs in animal studies. In another model, administration of human recombinant TNF to mice with severe but clinically inapparent lymphocytic chori-omeningitis virus infection caused rapid death. In contrast, TNF given earlier in the course of disease prevented mortality, and pretreatment protected against development of lethal disease [18].

TNF

Limitations of therapy with exogenous cytokines have to be recognised. These are associated with the inherent toxicity of such materials, their unclear pharmacological behavior and their pleiotropic effects. Efficacy of exogenous cytokines capable of potentiating normal host defence mechanisms may be curtailed in immunocompromised patients lacking pertinent effector cells or containing disease-related factors which prevent lymphocyte activation. Viral, bacterial, fungal and parasite adaptations to the presence of cytokines can pose new problems. Approaches that are based on cytokine intervention will have to take these factors into account. The exact molecular mechanisms underlying the manifestation of protective or antagonistic activities have to be elucidated before cytokines become established clinically as a broad therapeutic modality for microbial infections.

Mild plant and dietary immunostimulants

Michael J. Parnham

Introduction

Plants and minerals have been used since ancient times for the treatment of many ailments and diseases. Most were used for mystical reasons, and others relied on the "doctrine of signatures", which stated that the shape of the plant reflected its potential medicinal use. The root of the mandrake or ginseng, for instance, is shaped like that of the human body and has been used as a general tonic for a variety of illnesses [1]. It is claimed by herbalists to have immunostimulant properties. Siberian ginseng or taiga root (*Eleutherococcus senticosus*) is also used as a tonic and has been reported to exhibit immunostimulatory properties. The pharmacological bases of these actions are unclear, so that these plant medicines cannot be considered unequivocally as immunostimulants.

ginseng and tonics

In recent years, many folklore remedies have been subjected to pharmacological study and some have been shown to exhibit therapeutic immunostimulant properties. Antioxidant dietary constituents also have been shown to exert immunoprotective or immunostimulant properties and are widely sold as prophylactic nutritional supplements. Some of the compounds for which clear immunostimulatory actions have been described are discussed in this chapter. Combination products are not considered, since little scientific basis is available for their efficacy.

Plant immunostimulants

Purple coneflower (*Echinacea*)

History

The purple coneflower (Fig. 1) is indigenous to North America and was used by the American Indians of the Great Plains as a universal remedy,

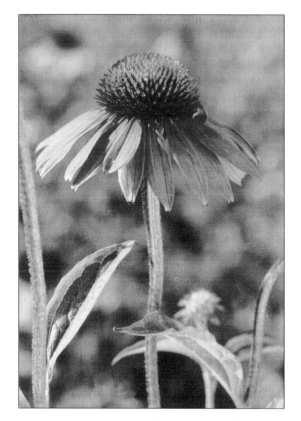

Figure 1 Purple coneflower (Echinacea purpurea)
Photo kindly provided by Madaus AG, Cologne, Germany.

particularly for colds, sore throats and pain [2]. Extracts of *E. angustifolia* (narrow-leaved purple coneflower) were introduced into medical practice in the United States at the end of the 19th century, becoming the most widely used medicinal plants by the 1930s. With the introduction of antibiotics, *Echinacea* fell into disuse. In Europe, *E. angustifolia* was introduced into homeopathic practice in response to publications from the United States. In 1937, a general lack of supplies subsequently led to the introduction of the common purple coneflower (*E. purpurea*) to Germany, where the squeezed sap was marketed. Most of the pharmacological studies on *Echinacea* have been performed in Germany on this preparation.

Chemical constituents

Compounds isolated from *Echinacea* species include caffeic acid derivatives, flavonoids, ethereal oils, polyacetylenes, alkylamides, alkaloids and polysaccharides [3]. Ingredients thought to contribute to the immunostimulatory properties of *Echinacea* include cichoric acid and an acid arabinogalactan.

Pharmacology

The squeezed sap of *E. purpurea* stimulates the phagocytic activity of neutrophils *in vitro* and *in vivo*. The response is moderate, but a significant increase in phagocytosis has been observed following repeated oral administration to healthy volunteers [3]. Stimulation of macrophages by *E. purpurea* has also been observed. The acid arabinogalactan isolated from the preparation is thought to be a major active component as it stimulates the cytotoxic actions of and transient cytokine release from mouse macrophages [3]. Release of cytokines probably accounts for the rise in body temperature observed in early studies on intravenous administration of *E. purpurea* [4], a route which is now rarely used. Other actions, such as stimulation of leukocyte adherence, also probably contribute to the oral activity of the preparation. Administered topically to the skin, the squeezed sap of *E. purpurea* enhances wound healing, probably by inhibiting hyaluronidase leading to increased hyaluronic acid secretion.

acid arabino-galactan and macrophage cytotoxicity

wound healing

Because of the uncertainty about the active constituent(s), no pharmacokinetic data are available on the squeezed sap of *E. purpurea*. Commercial preparations contain 60–80 g squeezed sap per 100 g.

Clinical indications

Nonhomeopathic preparations of *E. purpurea* (e.g. Echinacin, Echinaforce; Esberitox mono) are used orally for the adjuvant treatment of respiratory and urinary tract infections and topically for wound healing. Double-blind, controlled clinical trials have confirmed moderate efficacy in the treatment of mild respiratory infections [4]. Efficacy in the treatment of vaginal candidiasis has only been reported in open studies.

respiratory and urinary tract infections

Side effects

No adverse effects which are specific to *E. purpurea* have been observed, but as with all plant extracts, hypersensitivity responses have been reported which in rare cases can be severe.

Mistletoe (*Viscum album*)

History

Mistletoe (Fig. 2) has been used for centuries in Europe as a traditional herbal treatment for infections. In the last century, Rudolf Steiner, the originator of anthroposophy, suggested its use as a remedy for cancer. Biochemical analysis of mistletoe constituents led in the 1980s to the isolation and characterization of specific cytotoxic lectins which are responsible for the antitumor activity of the extract [5].

Chemical constituents

cytotoxic lectins

The main immunostimulatory constituents of mistletoe are the glycosylated lectins, ML-I, ML-II and ML-III. The major component is ML-I, which is used to standardize mistletoe extracts. It consists of two polypeptide chains linked by a disulphide bridge. Other constituents of mistletoe include flavonoids, viscotoxins and polysaccharides.

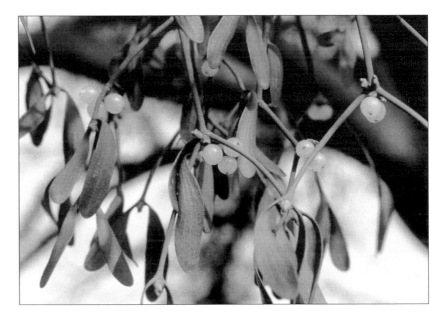

*Figure 2 Mistletoe (*Viscum album*)*
Photo kindly provided by Madaus AG, Cologne, Germany.

Pharmacology

ML-1 has a broad range of affinities for α/β-linked galactopyranosyl residues. High nanogram concentrations of all three mistletoe lectins are cytotoxic, ML-III being the most active. This action appears to be related to induction of apoptosis. At lower concentrations, ML-I and ML-I-standardized mistletoe extracts stimulate release of interleukins 1 and 6 and tumor necrosis factor α (TNFα) from peripheral blood mononuclear and skin cells [6]. Repeated doses of mistletoe extract at an ML-I equivalent of 1 ng/kg subcutaneously (s.c.) in cancer patients cause an increase in body temperature, increases in circulating helper T-cells and natural killer (NK) cells and enhanced expression of IL-2 receptors (CD25) on lymphocytes [7]. A direct stimulatory action on T-cells is likely. In mice, mistletoe extract reduces formation of melanoma metastases. Mistletoe extract is inactive on oral administration and only exhibits immunostimulatory activity on parenteral injection.

apoptosis

T-cell stimulation

Clinical indication

In German-speaking countries, ML-I-standardized mistletoe extract (e.g. Iscador, Lektinol) is administered intracutaneously at 0.5–1.0 ng/kg twice weekly for at least 3 months in cancer patients. Quality of life is reported to be improved in recent clinical trials.

cancer therapy

Side effects

Mistletoe extract can cause fever, headache, orthostatic hypotension and allergic reactions.

Dietary antioxidants

Several constituents of the normal diet help to protect against the damaging effects on lipid membranes of reactive oxygen species, such as superoxide anion, H_2O_2 and hydroxyl radical which are formed during a variety of physiological oxidation processes. Vitamin E is a lipid-soluble antioxidant which breaks the chain reaction of lipid peroxidation by scavenging peroxy radicals. The resulting vitamin E radical is transferred to water-soluble antioxidants, such as vitamin C (ascorbate), for excretion

glutathione peroxidase

in the urine. Selenium is an essential dietary trace element which is incorporated into the active site of the enzyme glutathione peroxidase (GSH-Px). GSH-Px catalyses the breakdown of hydroperoxides to hydroxy acid (oxidizing GSH to GSSG), thereby complementing the action of vitamin E (Fig. 3).

Among these nutrients, vitamin E and selenium have been shown to have clear immuno-stimulant/immunoprotective properties and play a role in disease prophylaxis.

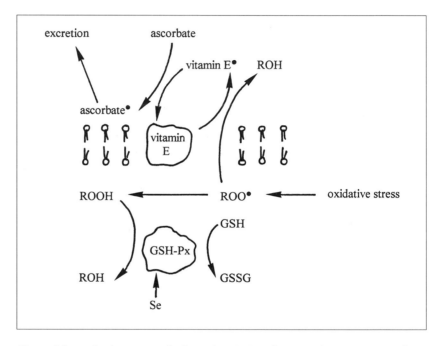

Figure 3 Interplay between selenium, vitamin E and vitamin C in protection of membranes from oxidative damage
(ROOH = lipid hydroperoxide, ROO·, hydroperoxy radical, ascorbate·, semidehydroascorbate radical, vitamin E·, vitamin E radical).

Vitamin E

History

Vitamin E was discovered in 1922 by H. Evans and K. Bishop as a dietary factor required for normal rat reproduction. It was officially recognized only in 1968. Vitamin E is a generic description for all tocol and tocotrienol derivatives exhibiting the biological activity of α-tocopherol.

Pharmacology

Lymphocytes and mononuclear cells have the highest vitamin E content of any cells in the body. Exposure of these cells to oxidative stress, such as that which occurs during inflammation or infection, leads to a loss of vitamin E and cellular dysfunction. Addition of vitamin E *in vitro* to lymphocytes which have been subjected to lipid peroxidation reverses immunosuppression, measured in terms of cell proliferation and antibody formation. This protective action of vitamin E is seen most clearly in experimental vitamin E deficiency in animals. Under these conditions, antibody titres and antibody-forming cells are severely depressed, T-cell responses, including proliferation and IL-2 production, are decreased, and mortality to various infections is enhanced [8]. In all cases, supplementation with vitamin E reverses the immunosuppression. Prolonged vitamin E supplementation of mice also partially reverses immunosuppression caused by retrovirus infection [9].

lymphocyte vitamin E and immunosuppression

Vitamin E deficiency in humans is rare, but can arise in preterm infants, in association with impaired neutrophil phagocytic capacity. Phagocytic activity can be restored by administration of vitamin E to newborn children, including those with glutathione deficiency [10].

neutrophil phagocytosis

Vitamin C is present at high concentrations in neutrophils and is required for optimal phagocytosis [8]. Little data is available, however, on the immunostimulant effect of combined vitamin C and E supplementation.

Clinical use

Vitamin E supplements are available for the treatment of deficiency symptoms and for the protection of muscles, blood vessels and the immune system from the effects of oxidation. The most convincing indication for clinical supplementation with vitamin E to achieve immunostimulation is the aging subject. The activities of antioxidant enzymes decrease with age, leading to a general increase in lipid peroxide tone in the body. In several double-blind controlled studies, supplementation of elderly subjects with vitamin E for several months augmented delayed-type hypersensitivity skin tests and proliferative responses of mononuclear cells to mitogen [11]. Whether this enhancement of immune responses by prophylactic vitamin E supplementation leads to an increase in resistance to infectious diseases in humans remains to be demonstrated. Epidemiological studies which suggest a protective effect of vitamin E against cancer cannot be interpreted solely on the basis of possible ef-

aging and immunosuppression

fects on the immune system, because protection against cell damage in general is also involved in the response to vitamin E.

Side effects

The evidence is compelling that intake of vitamin E above the recommended daily allowance (RDA) is of benefit to health. Vitamin E, given orally, has a very low toxicity. The RDA in the United States is 10 mg. At daily doses up to 3000 mg, vitamin E is without any side effects.

Selenium

History

liver damage

glutathione peroxidase

thyroxine metabolism

The element selenium was discovered in 1818 by the Swedish chemist Berzelius, who named it after Selene, the Greek goddess of the moon. A biological role for selenium was first demonstrated in 1957 by Klaus Schwarz, who found that selenium protected against dietary liver degeneration in rats. Subsequently, in 1973, Flohé in Germany and Rotruck in the United States showed that selenium is present at the active site of the enzyme GSH-Px. Two types of selenium-containing GSH-Px enzymes are now known, the classical GSH-Px and a phospholipid hydroperoxide-specific GSH-Px. In 1991, type I iodothyronine deiodinase, which converts thyroxine to its active metabolite, was found to be a selenocysteine-containing enzyme [12]. Because many geographical areas, particularly Finland, parts of China and New Zealand, have a low soil selenium content, nutritional supplementation with sodium selenite or selenium-enriched yeast is widespread.

Pharmacology

phagocytosis

Diet-induced selenium deficiency is associated with a variety of defects in neutrophil and lymphocyte functions in experimental and domestic animals which are reversed by selenium supplementation [13]. These defects are considered to be due to a reduction in the activity of protective GSH-Px in association with increased production of reactive oxygen species, such as that occurring during the oxidative burst of phagocytes. As a result, cells in the vicinity of actively phagocytosing cells are damaged. This process also occurs to some extent in selenium-adequate animals, in which GSH-Px activity decreases in cells at local sites of inflammation. In neutrophils from humans with a low selenium status, sodium selenite added *in vitro* is able to enhance the phagocytic and bactericidal activities of the cells [14], probably by protecting them from autolytic damage.

In addition to protecting phagocytes from damage, inorganic selenium administered to animals in nutritional excess has been shown to enhance antibody titres in response to vaccines or sensitization to erythrocytes. Studies on human lymphocytes *in vitro* suggest that sodium selenite selectively enhances the synthesis of immunoglobulin G (IgG) antibodies [15]. However, the effective dose range for selenium supplementation above nutritional requirements is relatively narrow, since increasing the dose leads to immunosuppression. Enhancement of cytotoxic lymphocyte activity is a consistent response to selenium supplementation of animals and humans in nutritional excess, with increased expression of IL-2 receptors on peripheral T-cells [13]. Administered to patients on hemodialysis, selenium supplementation (200–500 µg, 3 times weekly) enhanced T-cell responses to mitogens as well as delayed hypersensitivity responses [16].

antibody synthesis

enhanced T-cell responses

Clinical use

Sodium selenite or seleno-yeast is widely available as a nutritional supplement, providing 50–100 µg selenium/day. This is of benefit immunologically in subjects with inadequate selenium intake, including patients on total parenteral nutrition. Although serum selenium status is low in various inflammatory skin diseases and rheumatoid arthritis, clear therapeutic benefit of nutritional supplementation with selenium has yet to be demonstrated. Like vitamin E, selenium supplementation enhances lymphocyte proliferation responses in the elderly [17]. There is growing evidence that prolonged selenium intake in nutritional excess is associated with a reduced incidence of a variety of cancers.

Side effects

Selenium as sodium selenite or selenomethionine is considered to be nontoxic on repeated ingestion up to approximately 1000 µg of selenium per day. Above this dose, hair and nail loss and skin lesions can arise. At higher intakes, nervous system abnormalities, including numbness, convulsions and paralysis occur.

335

Emerging therapies

In addition to the search for the active immunostimulatory agents in extracts of *E. purpurea*, *V. album* and *Eleutherococcus senticosus*, a wide variety of plants are under investigation worldwide for immunostimulants, antibacterial and anticancer constituents. Plants are a rich source of novel compounds which can act as prototypes for synthetic substances.

ebselen

Based upon the role of selenium in GSH-Px, a benzisoselenazolone, ebselen, which has GSH-Px-like activity, is under clinical development as an antiinflammatory agent, specifically for cerebral ischemia; the discovery of this compound has stimulated a search for other antiinflammatory or immunomodulatory agents [18]. Ebselen and a variety of other selenoorganic compounds have been found to be cytokine inducers *in vitro* and *in vivo* and have been proposed as potential antiviral agents [19].

self-medication and mild immuno-stimulants

The immune system is subjected to a wide variety of stress factors in Western society. These include overwork, lack of exercise, air pollution and processed foods. Although it is often financially impracticable to perform extensive clinical studies on mild immunostimulants, it is widely agreed that in view of these stress factors, the benefit of dietary antioxidants in nutritional excess is probably greater than has been demonstrable as yet. It is likely that with increasing emphasis on self-medication to reduce health budgets, the commercial importance of plant and dietary immunostimulants for the therapy and prophylaxis of mild infectious disorders will increase. As a result, further scientific data on their pharmacological and clinical effects are expected in the future.

Immunosuppressives: transplant rejection inhibitors and cytotoxic drugs

Henk-Jan Schuurman, Gerhard Zenke and Max H. Schreier

Introduction

Suppression of immune reactivity can either be an undesirable effect or a situation which is specifically induced to the benefit of a patient. Examples of the first come from immunotoxicology, e.g. xenobiotics or environmental factors causing immunosuppression (see Chapter D1). Virus infections, as exemplified by human immunodeficiency virus, can cause severe immunodeficiency. Under clinical conditions suppression of the immune system is specially indicated in two indications: autoimmunity and organ transplantation [1]. Autoimmune diseases like rheumatoid arthritis are mainly treated by inhibition of the effector phase with antiinflammatory drugs like corticosteroids (see Chapter C9) but the use of T-cell immunosuppressants like cyclosporine, which was mainly developed for transplantation, has shown benefit in patients with autoimmune diseases.

why immuno-suppression?

In contrast, in organ transplantation there is a principal need for interference with the initiation of an immune response which is induced by the grafted organ. Generally, high-dose immunosuppression is needed in the first posttransplant period (induction treatment), or in the treatment of rejection episodes. To keep graft function stable, so-called maintenance treatment is given. Originally, when transplantation was introduced as a treatment of end-stage organ failure, there were few possibilities to prevent or treat allograft rejection. In the sixties and early seventies, this was mainly restricted to combinations of azathioprine, corticosteroids and cyclophosphamide. Combinations of these drugs were effective, but associated with severe side effects, mainly related to bone marrow depression (leukopenia, anaemia). The only more specific reagent, anti-lymphocyte globulin (ALG), became available in 1966 and was used in induction treatment immediately after transplantation. Based on these drugs, kidney transplantation developed slowly, and the lack of appropriate immunosuppressive regimens slowed down the introduction of heart transplantation in clinical medicine after it was first performed in 1963.

organ transplantation

Principles of Immunopharmacology, ed. by F. P. Nijkamp and M. J. Parnham
©1999 Birkhäuser Verlag Basel/Switzerland

xenobiotic immuno- suppression

The most widely used immunosuppressives at present are xenobiotics, i.e. orally active drugs produced by microorganisms or chemically synthesized molecules [2, 3]. A landmark in immunosuppression for transplantation was the introduction of cyclosporine (Sandimmmune, now Neoral) in 1983 [4]. Using cyclosporine as a basic immunosuppressant in combination with azathioprine and corticosteroids, 1-year graft survival in kidney transplantation increased to 80–90% and also heart transplantation reaches a 1-year patient survival of about 80%. In most transplant centres, induction immunosuppressive treatment during the first 2–4 weeks after transplantation nowadays includes either triple therapy, i.e. cyclosporine, azathioprine (Imuran) and corticosteroids, or quaduple therapy, in which antibody OKT3 (muronomab-CD3, Orthoclone OKT3) or another anti-lymphocyte antibody (ATG, anti-thymocyte globulin) are added to the immunosuppressive regimen. Cyclosporine treatment is monitored on the basis of blood concentration, and that of azathioprine on the basis of blood leukocyte counts. As cyclosporine side effects primarily concern the kidney, in a number of centres patients with a kidney transplant are first treated with cyclosporine after good kidney

induction and maintenance immuno- suppression

function is achieved. When patients show stable graft function, the induction treatment is gradually converted into maintenance treatment, in which lower cyclosporine doses are used, and another aim is to reduce corticosteroid and azathioprine treatment (so either triple treatment with low-dose cyclosporine, azathioprine and corticosteroids, or double cyclosporine-corticosteroid treatment). Rejection crises (documented by histopathology of a graft biopsy or biochemical markers in blood) are normally at first treated with high-dose intravenous corticosteroids (bolus injections on 3–5 successive days): so-called steroid-resistant rejections are to be treated at first by antibodies, either OKT3, ATG or in severe forms anti-lymphocyte globulin (ALG).

new immuno- suppressives

New immunosuppressants have nowadays been introduced like FK506 (tacrolimus, Prograf) and mycophenolate mofetil (RS-61443, Cellcept), 15-deoxyspergualin (gusperimus, Spanidin), and mizoribine (Bredinin), or are in an advanced stage of development (rapamycin or sirolimus, Rapamune; leflunomide, Arava) [5, 6] (Table 1, Fig. 1). Remarkably, most of these xenobiotic immunosuppressives originated from antiinfection or cancer drug development programmes; because of their failure in these indications or because immunosuppression was observed

Figure 1 (continued on next page)

Structures of cyclosporine, FK506, rapamycin, mycophenolate mofetil and mycophenolic acid, mizoribine, leflunomide and its active metabolite A 77 1726, brequinar, FTY 720, 15-deoxyspergualin, azathioprine, cyclophosphamide and methotrexate.

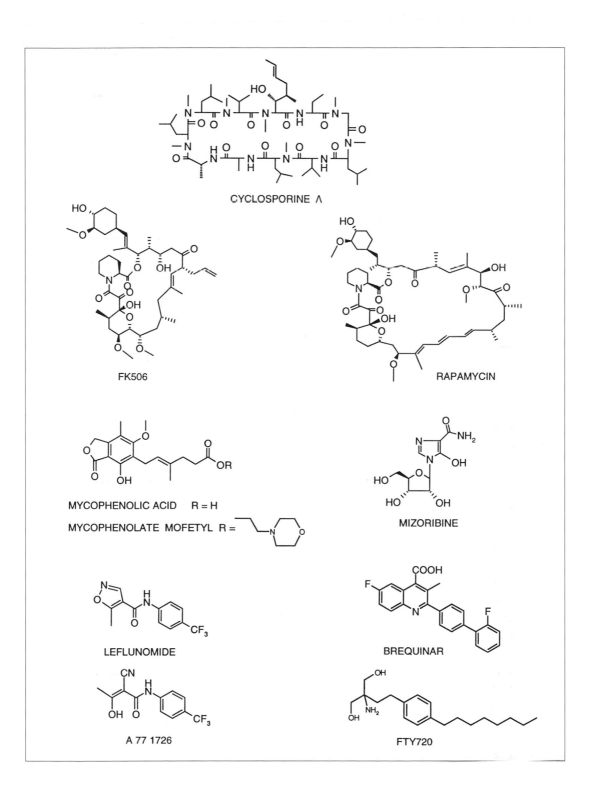

CYCLOSPORINE A

FK506

RAPAMYCIN

MYCOPHENOLIC ACID   R = H

MYCOPHENOLATE MOFETYL   R =

MIZORIBINE

LEFLUNOMIDE

BREQUINAR

A 77 1726

FTY720

339

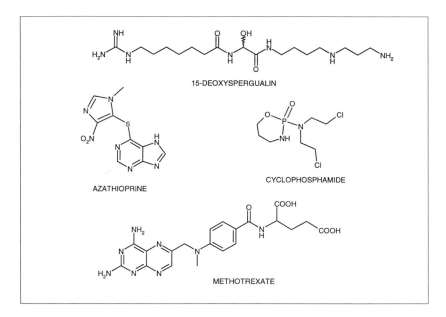

15-DEOXYSPERGUALIN

AZATHIOPRINE

CYCLOPHOSPHAMIDE

METHOTREXATE

Figure 1 (continued)

complications of immuno-suppression

as a "side effect", the drugs were subsequently developed as immuno-suppressants. Only FK506 was specifically developed as an immuno-suppressant and turned out to have the same mechanism of action as cy-closporine. All these drugs work intracellularly, by inhibition of early or late events in intracellular signalling after lymphocyte activation, or by inhibition of cell proliferation (direct interference in DNA/RNA synthe-sis) following activation. As these intracellular pathways are not truly se-lective for lymphocytes, these drugs have a quite narrow therapeutic win-dow. Their side effects can be reduced by combination treatment: ad-ministration at lower doses in combinations which are synergistic in immunosuppression can be associated with higher therapeutic windows. The different classes of drugs will be described further in the following sections.

With the present spectrum of immunosuppressants and extensive clinical experience with various drug combinations, the management of immunosuppression in patients with transplanted organs has markedly improved. However, major complications that are directly associated with immunosuppression still occur, such as drug toxicity, increased sus-ceptibility to infection and development of tumors, and in particular so-called posttransplant lymphoproliferative disease. On the other hand,

chronic rejection

long-term graft survival is hampered by graft dysfunction due to chron-

Table 1 Main immunosuppressants presently on the market or in advanced clinical development

Compound	Trade name	Mechanism of action
Xenobiotics		
Cyclosporine	Neoral	calcineurin inhibitor
FK506, tacrolimus	Prograf	calcineurin inhibitor
Rapamycin, sirolimus	Rapamune	inhibitor of growth factor-driven cell proliferation
Cyclophosphamide		inhibitor of cell proliferation
Methotrexate		inhibitor of cell proliferation: antiinflammatory
Azathioprine	Imuran	inhibitor of cell proliferation
Mizoribine	Bredinin	inhibitor of inosine monophosphate dehydrogenase
Mycophenolate mofetil	Cellcept	inhibitor of inosine monophosphate dehydrogenase
Leflunomide	Arava	inhibitor of dihydroorotate dehydrogenase
15-Deoxyspergualin	Spanidin	inhibitor of cell differentiation
Biologicals		
OKT3	Orthoclone-OKT3	T-cell depletion
CD25 antibody, basiliximab	Simulect	depletion of CD25$^+$ T-cells
CD25 antibody, daclizumab	Zenapax	depletion of CD25$^+$ T-cells
CD4 antibody		depletion of CD4$^+$ cells
CD52 antibody	Enlimomab	depletion of leukocytes
anti-TNFα antibody	Remicade	TNF blockade
CTLA4-Ig		inhibition of costimulation

ic rejection. This phenomenon not only relates to the immune response of the recipient to the graft, but also to intrinsic changes in the graft itself, mainly regarding the vasculature, so-called graft vessel disease or accelerated graft arteriosclerosis. This involves thickening of the intima of blood vessels of the graft and is ascribed to migration of smooth muscle cells to this site followed by cellular proliferation and extracellular matrix formation. With prolonged graft survival, chronic rejection is now a major cause of graft loss in long-term surviving patients. Drugs for the prevention or treatment of this condition are not yet available. Some new immunosuppressants (rapamycin, mycophenolate mofetil) are claimed to be effective, as these not only contribute to better immunosuppression (diminished host attack), but also inhibit the vascular response due to their inherent mechanism of action.

Since allograft rejection is a T-cell mediated process, the main target for immunosuppression in transplantation is the T-lymphocyte. But other cell types of the immune system like B-lymphocytes and macrophages are involved to a variable extent as well. The role of natural killer cells in graft rejection is still unclear. This might change in the future when xenotransplantation (transplantation of nonhuman organs into humans) will become available. The rejection of xenografts cannot be prevented by T-cell immunosuppressants since it involves not only T-cells but also B-lymphocytes, which are triggered in a T-cell independent way. This is also relevant in allotransplantation, because B-cell reactivity appears to be involved in chronic rejection as well. There are no specific B-cell drugs available as yet, but a number of immunosuppressants discussed below show both T- and B-cell inhibitory activity.

Calcineurin inhibitors

Cyclosporine

Cyclosporine (Cyclosporin A), is a cyclic undecapeptide isolated from the fungus *Tolypocladium inflatum gams*. Its biological activity *in vivo* was first dicovered in 1973 in a large microbiology screening programme, which included antibody formation to sheep red blood cells in mice [4]. Subsequently, it showed efficacy in kidney allotransplantation in rats and pigs (1977). This was followed by first clinical trials in human kidney transplant patients, and its introduction to clinical transplantation in 1983. Since cyclosporine is a highly lipophilic molecule, it is poorly soluble in water; for oral administration the first commercial formulation was an oil-based formulation with variable absorption. Since the drug shows a relatively narrow therapeutic window, the kidney being the first target for undesirable side effects, drug level monitoring proved necessary to control drug exposure in the therapeutic range without these side effects. Presently, a microemulsion formulation (Neoral) is marketed that shows improved absorption and far less inter- and intraindividual variation.

Cyclosporine shows immunosuppressive activity in a large spectrum of animal models of human immune-mediated diseases [7]. Its suppressive effect is mainly restricted to T-lymphocytes. T-cell-independent B-cell responses are not affected. At the time of introduction the mechanism of action of cyclosporine was largely unknown. A first insight into the mode of action of the compound came from the observation that the compound inhibits the production of IL-2, one of the first cytokines produced after T-cell activation. Subsequently it was demonstrated that cyclosporine inhibits interleukin-2 (IL-2) gene transcription by interfering with the calcium-dependent intracellular signalling mechanism [8] (Fig. 2). A family of cytoplasmic proteins called cyclophilins (CYP in Fig. 2) has been identified which strongly binds to cyclosporine. Cyclophilins are enzymes catalysing cis-trans isomerization of peptidyl-prolyl bonds (so-called proline isomerase or rotamase activity, important for proper folding of newly synthesized proteins *in vivo*). This inhibition of rotamase activity, however, does not cause the immunosuppressive effect, which is actually mediated by the binding of the cyclosporine-immunophilin complex to the serine/threonine phosphatase calcineurin (CNA, CNB in Fig. 2), which plays a pivotal role in calcium-dependent intracellular signalling.

cyclophilin binding

Activation of T-cells via the T-cell receptor results in a cascade of events that among others involves the activation of the protein tyrosine kinases $p56^{lck}$, $p59^{fyn}$ and zeta chain-associated protein 70 (ZAP-70), followed by phosphorylation of phospholipase Cγ1 resulting in generation of second messengers phosphatidyl inositol 1,4,5-triphosphate and diacylglycerol, which in turn yield an increase in cytoplasmic free Ca^{2+} and activation of protein kinase C. Free Ca^{2+} upon complexing with calmodulin activates the phosphatase calcineurin. The cyclosporine-cyclophilin complex upon binding to calcineurin inhibits its phosphatase activity. Calcineurin dephosphorylates the nuclear factor of activated T-cells (NFAT) which is then translocated to the nucleus, where it initiates together with other transcription factors (e.g. NF-κB and AP-1) expression of early T-cell activation genes, especially the IL-2 gene. Immunophilins and calcineurin are abundantly expressed in different cell types. The apparent T-cell selectivity of cyclosporine has therefore been related to the fact that Ca-dependent T-cell activation via the T-cell receptor uniquely involves the calmodulin-calcineurin pathway. There is as yet no unequivocal proof that potential side effects like damage to kidney tubules follow the same intracellular mechanism.

calcium dependent T-cell activation

In agreement with its mechanism of action, calcium-independent cell triggering is not affected by cyclosporine. For instance, T-cells can be activated via the costimulatory CD28 molecule on the cell surface which in combination with activated protein kinase C (see above) can yield lymphokine gene transcription and T-cell activation in the absence of calcineurin activation. It has therefore been hypothesized that this pathway is involved in T-cell activation and allograft rejection that is resistant to cyclosporine treatment.

cyclosporine-resistant pathway

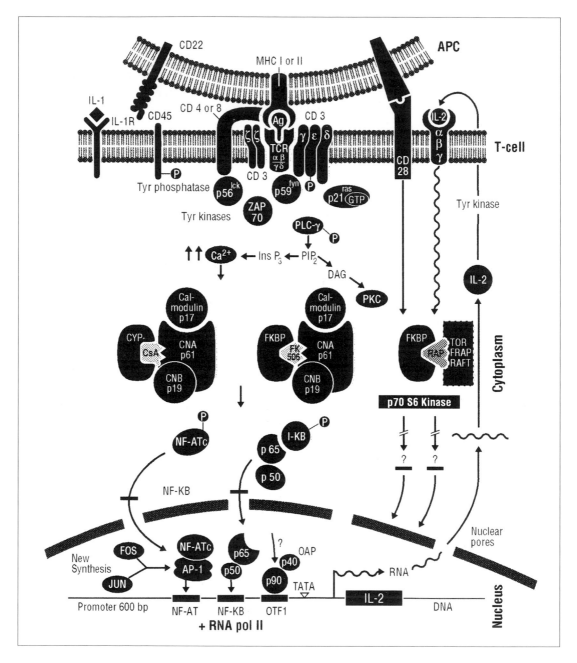

Figure 2

Intracellular signalling pathways and points of inhibition by cyclosporine (via binding to cyclophilin, CYP), FK506 (via binding to FKBP) and rapamycin (via binding to FKBP). Also cell surface molecules for biologicals (OKT3 binding to CD3; anti-IL-2 receptor antibodies) or those presently considered as potential drug targets (CD4, CD28, CD45) are shown. For explanations, see text.

FK506 (tacrolimus)

FK506 is a macrocyclic lactone isolated from the actinomycete *Streptomyces tsububaensis*. It was discovered in 1984 in an immunological screening programme specifically established to identify immunosuppressive compounds. Subsequently, its immunosuppressive activity was demonstrated in various animal models of transplantation (rat, dog). The spectrum of immunosuppressive activity appeared to be identical to that of cyclosporine, but remarkably at much lower doses than cyclosporine, both *in vitro* and *in vivo*. Also, therapeutic drug levels in the circulation appear to be much lower than those for cyclosporine. FK506 is very lipophilic and poorly soluble in water, resulting in variable absorption necessitating regular drug monitoring: for oral adminstration, a solid dispersion formulation in hydroxypropylmethyl cellulose is used. Major side effects are strikingly similar to those of cyclosporine but also involve the central nervous system as target organ. Difference from cyclosporine may at least in part be explained by differences in pharmacokinetics, as the mechanism of action appears to be the same. This does not hold for other side effects like the lack of gingiva hyperplasia and hirsutism of cyclosporine and the more pronounced diabetogenic effect of FK506.

discovery and development

The similarity between FK506 and cyclosporine regarding their immunosuppressive activity is based on the fact that both drugs inhibit calcineurin phosphatase activity and subsequent intranuclear events in T-cell activation (Fig. 2). However, in accord with the different molecular structure, FK506 does not bind to cyclophilins as cyclosporine does. A family of immunophilins with rotamase activity has been identified, called FK506 binding proteins (FKBPs). Of these, FKBP12 appears to be most relevant: upon binding to FK506, the complex binds to calcineurin at the same site as the cyclosporine-cyclophilin complex and thereby inhibits T-cell activation.

FK506 and cyclosporine: similar mechanism

The efficacy of FK506 in humans was first shown in liver transplantation. In liver disease, e.g. liver allograft dysfunction, the absorption of FK506 is increased and its metabolism decreased resulting in higher exposure, which is required in cases of rejection. Now the drug is widely used in patients that poorly tolerate cyclosporine treatment.

Inhibitors of growth factor modulation

Rapamycin (sirolimus)

discovery and
development

Rapamycin is a macrocyclic lactone, isolated from the actinomycete *Streptomyces hygroscopicus*, with a long history dating from the mid 1970s. It was first discovered as an antifungal compound, which was not further developed as side effects were encountered, including involution of lymphoid tissue. Subsequently, antitumor effects were documented, as well as immunosuppressive activity in rat models of autoimmune disease. After structural similarities between rapamycin and FK506 were identified, studies on the efficacy of the compound in rat and mouse organ allograft models were initiated and first reported in 1989. Since then, the compound has been developed for clinical use in transplantation. Launch is expected in 1999. A major complication was the development of a proper oral formulation with acceptable stability, bioavailability and predictability in absorption characteristics. The compound is very lipophilic and poorly soluble in water. In oily solution, as well as in microemulsion, the compound appears readily absorbed after oral administration.

mechanism of
action

Rapamycin proves to be an extremely potent immunosuppressant, affecting both T-lymphocytes and antibody production by B-lymphocytes, as demonstrated in a wide spectrum of experimental animal models, as well as in clinical trials in renal transplantation. This is achieved at relatively low blood levels *in vivo*. In animal models, the drug shows synergistic action in combinations with cyclosporine, which points to a difference in mechanism of action. Indeed, whereas cyclosporine and FK506 inhibit early events in T-cell activation, e.g. the expression of growth factors such as IL-2 in the G0–G1 stage of the cell cycle (see above), rapamycin inhibits progression of G1 to S phase of the cell cycle. At the molecular level, it has been demonstrated that rapamycin binds, like FK506, to immunophilins of the FKBP family, in particular FKBP12 (Fig. 2). The rapamycin-FKBP complex does not bind to calcineurin, but to target molecules called mTOR (mammalian targets of rapamycin; alternative names in literature are FRAP and RAFT, Fig. 2), proteins with a kinase activity. This rapamycin-FKBP-TOR complex inhibits, in an as yet undefined way, intracellular cytokine-driven cell proliferation, presumably via p70 S6 kinase, which is involved in translational control (Fig. 2). Apparently, this pathway is particularly relevant in lymphoid cells, underlying the peculiar imunosuppressive characteristics of the drug.

Since growth factor-driven cell proliferation applies to other cell types as well, the therapeutic window of the compound in immunosuppression is expected to be narrow. On the other hand, this antiproliferative action of the drug could be beneficial in chronic rejection of solid organ allografts. Indeed, it has been shown that rapamycin, in contrast to cyclosporine and FK506, inhibits the proliferation of smooth muscle cells *in vitro*, and in animal transplantation models the compound inhibits intima proliferation of blood vessels, as observed in chronic rejection. It remains to be seen whether this applies also to the clinical situation of patients with an organ allograft.

effect on chronic rejection

Cytotoxic drugs

The designation "cytotoxic drugs" is used here to describe drugs that directly interfere with DNA/RNA synthesis and as such affect cell proliferation.

Cyclophosphamide

Cyclophosphamide is one of the first immunosuppressive drugs described. It is an alkylating agent that was originally used as an anticancer drug. The compound inhibits cells from entering the S phase of the cell cycle, which is subsequently blocked at the G2 phase. The drug was used in initial trials in clinical transplantation around 1970, in particular in patients with azathioprine toxicity. Severe side effects were encountered, mainly bone marrow depression with severe leukopenia and anaemia. Since the introduction of more selective T-cell immunosuppressants, the drug has barely been used because of these side effects. However, cyclophosphamide is among the most powerful inhibitors of B-cells, and has received renewed interest for experimental animal research in xenotransplantation.

'old' but still potent immunosuppressant

Methotrexate

Methotrexate is a folate antagonist, which nowadays is mainly used in a low-dose treatment regimen (weekly administration) in subsets of patients with rheumatoid arthritis (see Chapter C10). Its mechanism of action under these conditions is not completely resolved. It has been suggested that low-dose methotrexate is converted into a polyglutamate that

immunosuppressive and antiinflammatory drug

347

inhibits transmethylation reactions, resulting in an increased release of adenosine and decreased synthesis of guanine. Although this condition affects purine metabolism, an antiinflammatory signal is delivered by the binding of adenosine to specific adenosine (A2) receptors. Thus, methotrexate at a low dose does not appear to be an immunosuppressant, but rather an antiinflammatory drug.

Azathioprine

'old' drug still used as adunct immuno-suppressant

Azathioprine is used from the early days of clinical immunosuppression, being introduced as an immunosuppressant for transplantation in 1961. Its development followed the pioneering work on 6-mercaptopurine as an antileukaemic agent in the 1940s. Nowadays the drug is still in use in conjunction with baseline immunosuppression (e.g. cyclosporine) in transplantation: its dosing and dose adaptations are based on the initial side effects, i.e. blood leukocyte counts. Despite its long clinical use, the exact mechanism of action is still not completely clear. The drug is converted by red blood cell glutathione to 6-mercaptopurine, which in turn is converted into a series of mercaptopurine-containing nucleotides which interfere with the synthesis of DNA and polyadenylate-containing RNA. One of the nucleotides formed is thioguanylic acid which can form thioguanosine triphosphate. This can be incorporated into nucleic acids and induce chromosome breaks as well as affecting the synthesis of coenzymes. As a general inhibitor of cell proliferation, azathioprine affects both T- and B-lymphocyte reactivity.

Mizoribine and mycophenolate mofetil

discovery and development

Mizoribine is an imidazole nucleoside, isolated as a potential antibiotic from the culture filtrate of the soil fungus *Eupenicillium brefeldianum*. Its immunosuppressive activity was demonstrated first by the inhibition of mouse lymphoma cell lines and subsequently by the inhibition of an antibody response in mice immunized with sheep erythrocytes. It was subsequently shown that the drug is phosphorylated intracellularly to the active form, mizoribine 5'-monophosphate, under the influence of adenosine kinase. This compound is a competitive inhibitor of the enzyme inosine monophosphate dehydrogenase (IMPDH), which is a rate-limiting enzyme in purine biosynthesis in lymphoid cells (Fig. 3). The drug has been in use in clinical transplantation since 1984, only in Japan, mainly as a replacement for azathioprine.

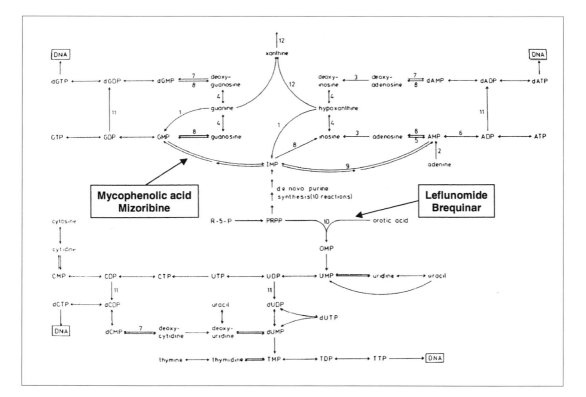

Figure 3 Purine/pyrimidine pathway and points of inhibition by mycophenolic acid, mizoribine, leflunomide and brequinar

For purine metabolism two pathways are shown, the salvage pathway (conversion of guanine into guanosine monophosphate, GMP, by hypoxanthine-guanine phosphoribosyltransferase, HGPRT) and the de novo pathway (conversion of inosine monophosphate into guanosine monophosphate, mediated by IMPDH). For pyrimidine metabolism the de novo pathway (conversion of orotic acid into uridine monophosphate, UMP) and the salvage pathway (conversion of uridine in UMP, and cytidine in cytidine monophosphate, CMP) are shown. Major enzymes involved are HGPRT (1), adenine phosphoribosyltransferase (2), adenosine deaminase (3), purine nucleoside phosphorylase (4), adenosine kinase (5), adenylate kinase (6), deoxycytidine kinase (7), 5'nucleotidase (8), adenosine monophosphate dehydrogenase (9), dihydroorotate dehydrogenase (10) and ribonucleotide reductase (11).

Mycophenolate mofetil is the morpholinoester of mycophenolic acid, a fermentation product of various *Penicillium* species, orginally isolated and purified in the early 1910s. Mycophenolic acid was originally studied for its antibacterial and antifungal activity, and subsequently its antitumor activity in the late 1960s, but these activities were not further followed up in clinical development. The compound was specifically selected as a drug inhibiting IMPDH in the mid-1980s: its selection was based on the fact that the compound is not a nucleoside, that it fails to require phosphorylation to become active, and that it does not show unwanted side effects of nucleosides such as induction of chromosome breaks and inhibition of DNA repair enzymes. Mycophenolic acid is a noncompetitive reversible inhibitor of IMPDH (Fig. 3). The morpholinoester of mycophenolic acid, mycophenolate mofetil, was developed as an immunosuppressant. It is rapidly hydrolysed by esterases to yield mycophenolic acid. The drug was introduced to the market in 1995 for the indication transplantation, mainly as a replacement for azathioprine.

IMPDH inhibition: selectivity

The fact that inhibition of IMPDH causes quite selective immunosuppression is related to the relevance of different pathways in purine metabolism in different cell types. Two pathways exist, the salvage pathway (conversion of guanine into guanosine monophosphate by hypoxanthine-guanine phosphoribosyltransferase, HGPRT) and the *de novo* pathway (conversion of inosine monophosphate into guanosine monophosphate, mediated by IMPDH). Lymphocytes highly depend on the *de novo* pathway and do not use the salvage pathway. In contrast, cells of the central nervous system highly depend on the salvage pathway. Cell types like smooth muscle cells, fibroblasts, endothelial cells and epithelial cells can use both pathways for purine synthesis. Hence, inhibition of IMPDH results in a quite selective inhibition of purine biosynthesis in lymphocytes. For mycophenolic acid, an additional selectivity has been documented for the two isoforms of IMDPH: the type I isoform is predominantly expressed in resting lymphocytes, and the type II is strongly expressed in lymphocytes after activation. This type II isoform is 4–5 times more sensitive to inhibition by mycophenolic acid than the type I isoform: hence mycophenolic acid is a more potent inhibitor of activated lymphocytes. As both T- and B-lymphocytes are affected by IMPDH inhibition, mizoribine and mycophenolate mofetil are effective inhibitors of both T- and B-lymphocytes. This has not only been demonstrated in rodent models but also for mycophenolate mofetil in pig-to-primate xenotransplantation models, where the suppression of xeno-antibody formation is a critical issue.

effect on cell adhesion

Apart from affecting RNA synthesis, IMPDH inhibition has other effects as well. IMDPH inhibition results in lymphocytes in depletion of guanosine triphosphate (GTP) (Fig. 3), which affects the transfer of fucose and mannose to glycoproteins, which include adhesion molecules on the cell surface. Examples of adhesion molecules whose expression is inhibited are very late antigen-4 (VLA-4) and ligands for selectins. On the basis of this mechanism, IMPDH inhibitors could affect the recruitment of inflammatory cells into tissue, and effector-target-cell interactions within tissue. This potential effect has been demonstrated by the inhibition of the adhesion of T-lymphocytes to endothelial cells *in vitro* when either T-cells or endothelial cells are pretreated with mycophenolic acid.

Finally, as IMDPH inhibition can affect cell growth in other cell types besides lymphocytes, it might have an effect in chronic rejection. Mycophenolic acid inhibits proliferation of human smooth muscle cells *in vitro*, and is effective in a rat vessel transplantation model, which mimics chronic rejection in solid organ allografts.

effect on chronic rejection

Leflunomide and brequinar

Leflunomide (HWA 486) is an isoxazole derivative, originally synthesized as part of a agriculture herbicide programme in the mid 1970s [9]. Its antiinflammatory activity was demonstrated in animal models of adjuvant arthritis and experimental allergic encephalomyelitis: first studies on its immunosuppressive action in models of autoimmune disease were documented in 1990. Since then, the compound has been extensively investigated in animal models of solid organ allo- and xeno-transplantation (rodents, dog, monkey): the compound proved to be a potent immunosuppressant both for T- and B-lymphocytes. Leflunomide has been clinically developed for rheumatoid arthritis. A major drawback for its development for the indication transplantation is the long half-life in humans (15–18 days): analogues (malononitriloamides) with a shorter half-life are in early development.

discovery and development

Leflunomide is a prodrug that under the influence of intestinal mucosa or liver is metabolized to the active isoxazole open-ring form (compound A77 1726, Fig. 1). The anti-proliferative action (entry into S phase of the cell cycle), although still not completely understood, is based on its inhibition of two different intracellular pathways. The first involves the enzyme dihydroorotate dehydrogenase (DHODH), which is the fourth rate-limiting sequential enzyme in the *de novo* pyrimidine biosynthetic pathway (Fig. 3). This pathway is particularly relevant for the proliferative response of lymphocytes, as limited intracellular pools of substrates restrict the use of the salvage pathway by these cells. Also, the intracellular concentration of DHODH is relatively low in lymphoid cells, so that this pathway is easily inhibited. Inhibition of DHODH results in depletion of intracellular pyrimidine nucleotides, which have several vital cellular functions, including synthesis of DNA, RNA, glycoproteins (adhesion proteins) and phospholipids. A second mechanism of action is inhibition of protein phosphorylation by inhibition of tyrosine kinase activity. The relevance of this mechanism for the immunosuppressive action of leflunomide is questionable, as kinase inhibition generally re-

DHODH inhibition: selectivity

tyrosine kinase inhibition

quires higher concentrations in *in vitro* experiments than the inhibition of DHODH.

T- and B-cell immunosuppression

Like inhibition of IMPDH, inhibition of DHODH affects not only T-cells but also B-cells; hence leflunomide has been been shown to be a potent drug affecting T-dependent and T-independent antibody synthesis. There are reports that leflunomide affects B-cells even more potently than T-lymphocytes. There are also claims that the drug might be effective in chronic rejection, as demonstrated by the *in vitro* inhibition of rat smooth muscle cell proliferation, and the efficacy *in vivo* in rodent vessel transplantation, a model mimicking vascular pathology in chronic rejection of solid organ allografts. This has not been followed up, since the drug is only developed for the indication rheumatoid arthritis. Apart from its immunosuppressive activity, the antiinflammatory action of the drug (inhibition of the production of inflammatory cytokines) might be relevant for this indication.

bredquinar

There is another drug with a similar mechanism of action as leflunomide, namely brequinar sodium (DUP 785). This is a substituted 4-quinolinecarboxylic acid analogue produced by organic synthesis. It was originally developed as an anticancer drug and subsequently as an immunosuppressant for the indication transplantation. It is a potent inhibitor of DHODH; like leflunomide it also inhibits protein tyrosine kinase but only at relatively high concentrations. Its clinical development has been halted because of a narrow therapeutic window and side effect profile (bone marrow depression, mainly thrombocytopenia).

Other immunosuppressive drugs

15-Deoxyspergualin (gusperimus)

discovery and development

15-Deoxyspergualin is a synthetic derivative of spergualin, an antibiotic isolated from the soil bacterium *Bacillus laterosporus* in a screening programme for anticancer drugs in the early 1980s. Its immunosuppressive activity in a mouse skin transplantation model was demonstrated in 1985, and the drug was subsequently developed for the indication transplantation. It has been available commercially in Japan since 1994. A major drawback in its clinical application is the low oral bioavailability of the drug, which means that it has to be administered parenterally.

T- and B-cell immunosuppression

15-Deoxyspergualin is a potent immunosuppressive compound in animal models of transplantation and autoimmunity. B-cells are equally inhibited as T-cells. However, the mechanism of action is less well understood than that of the compounds mentioned above. The compound affects the differentiation of stimulated lymphocytes into effector cells, e.g. cytotoxic T-cells or antibody-producing plasma cells, and the entry of cells from G0 or G1 into the S phase of the cell cycle. An inhibitory effect on macrophage activation has been claimed as well. At the molecular level, inhibition of polyamine biosynthesis and inhibition of DNA-polymerase activity has been documented. Also, binding of the compound to a cytosolic member of the heat-shock protein family, HSP70, has been described. Heat-shock proteins participate in the folding and unfolding of proteins and play a role in protein transport to intracellular organelles. The peptide-binding groove of this protein appears to be similar to that of MHC class I molecules. Therefore it has been suggested that 15-deoxyspergualin may compete for the peptide-binding groove and thereby inhibit antigen presentation.

heat-shock proteine binding

Biologicals

ALG/ATG/OKT3

Horse anti-lymphocyte globulin (ALG) and rabbit anti-thymocyte globulin (ATG) were originally introduced as immunosuppressants for induction treatment after transplantation or in treatment of rejection episodes. These reagents induce a severe but temporary depletion or inactivation of T-cells (in the case of ATG) or lymphocytes (ALG) from the circulation. OKT3 is a mouse immunoglobulin (Ig)G2a monoclonal antibody specific for the CD3 ε-chain of the T-cell receptor complex. Upon OKT3 binding to CD3, the entire receptor complex is modulated from the cell surface. This modulation results in depression of T-cell activity. The mechanism of action of OKT3 is not completely understood: there are claims that the antibody induces apoptosis of the cells.

history of development

OKT3 was the first monoclonal antibody to be approved for clinical application in the mid-1980s. Its use in either induction treatment, or treatment of steroid-resistant rejection, has shown the potential side effects of this class of biologicals. A major side effect is the so-called cytokine-release syndrome, which is related to the potent stimulatory activity of OKT3 (besides its depressing activity). This cytokine-release syndrome can emerge quickly upon first dosing and results in malaise, fever, myalgia, rigors, headache and diarrhoea, in more severe cases hypotension, wheezing and/or pulmonary edema. Also, a temporary rise in serum creatinine is part of this cytokine-release syndrome. A second side effect

OKT3

cytokine-release syndrome

is related to the fact that OKT3 is a mouse immunoglobulin, and thus can induce anti-mouse antibody formation. The presence of such antibodies in the circulation reduces the efficacy of OKT3 in subsequent courses of treatment.

new approaches: chimeric and humanized antibodies

In order to avoid the formation of anti-mouse antibodies and to restore the effector function of the specific monoclonal antibodies, later generation antibodies for clinical application are generated by genetic engineering. Two major approaches are followed: (1) chimeric antibody, in which the constant part of immunoglobulin heavy and light-chains in the mouse antibody molecule is replaced by human immunoglobulin sequences, and (2) humanized antibody, in which the sequence encoding the complementary determining regions of the variable part of the mouse antibody is inserted in the sequence encoding human immunoglobulin. The second approach may lead to a loss of binding affinity, as has been shown for the antibody daclizumab mentioned below. Engineered antibodies have the advantage that the half-life in the circulation can be substantially longer, e.g. from 24–48 h for a mouse antibody to 2–4 weeks for an engineered antibody. Although murine antigenic determinants are still present in the variable part of light and heavy-chains, albeit less so in the humanized antibody, the immunogenicity is strongly reduced.

Anti-IL-2 receptor antibodies

chimeric and humanized antibodies: first inclinics

The development of antibodies to the α-chain of the IL-2 receptor (anti-CD25 antibody) is based on the fact that this chain of the receptor is expressed on the surface of T-cells only after activation: in peripheral blood, CD25$^+$ cells are present in quite low numbers. Thus, CD25 antibodies are presumed to bind only activated T-cells. Two antibodies have recently been approved for the indication transplantation: one is a humanized antibody (daclizumab, Zenapax), and one is a chimeric molecule (basiliximab, Simulect). Both antibodies have been shown to reduce the incidence of acute rejection [10, 11] after kidney transplantation. There are no significant side effects, and CD25$^+$ T-cells are absent in circulation as long as receptor-saturating antibody levels are maintained.

New approaches and perspectives

For the development of novel immunosuppressants, several aspects have to be considered:

First, the major problem of current mainstream immunosuppressants is still toxicity (direct drug toxicity, increased susceptibility to infection, development of tumors). The development of drugs with fewer side effects may be most likely achieved by selecting targets for pharmacological intervention that are specifically relevant for the immune response and not for other (cell) biological processes. Besides selectivity, a critical aspect in the selection of new drug targets is the redundancy of potential targets. Nonredundancy of targets is demonstrated most convincingly by the phenotype of human primary immunodeficiencies and knockout mice. Interference with such targets is expected to be very effective. Specific for the immune system are different activation mechanisms which might be relevant for direct and indirect presentation of allograft antigens. Some of these new avenues in drug development will be discussed below: they concern either intracellular processes or cell surface interactions.

toxicity and selectivity

Second, for solid organ transplantation, chronic rejection is a major cause of chronic graft failure, and therefore there is a clinical need for drugs interfering with chronic rejection. Prevention or treatment of chronic rejection or graft vessel disease may require nonimmunological approaches in addition to improved novel immunosuppressants; these nonimmunologic approaches are not considered here.

chronic rejection

Third, specific drug targeting to the organ involved presents a possibility to cope with the systemic side effects of immunosuppressants. An example of this approach comes from lung transplantation, which generally requires strong immunosuppression and hence is associated with a rather small therapeutic window between immunosuppression and side effects. Using inhaled immunosuppressive therapy, for instance corticosteroids and cyclosporine, beneficial effects with more effective immunosuppression have been shown [12].

drug targeting

Fourth, the final goal in immunosuppression in transplantation and autoimmunity is the induction of tolerance, often referred to as the "Holy Grail", i.e. donor-specific unresponsiveness in the case of transplantation. Some examples of tolerance induction are given below.

tolerance

Finally, antisense technologies and gene therapy have developed during the last few years to such an extent that first applications in immunosuppression become feasible.

gene therapy

Antigen presentation to T-cells

Since the interaction between T-lymphocytes and antigen-presenting cells and the subsequent activation of T-cells are the central events leading to

costimulatory signalling

355

the activation of the immune system (in the case of transplantation to graft rejection), current approaches focus on molecules specifically involved in this process. Of special interest are molecules involved in the costimulation of T-cells, which according to the two-signal model are essential for T-cell activation (see Chapter A3). It is worth mentioning that compounds preventing T-cell costimulation have the potential to induce T-cell anergy or unresponsiveness, which could lead to antigen-specific tolerance.

targets and surface

One approach is to intervene at the cell surface with molecules intimately involved in antigen presentation using biologicals such as antagonistic monoclonal antibodies or soluble receptor antagonists. With respect to antibodies, purely blocking antibodies are distinguished from so-called depleting antibodies, which upon antigen binding destroy the corresponding cells via complement-mediated effects or antibody-dependent cellular cytotoxicity (ADCC). Surface molecules of special interest on the T-cell include, among others, CD2, CD4, CD28 and the related molecules CTLA4, CD45 and CD154 (CD40 ligand). Depleting

anti-CD4

and nondepleting anti-CD4 monoclonal antibodies have been studied most extensively. Encouraging results emerged from experimental organ transplantation in rodents and primates. In rodent transplantation, anti-CD4 antibodies have been used to induce donor-specific unresponsiveness. However, the mechanism responsible for this phenomenon is still unclear, especially for nondepleting antibodies. Moreover, application of these results in clinical transplantation has been of quite limited success. A humanized CD4 antibody is currently in development for the indication rheumatoid arthritis, however. Antibodies to CD2, which play an important role not only in T-cell activation but also in T-cell adhesion, have been shown to prevent allograft rejection in animal models. CTLA4-Ig, a fusion protein of the extracellular domain of CTLA4 and the constant domains of immunoglobulin, which prevents binding of the B7 molecules to CD28, one of the major T-cell costimulatory molecules, has been shown to be efficacious in several rodent and primate transplantation models. This biological is now in clinical trials. More recently, anti-CD154 monoclonal antibodies have been introduced, which especially in combination with CTLA4-Ig show very promising results in rodent transplantation models, including the prevention of chronic rejection. There is evidence now that anti-CD154 antibodies are effective in primate transplantation as well [13]. Monoclonal antibodies directed

anti-CD45

against the RB isoform of CD45, a lymphocyte-specific surface molecule with intracellular tyrosine phosphatase activity, have been described to prolong allograft survival in mice and monkeys.

On the antigen-presenting cell side, monoclonal antibodies to ligands of T-cell costimulatory molecules like CD80, CD86 and CD40 have been used successfully in transplantation models. Blocking CD40 is especially attractive, since CD40 is expressed not only on antigen-presenting dendritic cells but also on macrophages, B-cells and endothelial cells. It plays an important role in the activation of these cells with respect to upregulation of cell surface molecules involved in adhesion and costimulation of T-cells and of cytokine production. Further potential sites of intervention are at the level of antigen uptake, processing and assembly with major histocompatibility complex (MHC) class II molecules.

Drug discovery programmes are aimed at the identification of small molecular weight compounds which inhibit specific cell surface interactions. In contrast to the biologicals mentioned above, such inhibitors would have the advantage of being orally active. However, it might not be easy to identify small molecules which block the interactions of large protein surfaces.

low MW inhibitors

T-cell signal transduction

Present knowledge of T-cell transduction pathways (Chapter A3) has revealed potentially interesting targets for drug development. The signalling pathway emanating from the T-cell receptor includes, among others, T-cell-selective molecules such as protein tyrosine kinases of the src family (p56^{lck} and p59^{fyn}) and ZAP-70 (see also the section on calcineurin inhibitors above). The pivotal and selective role of ZAP-70 for T-cell activation is documented by the severe combined immunodeficiency phenotype of humans who lack functional ZAP-70. CD28 coreceptor signalling is less well defined and involves components of several pathways like JNK, PI3 kinase, p21^{ras} and p38 MAP kinase. The relative contribution of these cascades to overall CD28 signalling may depend on the state of activation of the T-cells and the level of CD28 activation. Interestingly, it has been reported that CD28 signalling may involve cyclosporine-resistant pathways (see above). All these kinases are potential targets for the development of new immunosuppressants. The major challenge here is to identify inhibitors with high selectivity which fail to inhibit other kinases, which are of critical importance in other cell types as well. A number of molecules that do not exhibit catalytic function act as specific adaptor molecules by mediating the interaction between different components of signal transduction pathways. Generally these proteins contain domains that are important for protein-protein interactions such as SH2/SH3 domains. These interactions are actively studied as potential drug targets as well. Here again, the major hurdle is to develop small molecular weight inhibitors which block the interaction of relatively large protein surfaces.

protein kinase

ZAP-70

CD28

Cytokines

cytokine redundancy

Immune cells communicate not only through direct contact of cell surface molecules, but also through cytokines (see Chapter A4). Recent cloning of cytokines and cytokine receptors, understanding of their function and elucidation of their signal transduction pathways has opened new possibilities for intervention (see anti-IL-2 receptor antibodies described above). However, especially in the field of cytokines, redundancy has to be considered. Of special interest is the paradigm of cytokines associated with T helper (Th)1/Th2 cells or immune deviation (see Chapter A3). It is suggested that transplant rejection may represent primarily a Th1 response, whereas transplantation tolerance may be favored by Th2 cells. However, it is unclear whether this hypothesis applies to allograft rejection in humans. Nevertheless, purified proteins, engineered proteins (antagonistic mutants), domains of proteins (soluble cytokine receptors) or antibodies are used to manipulate cytokine responses. Certain cytokines possessing intrinsic immunosuppressive properties, like IL-10 and transforming growth factor β (TGFβ), have been administered as such to treat rejection. Cytokines promoting Th2 responses (e.g. IL-4) or blockade of cytokines promoting Th1 responses (e.g. IL-12) might induce a beneficial deviation of the immune system towards a Th2 response. Interference with cytokines in the clinical setting so far has mainly been proved promising for an antibody to the inflammatory cytokine tumor necrosis factor α (TNFα) (Remicade), that is now in development for the indication rheumatoid arthritis [14].

Th1/Th2 pathways

TNFα antibody

JAK/STAT pathway

With regard to cytokine receptor signalling, the pathway involving Janus kinase (JAK) and signal transducer and activator of transcription (STAT) is of special interest. For transplantation, JAK3 seemed to be the most relevant since it is selectively associated with the common γ-chain of IL-2, IL-4, IL-7, IL-9 and IL-15 receptors. All the corresponding cytokines share T-cell growth-promoting activity. IL-7 is produced by stromal cells, and IL-15 by macrophages, endothelial and epithelial cells ,and their production is not affected by cyclosporine or FK506. Anti-γ-chain antibodies and JAK inhibitors are under evaluation. JAK activation upon ligand binding results in receptor phosphorylation. STATs are then recruited to the receptor and become phosphorylated by the JAKs. This induces STAT dimerization and translocation to the nucleus, where they activate STAT-responsive genes. All these interactions (STAT receptor, STAT dimerization, STAT-DNA) involve SH2 domains. With respect to immune deviation, the IL-12 receptor/STAT4 system seems to be an attractive target. In addition, Th1- and Th2-specific transcription factors have been described recently.

Cell traffic and adhesion

Another important paradigm for the modulation of the immune system is the regulation of leukocyte trafficking by adhesion. Adherence of leukocytes to the vascular endothelium is not only pivotal to an inflammatory process but also plays a role in transplant rejection since the graft endothelium is the major contact site for immune cells of the host. Several cell surface molecules are involved in the adhesion process, which is subdivided into several steps, i.e. rolling, firm adhesion and extravasation. Members of the selectin family mediate the first contacts via carbohydrate structures. Members of the heterodimeric integrin superfamily like Mac-1, LFA-1 and VLA-4 are involved in the later steps. Individual integrins are expressed on different cell types. They interact with their specific, widely expressed ligands that include not only surface molecules but also components of the complement system and the extracellular matrix, which all contribute to the activation of the graft endothelium. In addition to their function as adhesion molecules, VLA-1 and LFA-1 have a costimulatory activity for T-lymphocytes. All these features make these molecules attractive targets for the prevention of graft rejection, especially for chronic rejection. Biologicals, mainly monoclonal antibodies, are currently being evaluated for clinical application. However, administration of anti-LFA-1 and anti-ICAM-1 antibodies in first clinical transplantation trials has so far yielded no convincing results.

selectins
integrins

anti-LFA-1/ICAM-1
antibody

Recently, a new immunosuppressive drug, FTY720 (Fig. 1), has been identified that affects lymphocyte recirculation. It is a chemical analogue of the natural metabolite myriocin. FTY720 prolongs allograft survival with high potency and efficacy in mice, rats, dogs and monkeys. Its mechanism of action has not been fully elucidated but differs from that of other immunosuppressive drugs. It rapidly depletes T- and B-cells from the periphery, which at least in part is due to an increased rate of homing to mesenteric lymph nodes and Peyer's patches [15].

FTY720:
lymphocyte
recirculation

Tolerance

Tolerance can be relatively easily induced in rodent transplantation models, for instance in rats by using a short course of immunosuppression. This is not the case in humans or nonhuman primate models. In the clinic, blood transfusions (either from unrelated donors or donor-specific) have given a first indication that the immune system can be "modulated" in order to reduce alloreactivity towards the graft. There are a number of approaches in induction of transplantation tolerance that have

blood transfusion

shown promising results in primates and hence could be developed towards a clinical application:

costimulatory pathway

- induction of anergy by blocking costimulatory pathways. The focus has been on the CD28-B7 and the CD40-CD154 interactions: in a rhesus monkey kidney transplantation model the administration of an antibody to the CD40 ligand and CTLA4-Ig in the peritransplant period induced long-term allograft acceptance without the need for chronic immunosuppression [13];

CD3 immunotoxin

- severe T-cell depletion using an immunotoxin targeting of T-cells. A chemical conjugate between an anti-CD3 antibody and a mutated diphtheria toxin yielded long-term allograft survival of rhesus monkey kidney allografts when given in the peritransplant period. This result is ascribed to the severe T-cell depleting effect of the immunotoxin that not only included T-cell depletion from the blood circulation as observed with the anti-CD3 antibody but also depletion from lymphoid organs [16];

bone marrow chimerism

- bone marrow chimerism [17]. This includes the eradication of the immune system including stem cells in bone marrow by high-dose chemotherapy and/or irradiation, followed by bone marrow transplantation. In this situation, a condition of "mixed chimerism" is created, in which the individual accepts transplants from the bone marrow donor without the need of additional immunosuppression. This procedure has been shown to be effective in large animal transplantation models including pigs and nonhuman primates. This induction of "central tolerance" (tolerance at the level of precursors of lymphocytes) is now optimized in rodents with regard to minimizing the myeloablative regimen so that a clinical application may become feasible.

Corticosteroids

Julia C. Buckingham, Rod J. Flower and Nick J. Goulding

Introduction

The term *corticosteroids* refers to the family of steroid hormones secreted by the adrenal cortex. These hormones fall into three main groups, namely *glucocorticoids, mineralocorticoids* and *sex steroids*, which fulfil different biological functions and are produced by histologically distinct zones of the cortex. The mineralocorticoids, notably aldosterone, are secreted by the superficial *zona glomerulosa*; they have important actions on the kidney, promoting Na^+ retention and K^+ excretion, and thereby contribute to the regulation of water and electrolyte balance. The glucocorticoids (predominantly cortisol or corticosterone, dependent on the species) are derived mainly from the middle zone of the cortex, the *zona fasciculata*, and exert widespread actions in the body which are required for the maintenance of homoeostasis; their name reflects their prominent effects on carbohydrate metabolism which were amongst the first of their many properties to be recognised. The adrenal sex steroids comprise mainly androgens but also oestrogens, irrespective of the sex of the individual. They are secreted by the inner layer of the cortex, the *zona reticularis*, and they exert influences on functions as diverse as behaviour and the development and maintenance of secondary sex characteristics; increasing attention is focused on dehydroepiandrosterone (DHEA), which is the major adrenal androgen and which appears to oppose many of the actions of the glucocorticoids in the brain and periphery. In this chapter we will focus upon the glucocorticoids because these are the only steroid hormones which possess potent antiinflammatory and immunosuppressive properties.

The life-maintaining role of the adrenal cortex was first established over 100 years ago by Thomas Addison [1], who described the salient features of chronic adrenocortical insufficiency, a condition now termed Addison's Disease. However, some 50 years elapsed until, largely due to the pioneering work of Hans Selye, the fundamental requirement for glucocorticoids was recognised, and it is only relatively recently that the rea-

adrenal cortex
corticosteroids
- **glucocorticoids**
- **mineralo-**
  corticoid
- **sex steroids**

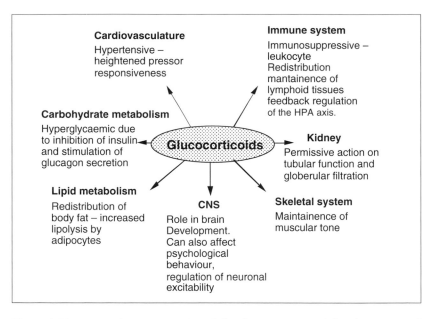

Figure 1 Diagrammatic representation of the diverse actions of the glucocorticoid hormones on multiple organ systems

**glucocorticoids
antiinflammatory
host defence**

son for this has been fully appreciated. In the 1980s, Allan Munck [2] evolved the notion that the hypersecretion of the glucocorticoids which occurs in conditions of physical (e.g. infections, tissue injury/inflammation) or emotional stress serves to check the body's "defence mechanisms" (e.g. the immune response, the inflammatory response, the release of opioid peptides, insulin and so on) which would normally be activated to protect the body. Without this chemical brake, these defence mechanisms could accelerate and become dominant, causing a potentially fatal collapse of homoeostatic physiology, an observation which has been verified by studies in adrenalectomised animals [3, 4].

Glucocorticoids have been used clinically for many years to combat inflammatory and autoimmune disease and to prevent rejection in transplant patients. The doses required, however, to produce a beneficial therapeutic effect are almost always "supraphysiological", and until comparatively recently, the possibility that endogenous glucocorticoids contribute to the regulation of immune/inflammatory cell function received scant attention. During the last decade, however, convincing evidence has emerged that the low levels of cortisol/corticosterone normally present in the blood exert a significant tonic influence on the activities of immune and inflammatory cells and thereby form an integral part of the body's defence weaponry. Disturbances in glucocorticoid secretion or action may therefore contribute to the pathogenesis of a variety of disease processes. In accord with this concept, the sustained elevations in serum cortisol caused by primary or secondary disorders of the hypothalamo-pituitary-adrenocortical (HPA) axis in humans are frequently associated with a decline in immunocompetence. In the same vein, numerous studies in experimental animals suggest that the persistent elevations in glucocorticoids caused by repeated stress may increase susceptibility to infections. For example, repeated restraint stress reduces the ability of mice to combat microorganisms such as influenza virus or mycobacterium; the hazardous effects of the stress are, however, attenuated by the concomitant administration of the glucocorticoid antagonist, mefepristone (RU486) [5]. Adrenocortical insufficiency on the other hand may be an important contributory factor to the aetiology of chronic inflammatory and autoimmune disease. Such arguments are supported by reports that acute inflammatory responses frequently progress to a chronic disease state in rodent strains (e.g. the Lewis rat), which fail to mount a normal adrenocortical response to stress, whereas in animals which release corticosterone normally, the acute inflammatory episode is terminated promptly [6]. Such variations in the activity of the HPA axis may also contribute to the formation of potentially pathogenic autoantibodies in chronic diseases in humans as well as underlying disorders such as rheumatoid arthritis [7, 8].

HPA axis disease

Studies on the mechanisms responsible for the secretion and biological actions of the glucocorticoids must therefore take account of the fact that these steroid hormones are extremely powerful antiinflammatory and immunosuppressive substances which fulfil a significant physiological role in the control of host defence processes and which have served for over half a century as the basis for an entire armoury of potent antiinflammatory and immunosuppressive drugs. For the purposes of this particular book, we will divide the actions of the glucocorticoids into two broad categories, (i) antiinflammatory and immunosuppressive effects and (ii) effects on metabolism and on the neuroendocrine system.

Regulation of glucocorticoid homoeostasis

Synthesis, release and metabolism

The synthesis of the glucocorticoids is driven by the anterior pituitary hormone, corticotrophin (adrenocorticotrophic hormone, ACTH), which acts via membrane-bound receptors to activate the rate limiting enzyme in the steroidogenic pathway and thereby increase the conversion of the precursor cholesterol to pregnenolone. The newly synthesised steroid is not stored but released immediately into the bloodstream where approximately 95% of it is bound to a specific binding protein, *corticosteroid binding globulin* (CBG, a protein structurally related to the serpin family of serine protease inhibitors), and to albumin. In principle, only the free steroid has ready access to the target tissues. However, some cells (e.g. leukocytes) have receptors for CBG and may therefore trap the bound steroid; this process appears to facilitate the hydrolysis of CBG by local serine proteases and to cause the concomitant release of cortisol; it may therefore provide an important local mechanism of facilitating drug delivery, particularly at sites of inflammation where leukocytes are found in abundance [9]. In context, it is interesting to note that in normal circumstances the total cortisol level (a.m.) in the blood is 4–16 µg/100 ml, although in the clinic doses equivalent to about 100 µg/100 ml are normally required to produce a full range of beneficial antiinflammatory/immunosuppressive actions. The metabolic half-life of the endogenous glucocorticoids is approximately 90 min; metabolism, which importantly involves reduction of the A ring and subsequent conjugation, occurs in the liver, with the resulting metabolites being excreted in the urine and the bile [8].

Control of glucocorticoid secretion

glucocorticoids and the HPA axis

The glucocorticoids are the end products of the HPA axis (Fig. 2). Their secretion is thus triggered by stimuli which converge upon the hypothalamus to cause the release of the hypothalamic releasing hormones, corticotrophin-releasing hormone (CRH) and arginine vasopressin (AVP), which are transported via the hypophyseal portal system to the anterior pituitary gland where they act synergistically to initiate the release of ACTH, the primary trigger to steroidogenesis. Oversecretion of the glucocorticoids is prevented by a complex negative feedback system through which the steroids act at multiple sites in the axis to suppress the release of ACTH and its hypothalamic releasing factors. Increased levels of glucocorticoids in the blood can also suppress the release of other pituitary hormones such as growth hormone, prolactin, thyrotrophin and the gonadotrophins [7, 8].

In mammalian physiology, the secretion of glucocorticoids follows a diurnal pattern with maximal release occurring towards the end of the main sleep phase. In addition, pronounced increases in glucocorticoid release are triggered at times of psychological and/or physical (e.g. infection, injury) stress. These responses are orchestrated by the hypothala-

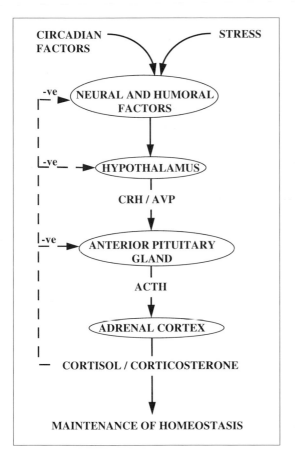

Figure 2 Schematic diagram illustrating the hypothalamo-pituitary-adrenocortical axis *CRH, corticotrophin releasing hormone; AVP, arginine vasopressin; ACTH, adrenocorticotrophic hormone. Reprinted from the International Journal of Tissue Research, with permission of the publishers.*

mus, which receives and integrates neural and humoral information from many sources and adjusts the output of CRH/AVP accordingly. The hypothalamus thus provides a vital link between the perception of physical and/or emotional stress and the regulation of crucial homoeostatic mechanisms such as immune and inflammatory responses and many important metabolic control systems [4, 5].

Molecular basis of glucocorticoid action

Genomic actions

The molecular basis of glucocorticoid action has puzzled and intrigued scientists and clinicians for many decades. It is now generally accepted that most, although not all, of the actions of these hormone drugs may be explained by interactions with intracellular cytoplasmic receptors and subsequent up- or downregulation of specific target genes [10–12]. Glucocorticoids, being relatively lipophilic, enter cells readily to gain access to these receptors [13]. On binding the steroid, the receptors undergo dimerisation and allosteric changes which release associated chaperone molecules (hsp90) [10]; the steroid-receptor complex than transmigrates to the cell nucleus and interacts with certain sequences (termed glucocorticoid response elements, GREs) which are located in the promoter regions of the target genes [11]. This genomic action, which may be discretely modulated by a variety of transcription factors such as members of the "leucine zipper" family including AP-1, CREBs and ATFs [12], alters the rate of transcription of specific target genes and thus enables the expression of specific proteins to be downregulated or upregulated. The cross-talk between glucocorticoid receptors and other DNA binding proteins provides the potential for an extremely complex series of interactions and nuances in the regulation of cellular response to glucocorticoids.

Corticosteroid receptors

two forms of the glucocorticoid receptor (α, β)

There are two main types of receptors in the body which recognise glucocorticoids; these are called the mineralocorticoid receptors (MRs) and the glucocorticoid receptors (GRs) respectively [11]. The MR has a high and approximately equal affinity for aldosterone and for the endogenous glucocorticoids, cortisol and corticosterone ($K_d \sim$ 1–2 nM); it has a discrete tissue distribution but is expressed in abundance in the kidney and the hippocampus. By contrast, the GR is a low-affinity receptor (K_d cortisol/corticosterone $\sim$ 10–20 nM) which bind aldosterone only very weakly and is thus glucocorticoid selective. GRs are expressed by virtually all nucleated cells in the body with estimated cellular concentrations in the region of 1×10^3–1×10^4 molecules/cell. Cloning studies have revealed that the human GR exists in two forms [10], designated *alpha* and *beta*, which represent alternate splice variants of a single gene. The alpha form (777 amino acids) has the capability to bind ligand and to interact with DNA. The beta form by contrast (742 amino acids) lacks the C-terminal ligand binding domain and appears to be a "silent" or "decoy" receptor; its function is not entirely clear, but it has been proposed that it may contribute to the phenomenon of "steroid resistance".

Intracellular regulation of glucocorticoid access to the receptors

In many tissues the intracellular delivery of glucocorticoids to their receptors is regulated by two isozymes, (termed 11β-hydroxysteroid dehydrogenase/reductase (11βHSD-2/11βHSD-1), which control the interconversion of cortisol/corticosterone to their inactive metabolites cortisone/11-keto-corticosterone (Fig. 3) [14]. 11βHSD-2 is particularly prevalent in peripheral cells which express the MR (e.g. kidney) where, by inactivating endogenous glucocorticoids, it permits selective access of aldosterone to its receptors; it is also abundant in the placenta, where it acts as a scavenger for maternal glucocorticoids and thus plays a key role

11βHSD-2

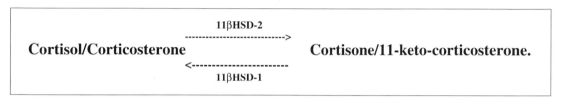

Figure 3 Intracellular metabolism of cortisol and corticosterone by 11β-hydroxysteroid dehydrogenase/reductase (11βHSD-2, 11βHSD-2)

in protecting the developing foetus from the potentially harmful effects of these steroids [15]. Inhibition of the expression or activity of 11βHSD-2 leads to MR overstimulation, Na^+ retention and hypertension; in addition, blockade of the placental enzyme may predispose the developing foetus to hypertension and diabetes in adult life. The second isozyme, 11βHSD-I, is widely expressed in many tissues, especially liver and brain, and mainly serves to generate biologically active glucocorticoids from preexistent substrates. Suppression of 11βHSD-1 expression leads to falls in blood glucose through a reduction in liver gluconeogenesis [14].

Target genes

In seeking to explain further the mechanisms by which the steroids produce their actions, we must seek to identify those genes which are regulated by glucocorticoids. This is an awesome task, since it is estimated that as much as 1% of the genome may be influenced by these hormones, a figure which is not perhaps surprising when one considers the extra-

**glucocorticoid
effects on
cytokines and
enzymes**

ordinary diversity of glucocorticoid action in the body (see Fig. 1 for more details). Nonetheless, considerable headway has been made, particularly in the identification of genes which are crucial to the development of immune and inflammatory responses. The majority are down-regulated by glucocorticoids and include, for example, the expression of various proinflammatory cytokines [e.g. interleukin-1 (IL-1), tumour necrosis factor α (TNFα)] [16] and their receptors (e.g. IL-2 receptors) and for enzymes which facilitate the release of inflammatory mediators [e.g. the "inducible" forms of cyclo-oxygenase (COX-2) [17] and nitric oxide synthase (iNOS)] [18]. However, a limited number of genes which code for potent antiinflammatory proteins (e.g. protease inhibitors) and are upregulated by glucocorticoids have also been identified. One such protein is lipocortin 1 (annexin I), which plays a prominent part in many of the antiinflammatory actions of glucocorticoids and also contributes to the regulatory actions of the steroids on the HPA axis itself [19] and will be discussed in detail below. The combination of these many inhibitory actions of the glucocorticoids on immune and inflammatory processes makes these drugs very powerful immunosuppressive and antiinflammatory agents; however, their promiscuity of actions on other systems gives rise to a spectrum of effects, many of which may prove harmful to the individual in the long term (see below).

Synthetic glucocorticoid drugs

**dexamethasone
prednisolone**

Many of the corticosteroids produced by the adrenal cortex exhibit both mineralocorticoid and glucocorticoid activities in varying degrees. Thus, aldosterone (the main endogenous mineralocorticoid) acts predominantly at the MRs, producing Na$^+$ retention and K$^+$ loss in the kidney, but it also has weak effects on GRs and thus on carbohydrate metabolism. On the other hand, cortisol (the main glucocorticoid in humans) has potent effects on immune and inflammatory cells and on carbohydrate metabolism (both GR-mediated) but shows only moderate mineralocorticoid activity. In developing synthetic glucocorticoid drugs, attempts have been made to separate the antiinflammatory actions from the unwanted mineralocorticoid effects. In Table 1 the mineralocorticoid and antiinflammatory potencies of various corticosteroids are compared, taking the activity of cortisol as a standard. It can be seen that, in some cases, the separation of these activities has been successful and that some glucocorticoids (e.g. dexamethasone) act selectively at GRs and are virtually devoid of mineralocorticoid activity. However, attempts to separate the

Table 1 Comparison of common glucocorticoids in terms of dose equivalents and potency

Steroid drug	Dose equivalents (mg)	Anti-inflammatory potency	Potency of sodium retention	Biological half-life (h)
Hydrocortisone	20	1	1	8–12
Cortisone	25	0.8	0.8	8–12
Prednisolone	5	4	0.8	12–36
6α-Methylprednisolone	5	5	0.5	12–36
Triamcinolone	4	5	0	12–36
Betamethasone	0.75	25	0	36–72
Dexamethasone	0.75	25	0	36–72

antiinflammatory, metabolic and many other GR-mediated actions of the steroids have not been successful. Hence, administration (particularly if prolonged) of these drugs as antiinflammatory agents, is frequently associated with a plethora of unwanted actions, including alterations in carbohydrate, protein and fat metabolism as well as potentially fatal suppression of the HPA axis. Abrupt cessation of therapy is thus likely to leave the patient in a dangerous state of adrenocortical insufficiency.

glucocorticoid therapy

Another reason for developing synthetic analogues of hydrocortisone (apart from the obvious benefits of producing a novel patentable drug) is to improve the duration of action of the steroid. Table 1 shows that the biological half-life of hydrocortisone is short but that the duration of action of some of the synthetic analogues is very long indeed. This has been achieved by synthesising derivatives (often fluorinated) of hydrocortisone which have a greater affinity for the receptor, which are metabolised only slowly by the body and which are not bound to CBG. Synthetic analogues of cortisol offer advantages in terms of convenience of dosage as well as rapidity and duration of therapeutic action.

Clinical use of glucocorticoids

Apart from replacement therapy in conditions of adrenocortical insufficiency (e.g. Addison's disease, congenital adrenal hyperplasia), the glucocorticoids are used therapeutically mainly for their antiinflammatory and immunosuppressive actions. They are used for the treatment of inflammatory diseases such as asthma, rheumatoid arthritis, inflammatory bowel disease and vasculitis as well as skin disorders such as psoria-

**glucocorticoid
side-effects**

sis and eczema. They are also useful for suppressing rejection after transplant surgery and in the treatment of allergy and other conditions associated with inappropriate immune responses, e.g. multiple sclerosis and autoimmune diseases such as systemic lupus erythematosus. Glucocorticoids are extremely valuable, sometimes even life-saving drugs. However, when used as antiinflammatory agents, their action is to suppress the manifestation of inflammation without necessarily eliminating the underlying cause. There is a danger that the host defence response to infections might also be suppressed, and latent infections such as tuberculosis become active.

Generally speaking, glucocorticoids are well tolerated when given acutely, even if the doses are high. With chronic treatment, however, problems arise, and in addition to the decreased resistance to infection (which is caused by the same depression of leukocyte and immune function that is the basis of much of the antiinflammatory effect), a broad spectrum of unwanted effects frequently emerges; these may include changes in carbohydrate, lipid and protein metabolism (giving rise to iatrogenic Cushing's syndrome), suppression of the HPA axis, hypertension, peptic ulceration, impaired glucose tolerance, myopathy, glaucoma, osteoporosis, osteonecrosis, cataracts, mood changes, hirsutism, irregular menstrual cycles and growth suppression in children. In practice, therefore, it is important to titrate the dose and frequency of administration to achieve the minimum and least-frequent dosage necessary to maintain a beneficial clinical effect and to take advantage of the possibility of local administration, e.g. by inhalation in asthma or by intraarticular injection for local inflammation in joints.

titering doses

Components of the inflammatory response which are modified by glucocorticoids

**transcription
translation
post-translation**

Glucocorticoids act at multiple points to inhibit the inflammatory and immune responses. The synthesis and release of many *mediators* is depressed, e.g. eicosanoid and nitric oxide production, histamine synthesis and release as well as cytokine [IL-1, IL-2, IL-3, IL-6, IL-8, IL-10, TNF, colony-stimulating factor (CSF) and plasminogen activator] generation. These effects are not only brought about by actions on the transcription of the relevant genes but may also involve posttranscriptional activities, including inhibition of protein processing, secretion and action of the cytokine in question [16, 20].

Glucocorticoids also affect the *cellular component* of inflammation; they profoundly influence the disposition of circulating inflammatory blood cells, provoking a profound blood neutrophilia and a reduction in neutrophils at inflammatory sites. Circulating monocytes are reduced, chemotaxis and superoxide anion production is inhibited and surface adhesion molecule expression is downregulated. Glucocorticoids reduce dramatically the number of circulating eosinophils and decrease eosinophil adherence and chemotaxis, they deplete peripheral basophil and mast cell numbers, inhibit granule release and reduce histamine content [21, 22]. In the immune system, glucocorticoids inhibit immunoglobulin production, antigen-induced proliferation of lymphocytes, reduce the mitogenic response, suppress production of lymphokines and inhibit other cell-cell interactions [20]. Glucocorticoids are potent inducers of lymphocyte cytolysis in animals but not in humans; however, they do have significant influence on rates of apoptosis (programmed cell death) in many types of human cells. In general, glucocorticoids enhance the rate of apoptosis, but the opposite effect is seen in neutrophils [23]. The intracellular signals culminating in apoptosis are dependent on GR binding and result in the calcium-dependent enzymatic degradation of internucleosomal DNA. Nuclear transcription factors have been implicated in these processes. Repression of the intracellular oncogene c-*myc* by glucocorticoids is one mechanism by which apoptotic events can be induced. Conversely, elevated expression of another oncogene, *Bcl-2*, can overcome glucocorticoid-induced apoptosis in B-lymphocyte lines.

cell-trafficking

immunity

apoptosis

The role of lipocortin 1 in glucocorticoid action

Chemistry, distribution and regulation of expression

Lipocortin 1 (also called annexin 1) is a 37-kDa member of the *annexins*, a superfamily of proteins found in a wide range of organisms (vertebrate, invertebrate and plant; see refs 19 and 24 for a comprehensive review). Members of this family are characterised by a highly homologous core domain which normally comprises a fourfold repeat of some 70 amino acids and gives the proteins a special ability to bind Ca^{2+} and negatively charged phospholipids. Attached to the core is an N-terminal domain which is unique in length and sequence for each member of the family and which often contains phosphorylation motifs (see Fig. 4 for the structure of lipocortin 1). It is widely believed that the N-terminus confers the biological specificity of individual annexins and thus enables

lipocortin 1

calcium binding protein

371

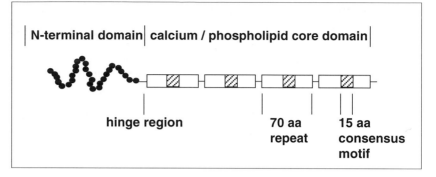

Figure 4 Schematic representation of the lipcortin 1 molecule
A member of the annexin family of calcium binding proteins, lipocortin 1 contains one copy of a characteristic "core" domain of a fourfold 70 amino acid repeat. A 15 amino acid consensus motif is located within each repeat. Lipocortin 1 is distinguished from other members of the family by a unique 30-amino acid N-terminal domain.

lipocortin 1
- **distribution**
- **induction**
- **export**

the proteins to exert distinct and specific actions on or in their respective target cells [19].

Lipocortin 1 is widely distributed throughout the body, although it is often concentrated in discrete cell types. In particular, it is associated with specialised glandular secretory epithelial cells such as those of the prostate and salivary gland [25]. It is found mainly in differentiated cells, and in some it may constitute an appreciable fraction of the total cell protein mass. From the point of view of this chapter, it is of interest to note that many cells involved in the inflammatory response (e.g. macrophages, polymorphonuclear monocytes etc.) have substantial amounts of the protein, as also do cells of the neuroendocrine system (e.g. the anterior pituitary, the hypothalamus) [26–28]. The subcellular distribution of lipocortin 1 is unusual. It is abundant in the cytoplasm, but it is also observed on the external surface of cell membranes, where it is attached by Ca^{2+}-dependent linkages to binding proteins; it may also be found attached to the inner leaflet of the cell membrane, and cell fractionation studies suggest that there is an integral membrane pool of lipocortin 1.

Lipocortin 1 aroused interest initially because the glucocorticoid (but not mineralocorticoid or sex steroid) hormones increase its synthesis and alter its subcellular disposition. An early observation, now confirmed many times, is that treatment of differentiated cells with natural or synthetic glucocorticoids *in vivo* or *in vitro* increases the amount of the protein found on the external plasma membrane (see [19] and [29] for a review). The mechanisms by which lipocortin 1 crosses the membrane are unclear as, unlike polypeptides released by exocytosis, it lacks a signal sequence. Nonetheless, this process of exportation (or "externalisation" as it is frequently called) appears to be an important facet of lipocortin 1 biology because, as we shall see later, it enables the protein to reach specific binding proteins on the outer cell surface which may be critical to its actions. It occurs relatively rapidly, usually within 0.5–2 h of steroid administration, and it is normally followed by increased *de novo* intracellular synthesis of the protein itself. Thus glucocorticoids exert a dual action on lipocortin 1, causing the initial exportation of the protein from the cells and subsequently the replenishment of the depleted stores. As one might predict, lipocortin 1 messenger RNA (mRNA) and protein levels are reduced substantially in adrenalectomised animals but are readily restored by maintenance doses of the glucocorticoids [30]. Administration of the glucocorticoid antagonist, mifepristone, also lowers the resting levels of the protein [31].

Studies on the promoter region of the lipocortin 1 gene have indicated that several factors other than glucocorticoids may also regulate the biosynthesis of the protein, including IL-6 and phorbol esters, which exert positive influences [29]. The apparently complementary actions of IL-6 and the steroids are particularly interesting since these substances have been shown to act cooperatively in some other biological systems, e.g. the generation of acute phase proteins by the liver.

Antiinflammatory action of lipocortin 1

Lipocortin 1 has been implicated, along with other proteins, in the regulation of the inflammatory response. Its antiinflammatory actions seem to be due, at least in part, to its ability to inhibit the release of arachidonic acid and thus the generation of lipid mediators of inflammation, such as prostaglandins and leukotrienes, but some other actions (e.g. the inhibition of leukocyte migration) do not seem to be accounted for in this way. Early work in the field (reviewed in [32]) suggested that lipocortin 1 may directly inhibit the enzyme phospholipase A_2 (PLA$_2$). Findings from several other laboratories have challenged this (e.g. [33]), and although inhibition of arachidonic acid release secondary to a reduction in cytosolic PLA$_2$ activity can be readily demonstrated in a number of preparations [34], it has not yet been possible to pinpoint the exact mechanism whereby lipocortin 1 produces its inhibitory actions. An effect on signal transduction is a distinct possibility.

lipocortin 1 inhibits phospholipase H$_2$

The extracellular mode of action of lipocortin 1 on cell function is still a matter of speculation, but there is increasing evidence that specific lipocortin 1 binding proteins located on the surface of human blood monocytes, macrophages and neutrophils may play an important role in the antiinflammatory properties of this protein [35]. Blood leukocytes isolated from patients with rheumatoid arthritis have been shown to have reduced lipocortin 1-binding capacity, as have cells isolated from sites of inflammation [35].

lipocortin 1 cell surface binding proteins

Evidence to support the notion that lipocortin 1 or peptide fragments of lipocortin 1 [36] possess antiinflammatory activity has come from studies in several different experimental models of inflammation. For example, the administration of human recombinant lipocortin 1 substantially inhibits the development of experimentally induced paw edema in the rat [37], fever in rats and rabbits [38, 39], neutrophil migration in the mouse air pouch [40] and even ischaemic brain damage in the rat [41]. Conversely, passive immunisation of animals with neutralising anti-lipocortin 1 antisera quenches the ability of the glucocorticoids to suppress edema formation and neutrophil migration in some models of inflammation [40] and may also exacerbate the brain damage caused by unilateral ligation of a carotid artery [41]. Similarly, antisense oligodeoxynucleotides directed against sequences specific to the lipocortin 1 gene have been shown to prevent some actions of the glucocorticoid action *in vitro* [42].

While corticosteroids are effective in most, if not all, experimental modes of inflammation, the same does not hold true for lipocortin 1. This is congruent with our ideas concerning the selective nature of steroid action. For example, antiinflammatory steroids inhibit the development of both carrageenin- and histamine-induced paw edema in rats; lipocortin 1 also blocks carrageenin-induced oedema, but it does not suppress the responses to histamine [37], pointing to the existence of two distinct mechanisms of steroid action in the control of these phenomena, one of which is dependent on lipocortin 1.

lipocortin 1 autoantibodies

Interestingly, autoantibodies to lipocortin 1 have been found in the serum of some patients with chronic inflammatory diseases such as rheumatoid arthritis and systemic lupus erythematosus. Moreover, there is evidence of a causal relationship between the antibody titres and the incidence of certain types of relative "steroid resistance", particularly those in which higher doses of the steroid are required over the long term to suppress the symptoms of the disease [43, 44].

Role of lipocortin 1 in the neuroendocrine system

As well as mediating some of the peripheral actions of glucocorticoids, increasing evidence suggests that lipocortin 1 plays a key role in the regulation of glucocorticoid *secretion* by serving as a mediator of the powerful negative feedback actions of the steroids in the pituitary gland and hypothalamus. For example, *in vitro* recombinant lipocortin 1 mimics, whereas anti-lipocortin 1 antisera specifically reverse, the inhibitory actions of glucocorticoids on the release of CRH and ACTH from the hypothalamus and anterior pituitary gland, respectively [45–48]. Similarly, *in vivo* passive immunisation of rats against lipocortin 1 overcomes the ability of dexamethasone to block the overt increases in HPA activity caused by antigenic challenge (Fig. 5) [47], whereas central injections

feedback suppression of HPA axis activity

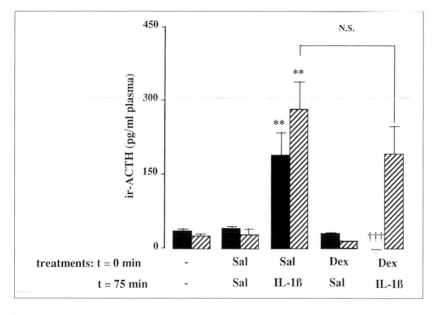

Figure 5

Passive immunisiation of rats against lipocortin 1 (LC1) specifically reverses the inhibitory actions of dexamethasone (DEX, 100 µg/kg, i.p.) on the ability of interleukin 1β (IL-1β, 3 µg/kg, i.p.) to stimulate the release of ACTH in adult conscious rats. Vehicle controls received equal volumes of sterile saline (SAL, 1 ml/kg, i.p.). Black columns, controls (1 ml/kg non immune sheep serum/day for 2 days, s.c.); Hatched columns, anti-LC1 polyclonal antiserum (raised in sheep, 1 ml/day for 2 days, s.c.). Measurements were made on day 3, 1 h after the injection of IL-1β. Values represent the mean ± SEM (n = 6–8). **P < 0.01 versus IL-1β-free; †††, P < 0.001 versus corresponding dexamethasone-free group (analysis of variance (ANOVA) and Scheffe's test). Reprinted from [47] with permission of the publishers.

of lipocortin 1 abolish the rises in glucocorticoid secretion provoked by injection of IL-1 or IL-6 [48]. Complementary studies suggest that lipocortin 1 may also play a key role in effecting the inhibitory actions of the steroids on the release of other pituitary hormones, notably prolactin [49], growth hormone [50] and thyrotrophin [51].

Lipocortin 1 is readily detectable in the hypothalamus and pituitary gland, and as in other tissues, it is exported from the intracellular compartment to the outer surface of the cells in response to a steroid challenge where it is retained by a Ca^{2+}-dependent mechanism. The mechanism by which lipocortin 1 traverses the cell membrane is unknown, but the fact that the protein does not contain a signal sequence and that the "externalisation" is unaffected by drugs which block the classical pathway of protein secretion suggest the process differs from conventional exocytosis [52]. Current evidence suggests that the cellular exportation of lipocortin 1 is critical for its actions as it enables the protein to target-cell surface "receptors" and, thus, to suppress peptide release; lipocortin 1 may therefore act as an autocrine or paracrine agent in the neuroendocrine system. This hypothesis is supported by observations that, on a temporal basis, exportation of the protein parallels the onset of inhibition of ACTH release induced by the steroids, and both actions of the steroids, are dependent on *de novo* protein synthesis, blocked by cycloheximide and specifically inhibited by treatment of the tissue with LC1 antisense oligonucleotides or neutralising antibodies [46, 53]. Moreover, using fluorescence-activated cell analysis and sorting, we have observed high affinity lipocortin 1 binding sites on the surface of a variety of pituitary cell types, including the corticotrophs, somatotrophs and lactotrophs [54]. Since lipocortin 1 is expressed predominantly by non-secretory cells of immunological lineage in the anterior pituitary gland (folliculostellate cells) and brain (microglia), it seems likely that it functions predominantly as a paracrine agent in these tissues; it may thus contribute to the complex interplay between the immune and neuroendocrine systems and thus be an important facet of the host defence processes [7].

lipocortin1 in neuroendocrine tissue
- **distribution**
- **externalisation**
- **binding site**

Other actions of lipocortin 1

In addition to its actions in the immune/inflammatory and neuroendocrine systems, lipocortin 1 has been shown to have several other properties, including the ability to prevent the growth of certain cells (e.g. A549 cells [55]), the differentiation of other cell types and even the apparent regulation of genes such as the induceable form of NOS [56].

Other effects of glucocorticoids

Although the general metabolic actions of the glucocorticoids are not specifically relevant to their antiinflammatory actions, they are important in understanding the side effects of these drugs (Fig. 1).

The glucocorticoids have profound effects on carbohydrate metabolism, causing decreased uptake and utilisation of glucose, increased gluconeogenesis and increased glycogen storage. They thus tend to raise blood sugar and, in excess, may precipitate "steroid diabetes". Glucocorticoids also have important effects on protein metabolism, causing decreased synthesis and an increased protein catabolism resulting in a negative nitrogen balance. In addition, they influence fat metabolism, promoting lipolysis through a permissive effect on the action of other lipolytic hormones (e.g. catecholamines) and cause the redistribution of body fat typical of Cushing's syndrome. Overall, the role of glucocorticoids is to maintain glucose homoeostasis at the expense of other substrates such as glycogen, protein and fat.

Glucocorticoids also affect water and electrolyte balance and, in excess, they may provoke hypertension, partly through their actions on MR, which lead to Na^+ retention, but also through modulation of vasoactive mediator action. Glucocorticoids are important in the control of musculo-skeletal physiology such that a deficiency in glucocorticoids leads to muscle weakness, whereas an excess precipitates muscle loss and osteoporosis. They are also concerned with the regulation of the activity of the central nervous system, and in addition to their important influence on neuroendocrine function, they also exert significant effects on mood and behaviour. Recent studies [57] have revealed a key role for steroids in brain development, and through these and other actions in the periphery, they may influence long-term "programming" in the foetus and neonate of a variety of physiological functions. High doses of glucocorticoids may be neurotoxic, and indeed a number of workers now consider that the elevations in serum glucocorticoids evident in ageing subjects may be a significant contributory factor in the pathogenesis of neurodegenerative disease.

metabolism

• **carbohydrste**

• **protein**

• **fat**

hypertension

CNS activity

brain development

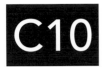

Disease-modifying antirheumatic drugs

*Clarissa Bachmeier, Malcolm L. Handel, Phillip G. Conaghan,
Kenneth M. Williams, Garry G. Graham, Peter M. Brooks and
Richard O. Day*

Introduction

Although rheumatoid arthritis (RA), the classic inflammatory arthritis, was first described 200 years ago, its pharmacological treatment is still problematical, and as yet there are no reliably curative or disease-remitting therapies. RA often inexorably progresses to disability, and many RA patients eventually suffer from deformity and increased mortality. Drug therapy relieves symptoms but perhaps only delays the damage and disability. However, it is accepted that RA sufferers require pharmacological therapies unless there are exceptional circumstances. Nonpharmacological approaches, including physiotherapy, joint splinting and psychosocial support, are undervalued but very important.

pharmacological treatment of RA

First-line pharmacological therapy for all inflammatory arthritides is a nonsteroidal inflammatory drug (NSAID). The NSAIDs are useful symptomatically but have no easily discernable effect on the progression of RA. Virtually all patients will require the addition of a second-line therapy, and these therapies have been termed disease-modifying antirheumatic drugs (DMARDs) or second-line agents (SLAs). This class of drugs is also known as slow-acting antirheumatic drugs (SAARDs), as their onset of effect is generally slow. There is debate on their true ability to modify critical disease parameters such as bony erosions to a significant extent, hence the range of acronyms. However, it is now believed that it is important to commence DMARDs as soon as a diagnosis of RA is made in order to have the maximal effect on slowing the progress of the disease. This approach contrasts to that of 5–10 years ago when DMARDs were only commenced on the appearance of bony erosions on joint X-rays. Evidence is now accumulating that the new aggressive approach to the early introduction of DMARD therapy is beneficial in slowing the progression of this disease. Many patients with RA and some other inflammatory arthritides also require the additional use of in-

NSAIDs

glucocortico-steroids

traarticular and/or oral glucocorticosteroids, there being a swing back to the use of low-dose, oral glucocorticosteroids in recent years.

Current pharmacological therapies

Glucocorticosteroids

The first report by Hench et al. of glucocorticosteroid usage in patients with RA dates from 1949. In addition to their wide use in the treatment of patients with RA, glucocorticosteroids are used for all inflammatory arthritides and conditions such as vasculitis and polymyalgia rheumatica. Corticosteroids effectively and rapidly suppress systemic and local signs of synovitis in RA patients. Relatively low doses of oral corticosteroids are used (usually 10 mg daily or less of prednisone or prednisolone) and are well tolerated in the short term, but higher doses and long-term use are associated with significant side effects. Patients with severe RA, vasculitis or active systemic lupus erythematosus (SLE) may require intravenous corticosteroids (e.g. 1 g of methylprednisolone daily for a few days). Intraarticular corticosteroid injections are an important treatment for monoarticular inflammatory synovitis or for single joints that are difficult to control in the polyarthritic patient. The long-term effects of intraarticular therapy are unclear, with animal studies suggesting both beneficial and detrimental effects on articular cartilage. Generally, an individual joint may be injected up to 3 to 4 times per year but no more in weight-bearing joints.

vasculitis
polymyalgia
rheumatica

intraarticular
corticosteroids

Efficacy

Corticosteroids are significantly better at improving clinical symptoms in RA patients than placebo, and they are superior to NSAIDs. The effect is rapid and most pronounced in the first weeks of administration. Corticosteroids have not traditionally been classified as DMARDs; however, a recent placebo-controlled study in patients with early RA reported a reduced rate of joint destruction in the prednisone-treated group after 2 years [1] as assessed radiologically. Pulse intravenous therapy has a beneficial effect for at least several weeks, and only few adverse effects are reported [2].

Mechanism of action (Fig. 1)

The glucococorticoid receptor is a transcription factor that is activated by glucocorticosteroids. The classical mode of action is for activated re-

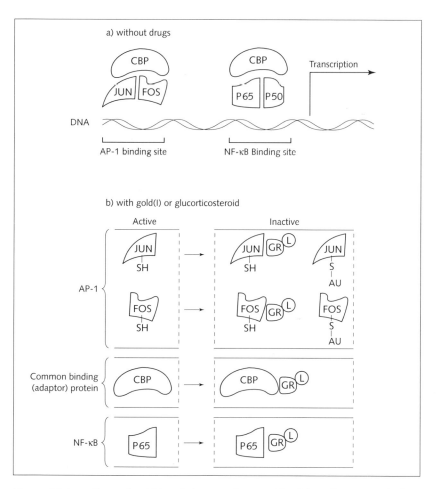

Figure 1 Interactions of gold I and glucocorticosteroids with nuclear transcription factors

(a) Formation of the Jun-Fos heterodimer associating with the CBP protein and binding to the AP-1 sites on DNA. Similarly, the formation of the NF-κB protein complex of P-65, P-50 and CBP proteins enabling binding to the NF-κB sites is depicted, both processes influencing transcription of genes important in the inflammatory and rheumatic diseases. (b) Gold-(I) (AU) binds to Jun and Fos via a sulphydryl (SH) group rendering AP-1 inactive. The binding of glucocorticosteroid ligand (L) to the glucocorticosteroid receptor (GR) allows the receptor complex to migrate to the nucleus and bind to Jun, Fos, CBP and P-65, thereby rendering AP-1 and NF-κB inactive.

glucocorticoid response element

Cushing's syndrome phospholipase A$_2$

ceptor to enter the nucleus and bind to specific DNA sequences termed glucocorticoid response elements (GREs), resulting in transcription of genes bearing a GRE in their promoter region. This positive regulation of gene expression accounts for many, and probably most, of the metabolic and endocrine effects of glucocorticosteroids that in excess are recognised as Cushing's syndrome. In particular, glucocorticosteroids enhance the expression of the protein lipocortin, which in turn downregulates phospholipase A$_2$ expression and leukocyte transmigration [3]. An effect of lipocortin leading to decreased synthesis of proinflammatory prostaglandins and leukotrienes has also been demonstrated [4]. In addition to their positive regulation of gene expression, glucocorticosteroids inhibit the expression of a wide variety of important proinflammatory genes that do not contain a recognizable GRE in their promoter regions.

Many of the important mediators of inflammation are proteins that are coded by genes containing promoter sites for the transcription factors AP-1 and NF-κB. AP-1 (activator protein-1) is a dimer of the nuclear proteins Jun and Fos. NF-κB (nuclear factor-κ B) was discovered as a transcription factor for the expression of immunoglobulin κ light-chain in B-lymphocytes. A major step in understanding the antiinflammatory mechanism of glucocorticosteroids was the finding that their activated receptors inhibit AP-1- and NF-κB-mediated transcription (reviewed in [5]). For example, glucocorticosteroids inhibit the NF-κB-mediated expression of adhesion molecules (ICAM-1 and ELAM-1), cytokines [interleukin (IL)-2, IL-6 and IL-8] and enzymes inducible nitric oxide synthase (iNOS) and cyclooxygenase-2 (COX-2). Glucocorticosteroids also inhibit the AP-1-mediated expression of collagenases I and IV.

AP-1, NF-κB, Jun, Fos

Several mechanisms of antagonism of AP-1 and NF-κB by glucocorticosteroids have been proposed [5]. Glucocorticoid receptor may inhibit AP-1-mediated transcription by directly binding Jun and Fos or by competing for a third protein of mutual importance for transcriptional activity [6]. Competitive antagonism by "protein-protein" interaction between glucocorticoid receptor and NF-κB may also take place [7]. In addition glucocorticosteroids mediate increased expression of IκBα, the cytoplasmic inhibitor of NF-κB [8, 9].

IκBα

Pharmacokinetics

The most widely used oral glucocorticosteroid in the treatment of the rheumatic diseases is prednisolone. Prednisolone is well absorbed, although there is some variation between formulations. The plasma half-life is short, in the order of 2–3 h, but the half-life of its pharmacodynamic effect is longer, and prednisolone is administered once or twice a day. Protein binding in plasma is saturable. There has been little relationship demonstrated between plasma concentrations or pharmacokinetic variables and the effect of prednisolone. The variability between individuals in efficacy and adverse effects for given doses of prednisolone has not been explained to date.

Toxicity

Corticosteroid therapy is commonly associated with side effects, and there is a broad range of possible adverse effects (Table 1). Corticosteroids induce bone loss, influencing both bone formation and bone re-

bone loss induced by corticosteroids

Table 1 Side effects of systemic corticosteroid therapy

Endocrine-metabolic	Dermatologic
obesity	striae
glucose/protein/lipid metabolism	acne
electrolyte imbalance	bruising
secondary adrenal insufficiency	skin atrophy
Musculo-skeletal	Growth retardation
myopathy	
osteoporosis	Susceptibility to infections
osteonecrosis	
Ophthalmic	
cataract	
glaucoma	
Gastrointestinal	
peptic ulcer disease	
pancreatitis	
Neuropsychiatric	
depression	
psychosis	
benign intracranial hypertension	

osteoporosis

sorption, which results in an increased bone fracture rate. The catabolic effect of corticosteroids on the bone is strongest in the first 6–12 months after initiation of the drug; there may be some reversibility of corticosteroid effect after cessation of treatment, but again, there is a significant degree of individual variation. Interestingly, recent work indicates that the osteoporotic effect of corticosteroids is less pronounced in RA patients than expected, perhaps because relief of symptoms allows more weight-bearing exercise to be undertaken, a factor that opposes bone loss. It is recommended that a dose equivalent to the physiological replacement dosage of cortisol (7.5 mg of prednisolone per day) not be exceeded if possible, as there seem to be increased side effects with increasing dose [10]. This is often possible in RA, but larger doses are often needed in other inflammatory rheumatic conditions such as polymyalgia rheumatica. The risk of hypothalamic-pituitary adrenal suppression by daily usage of corticosteroids is reduced by administration in the morning. If possible, alternate day administration reduces the suppressive effect further, although this is often not possible in RA patients due to the intensity of symptoms. Abrupt cessation of corticosteroids after long-term therapy may induce a corticosteroid "withdrawal" syndrome involving fatigue, myalgia, anorexia and weight loss. More dramatic symptoms such as hypotension and electrolyte imbalances can also occur, particularly in stressful situations such as emergency surgery. The dose of prednisolone must be reduced slowly, particularly when dosage is below 10–15 mg per day.

hypothalamic-pituitary adrenal suppression

Disease- modifying antirheumatic drugs

bony erosion

Although there is much evidence for the short-term control of disease by DMARDs, evidence of effects on long-term disease outcome is sparse. A recent study, however, demonstrated a positive association between a greater and earlier DMARD use and a better disability index value [11]. The current approach to RA treatment stresses the early commencement of DMARDs, generally within 3 months of the onset of RA. The rationale for early initiation of therapy is the evidence that many of the deleterious effects of RA such as bony erosions occur within the first 1–2 years of disease. The DMARDs most commonly used are methotrexate, antimalarials, sulphasalazine and gold injections. Clinically useful combinations of DMARDs are only now being identified, and biologic agents are still largely experimental, although promising efficacy in RA is appearing.

clinical guidelines for RA management

Clinical guidelines for the management of RA were recently published by the American College of Rheumatology [12]. There is no universally

Table 2 Overview of DMARDs used in the treatment of RA

Drug	Approximate time to benefit	Usual maintenance dose	Toxicity
Hydroxychloroquine	2–4 months	200 mg twice daily	infrequent rash, diarrhea, rare retinal toxicity
Sulphasalazine	1–2 months	1000 mg two or three times daily	rash, infrequent myelo-suppression, GI intolerance
Methotrexate	1–2 months	7.5–15 mg per week	GI symptoms, stomatitis, rash, alopecia, infrequent myelosup-pression, hepatotoxicity, rare but serious (even life threaten ing) pulmonary toxicity
Injectable gold salts	3–6 months	25–50 mg IM every 2–4 weeks	rash, stomatitis, myelo-suppression, thrombocytopenia, proteinuria
Oral gold	4–6 months	3 mg daily or twice daily	same as injectable gold but less frequent, plus frequent diarrhea
Azathioprine	2–3 months	50–150 mg daily	myelosuppression, infrequent hepatotoxicity, early flu like illness with fever, GI symptoms, elevated LFTs
D-penicillamine	3–6 months	250–750 mg daily	rash, stomatitis, dysgeusia, proteinuria, myelosuppression, infrequent but serious auto-immune disease

GI, gastrointestinal; IM, intramuscularly; elevated LFTs, elevated results on liver function tests.
For more detailed information on monitoring the symptoms and signs of toxicity, see the American College of Rheumatology Guidelines for Monitoring Drug Therapy in Rheumatoid Arthritis [13].

accepted scheme for therapeutic progression in the management of RA. Most patients discontinue an individual agent because of inefficacy or toxicity, and patients with severe disease often have used all current DMARDs. Hydroxychloroquine and sulphasalazine are usually used for milder disease, whereas methotrexate and gold are used for moderate to severe disease. An overview of DMARDs used in the treatment of RA is shown in Table 2.

The mechanism of action of DMARDs is not well understood, but they have a well-described toxicity profile, and there are guidelines for monitoring drug therapy in RA [13]. Patient education is very important

monitoring drug therapy

in the safe and effective administration of DMARDs, and patient organisations such as the Arthritis Foundation in Australia and the equivalent in other countries are invaluable in their support and service to arthritis sufferers.

Methotrexate

psoriatic arthropathy

Low-dose methotrexate (up to 25 mg given as a once-weekly oral or intramuscular dose) is an established DMARD for RA, psoriatic arthropathy and other inflammatory joint diseases. Its usage in RA patients was first reported in 1951. Since the 1980s methotrexate has become the most widely used antirheumatic drug due to its favourable efficacy and toxicity profile. Patient withdrawal from using this drug is less compared with other DMARDs, with up to 75% of patients still taking methotrexate 6 years after initiation of the treatment [14].

Efficacy

joint destruction

Although a complete remission is rarely seen, a meta-analysis of four randomised studies showed a 26% improvement in pain and a 39% improvement in the inflamed joint count in RA patients treated with methotrexate compared with placebo [15]. Sustained response to this DMARD of up to 7 years has been reported, as well as a corticosteroid-sparing effect. In comparative studies of efficacy, methotrexate is rated superior to auranofin, azathioprine and cyclosporin A. Joint destruction may be retarded by methotrexate. Importantly, the progression of joint erosions and joint space narrowing in RA patients was less pronounced in methotrexate-treated patients when compared with patients receiving auranofin [16] or azathioprine [17].

Mechanism of action

dihydrofolate reductase

folic acid and folinic acid

Methotrexate is a known cytotoxic agent. Its cytotoxic effects are related to the competitive inhibition of the enzyme dihydrofolate reductase by the drug, its oxidative metabolite 7-hydroxymethotrexate and the polyglutamated metabolic derivatives of both methotrexate and 7-hydroxymethotrexate. This inhibition results in reduction of the availability of reduced folate, which is an important requirement for the proliferation of cells (Fig. 2). Interestingly, folic acid or folinic acid is used as

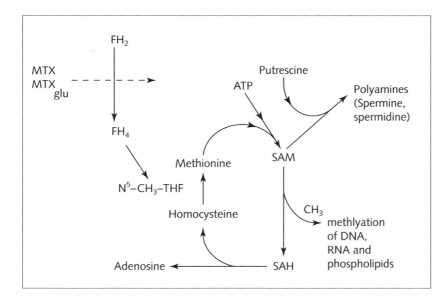

Figure 2 Some actions of methotrexate likely to be relevant to its mode of action
Inhibition of transmethylation reactions and polyamine formation by MTX. MTX promotes adenosine release by other mechanisms [18]. MTX, methotrexate; MTXglu, methotrexate polyglutamate; FH$_2$, dihydrofolate; FH$_4$, tetrahydofolate; N^5-CH$_3$-THF, N^5-methyltetrahydrofolate; SAM, S-adenosylmethionine; SAH, S-adenosylhomocysteine. Redrawn with permission of author and publisher [18].

an antidote to some of the adverse effects of low-dose methotrexate, particularly mouth ulcers and nausea. If the dose of these agents is too high, then methotrexate efficacy is, however, lost [18].

There is data that suggests an effect of methotrexate on the availability of several cytokines involved in rheumatoid arthritis, particularly IL-1, tumour necrosis factor α (TNFα), IL-6 and IL-8. Whether these effects are causal or simply epiphenomena remains unknown. At the molecular level, the inhibition of transmethylation reactions and drug-induced increases in adenosine concentrations are possible mechanisms of antiinflammatory and antirheumatic effects of this drug [18].

transmethylation
adenosine

Pharmacokinetics

The oral bioavailability of methotrexate is moderate, at about 65%. The intramuscular route can be used if excessive nausea occurs when the drug is taken orally and is not controlled by folic acid treatment. The plasma

bioavailability of
methotrexate

half-life is biphasic and possibly even triphasic, the initial half-life being short, of the order of 2–3 h, followed by the dominant half-life of the order of 7 h [19]. Plasma concentrations are difficult to measure beyond 24 h, although increasingly sensitive analytical techniques indicate a terminal half-life of days. The drug is oxidised in the liver to 7-hydroxymethotrexate. The drug is taken up by cells by an active transport process and is polyglutamated. The polyglutamated metabolite has a half-life much longer than that of the parent drug and is also a potent inhibitor of dihydrofolate reductase. Methotrexate is excreted unchanged in the kidneys in large part via the weak acid secretory pathway in the proximal renal tubule, this route accounting for over half of the clearance of the drug. The drug is therefore retained in renal impairment which is important in dosing, particularly in the elderly. There are competitive excretion interactions at the weak acid secretory pathway in the proximal tubule particularly with aspirin and other NSAIDs, but these only become clinically significant when methotrexate is given in higher doses and/or there is accompanying renal impairment.

polyglutamated metabolite

Toxicity

Adverse effects are the main reason for methotrexate discontinuation. Toxicity is not uncommon and may occur at any time in the course of the treatment [20]. Gastrointestinal side effects such as stomatitis, anorexia, vomiting and diarrhoea are the most frequent toxicities, occuring in up to 60% of methotrexate-treated patients but are usually quite mild. These adverse effects usually are responsive to dosage reduction, temporary drug discontinuation or usage of folic or folinic acid. Folate supplementation should be considered in all patients treated with methotrexate. Folic acid is cheaper than folinic acid and most commonly employed.

stomatitis

Renal function is very important in the selection of the dosage of methotrexate. A lower dose or cessation of therapy should be used in patients with chronic renal impairment or at times of volume depletion (such as perioperatively). Indeed, many of the listed toxicities have been reported associated with renal impairment. Older age may predispose to toxicity, again related to renal impairment. Abnormal plasma liver enzyme levels are frequently seen with methotrexate use; however, clinically significant liver disease with fibrosis and cirrhosis is uncommon. This serious liver complication may be associated with concomitant use of alcohol or preexisting liver disease. Cytopenias are reported in approximately 5% of methotrexate-treated patients, but severe myelodepression is uncommon. An elevated mean corpuscular volume may precede

renal function

cirrhosis

myelodepression

haematological toxicity. Interstitial pneumonitis is a serious and potentially fatal complication of methotrexate treatment, with occurrence rates reported to be from 0.3% to 11.6% [20]. Histological findings range from lymphocytic interstitial infiltrates to interstitial fibrosis. Many reported cases may have been due to infection, which must always be excluded. Methotrexate-induced pneumonitis is treated with methotrexate withdrawal and supportive care. Due to the teratogenic potential of methotrexate, pregnancy is contraindicated during usage. Treatment with DMARDs and methotrexate can often be stopped successfully during pregnancy because of the improvement in the activity of the RA associated with pregnancy.

interstitial pneumonitis

teratogenic potential

Monitoring

Methotrexate therapy should be avoided in patients with preexisting liver disease or a significant lung condition. Alcohol abstinence is usually recommended. Liver function tests are recommended every 4–8 weeks. In patients with persistently abnormal liver function tests, discontinuation of therapy and liver biopsy should be considered [21]. The following baseline evaluations are recommended: a complete blood count, a chest radiograph, hepatitis B and C serology in high-risk patients, aspartate aminotransferase (AST), alanine aminotransferase (ALT), albumin, alkaline phosphatase and creatinine. The complete blood count, AST, albumin and creatinine should be monitored every 4–8 weeks in the course of the treatment.

liver function tests

Sulphasalazine

Sulphasalazine consists of a salicylate and an antibacterial component, sulphapyridine, joined by an azo bond. This drug was synthesised in the late 1930s and originally developed and used on the basis of a belief in an infectious origin of RA. Sulphasalazine is a well tolerated and relatively safe drug compared with other DMARDs. It is commonly used for the treatment of ankylosing spondylitis and HLA B27-related arthropathies and RA. Usual maintenance dosage for RA patients is 1 g twice a day [22].

ankylosing spondylitis and HLA B27-related arthropathies

Efficacy

Sulphasalazine has been shown to be effective in several placebo-controlled double-blind trials demonstrating a significant improvement in clinical and laboratory outcome measures in RA patients. Its antirheumatic properties are equivalent to gold and penicillamine with only slightly less effect but a quicker onset of action, being measurable after 1–2 months. Cesssation rates are similar to, or somewhat less than, those observed with gold and D-penicillamine, most commonly related to insufficient efficacy and less commonly to toxicity. Sulphasalazine tends to slow joint destruction compared with placebo and hydroxychloroquine [23]. RA patients receiving sulphasalazine and hydroxychloroquine in combination do no better than sulphasalazine alone. Sulphasalazine has also proven effective in patients with ankylosing spondylitis [24] and an open study in patients with HLA-B27-associated asymmetrical oligoarticular arthritis suggests benefit for this condition.

joint destruction

Mechanism of action

sulphapyridine

The antirheumatic activity of sulphasalazine is thought to be related to its metabolic products sulphapyridine and aminosalicylate. There is some belief that the parent drug can affect the lymphocytes in the immunological tissue in the intestine and thus the gut immune response. This particularly relates to the theory that some inflammatory rheumatic conditions, in particular bowel-associated inflammatory arthritis such as is seen with ulcerative colitis and Crohn's disease, is caused by an aberrant immunological response to bowel microorganisms.

There is some data that suggests that systemic concentrations of sulphapyridine are more likely related to the antirheumatic effects of the drug. It is believed that the aminosalicylate metabolite, which is largely retained in the colon, is responsible for the antiinflammatory effects in the colon and thus the efficacy of the drug in inflammatory bowel diseases. Interestingly, uncontrolled data suggest that olsalazine, which is a dimer of salicylic acid molecules joined by an azo bond, may be effective in ankylosing spondylitis.

olsalazine

Pharmacokinetics

The drug is administered orally, and upon reaching the large bowel the azo bond is reduced by colonic bacteria. Sulphapyridine is absorbed, whereas aminosalicylate remains in the large intestine. Sulphapyridine is subject to oxidative and acetylation metabolic reactions in the liver [22].

Toxicity

Although there is a wide range of potential side effects, sulphasalazine is among the group of the best-tolerated DMARDs, along with hydroxychloroquine, methotrexate and auranofin. Toxicity is most frequent in the first 2–3 months of usage, but its likelihood can be reduced by gradually increasing the dosage and the use of enteric-coated formulations. Maintenance sulphasalazine dosage is usually 1 g two or three times daily. Serious side effects are rare, and most adverse effects are eliminated if the dose is reduced. Nausea and upper abdominal discomfort are the most frequent side effects at the start of the therapy. Leukopenia is very uncommon but can develop rapidly and at any time; it is most likely to occur in the first 6 months of therapy. Sulphasalazine should be avoided at around the time of conception and pregnancy, although no teratogenicity has been reported for this drug. It can induce a reversible reduction in sperm count.

leukopenia

teratogeneicity

sperm count

Monitoring

The main aim of monitoring is the early detection of haematological side effects. It is recommended that at baseline a complete blood cell count be performed as well as analysis of the glucose 6-phosphate dehydrogenase level, as this enzyme deficiency is associated with haemolysis with sulphasalazine. For the follow-up visits, complete blood cell counts every 2–4 weeks for the first 3 months are suggested. Baseline measurement of AST or ALT is advised in patients with known or suspected liver disease.

Antimalarials

Since the early 1950s hydroxychloroquine and chloroquine have been prescribed to treat various rheumatic disorders, mainly RA and systemic lupus erythematosus. Antimalarials are generally considered to be mild antirheumatic agents. Compared with other DMARDs, antimalarials are relatively safe drugs, which makes them attractive for use in the early stages of RA or in combination with other DMARDs. The usual daily doses for adults of normal weight are 200–400 mg/day for hydroxy-chloroquine and 250 mg for chloroquine [25].

Efficacy

A recent randomised, double-blind placebo-controlled study of 120 patients with early RA showed a beneficial effect of hydroxychloroquine in 60–80% of patients within the 36 weeks of study duration. Significant improvements were seen in pain, physical function and a joint index [26]. A study comparing sulphasalazine with hydroxychloroquine found sulphasalazine to be more effective in retarding the formation of bony erosions [27].

Mechanism of action

acidic sphingo-myelinase

NF-κB

phospholipase A$_2$

Aminoquinolines, chloroquine and hydroxychloroquine, are weakly basic drugs that accumulate in acidic organelles, particularly lysosomes, where they raise the pH. This may affect the function of acidic organelles or, more specifically, inhibit lysosomal enzymes such as lysozyme. Acidic sphingomyelinase is located within the lipid membrane of lysosomes and is an important mediator in the signal transduction pathway between the TNFα p75 receptor on the cell surface and activation of transcription factor NF-κB in the nucleus [28]. Raising the pH of lysozomes inhibits acidic sphingomyelinase activity, consequently inhibiting NF-κB activity and proinflammatory gene expression [28]. Antimalarials have also been reported to inhibit the production of interleukin-1 and the activity of many other enzymes, including phospholipase A$_2$. It is difficult to determine the relative importance of these phenomena in the many immunological and clinical effects ascribed to antimalarials.

Pharmacokinetics

The bioavailability of hydroxychloroquine is very variable, ranging from below 20% up to 100%, but the bioavailability appears to remain constant within an individual. The variable bioavailability may be responsible for much of the interpatient differences in the response to hydroxy-chloroquine [29].

Another important feature of the pharmacokinetics of hydroxy-chloroquine and chloroquine is the extremely long half-life of about 40 days. This means that steady-state concentrations may not be achieved until after 3–6 months of daily dosing. It has been hypothesised that achieving plateau concentrations earlier by loading regimens may decrease the time until the onset of effect of hydroxychloroquine, which is considered to be slower than sulphasalazine, for example [25].

A relationship between blood hydroxychloroquine concentrations and efficacy has been revealed in a cross-sectional study in rheumatoid arthritis patients. This suggests that there may be some value in measuring blood hydroxychloroquine concentrations to optimise dosing regimens in individual patients [30].

blood hydroxy-chloroquine concentration

Toxicity

Compared with other DMARDs, antimalarials are recognised as the least toxic, and they lack life-threatening toxicity. Most adverse effects are transient, and cessation of the drug is usually not required. Hydroxychloroquine and chloroquine have a very similar range of adverse effects, but in usual doses hydroxychloroquine is associated with less toxicity than chloroquine. Adverse reactions include gastrointestinal symptoms, myopathy, abnormal skin pigmentation and peripheral neuropathy although the latter three are rare. Of most concern is a rare, irreversible retinopathy, resulting in permanent visual loss. It is almost unknown with hydroxychloroquine with most cases being due to chloroquine. This effect can be avoided by limiting daily dosing measured on a weight basis. Thus dosing with hydroxychloroquine should not exceed 6.5 mg/kg daily.

abnormal skin pigmentation

irreversible retinopathy

Monitoring

It is recommended that there should be a baseline eye evaluation and fundoscopic and visual fields examinations every 6–12 months.

Gold

Gold treatment of patients with RA was first reported in 1929 by Forestier. Gold therapy is mainly used for RA and less frequently for psoriatic arthritis, particularly the nonspondylotic form. Initial dosage is oral (auranofin – up to 6 mg daily in divided doses) or intramuscular (aurothiomalate, aurothioglucose – 10–25 mg weekly). The short-term value of gold complexes for the treatment of RA is generally accepted. Gold

psoriatic arthritis

therapy may be maintained (10–50 mg intramuscularly every 2–4 weeks, or 3 mg orally once or twice daily) indefinitely while there is benefit.

Efficacy

Injectable gold compounds have shown short-term efficacy in improving clinical and laboratory parameters in RA patients, and their efficacy is similar to sulphasalazine, methotrexate and D-penicillamine [31]. An excellent response occurs in about a third of the patients treated with intramuscular gold compounds within the first year. A recent study suggested that aurothiomalate promoted the repair of bony erosions in early RA **erosions** [32]. As assessed by microfocal radiography, a new X-ray technique, RA patients receiving aurothiomalate showed less progression of erosions and a higher rate of erosion repair than patients without gold treatment. However, the long-term benefits of gold compounds are less impressive.

The short-term efficacy of auranofin has been demonstrated several times in RA patients. This oral gold compound is less efficacious than injectable aurothiomalate, and less effective than methotrexate and D-penicillamine [31]. A clinical benefit is often not maintained over time, and significant numbers of patients withdraw from treatment due to inefficacy.

Mechanism of action (Fig. 1)

thiol, cyanide The inorganic biochemistry of gold(I) salts is dominated by the high affinity of gold(I) for thiols, including cysteine residues and for cyanide. Several "proinflammatory" transcription factors, including AP-1 (Jun and Fos) and NF-κB have cysteine residues within their positively charged DNA binding domains. This unusual electrostatic environment favours the formation of a thiolate anion within the cysteine residue and enhances gold(I) affinity. As a consequence, low concentrations of gold(I) thiolates (5 μM) significantly inhibit AP-1 DNA binding in nuclear extracts [33], whereas the inhibition of any enzyme system reported to date requires at least a 10-fold higher concentration. Furthermore, the concentration of gold(I) thiomalate (10 μM) that inhibits AP-1-mediated transcription is within the concentration range of gold(I) achieved in the serum of RA patients treated with intramuscular gold salts. Gold(I) thioglucose has also been shown to inhibit the IL-1 induced expression of NF-κB and AP-1-dependent reporter genes and to inhibit DNA-binding activity of NF-κB *in vitro* [34]. Consistent with these effects on proinflammatory transcripton factors is the observation that gold(I) thiomalate inhibits expression of the adhesion molecules ICAM-1 and VCAM-1 in vascular endothelial cells [35].

ICAM-1, VCAM-1

Metabolism and pharmacokinetics

Gold complexes of albumin are the most significant complexes in plasma, and the total gold concentration is eliminated from plasma with an initial half-life of about 5 days [36]. Much of the gold following injection is excreted in urine, but some accumulates, particularly in the lysosomes of synovial lining cells, where gold is present for many years following the last dose of gold. Much gold appears in faeces when oral gold is administered. Only a very small amount of gold appears in breast milk, thus posing little risk to breast-fed infants.

gold

The bioavailability and disposition of gold is dependent on the administered formulation and the route of administration, reflecting differences in the lipid solubility of the forms. Thus, auranofin is bioavailable following oral administration as it is much more lipid soluble than aurothioglucose or aurothiomalate. A common metabolite of the injectable gold drugs is aurocyanide, $Au(CN)_2^-$. Aurocyanide is formed through the oxidation of thiocyanate, SCN^-, by myeloperoxidase, an important enzyme in the oxidative burst of neutrophils and monocytes. Thiocyanate is a normal body constituent which is oxidised, in part, to hydrogen cyanide which then reacts with gold complexes to yield aurocyanide. This gold complex is a potent inhibitor of the oxidative burst of neutrophils and also of the proliferation of lymphocytes. It may mediate many of the antirheumatic and adverse effects of the gold complexes [37]. Small amounts of hydrogen cyanide (60 to 250 µg per cigarette) are inhaled by cigarette smokers, but the response and adverse reactions are probably not affected by smoking, the local production of cyanide by neutrophils appearing to be more important than the inhalation of hydrogen cyanide.

aurocyanide

Toxicity

Adverse effects of injected gold therapy are common, involving up to 40% of patients. Toxicity, however, is generally minor and manageable if dosing is adjusted early upon appearance of adverse effects, although adverse effects are a common cause of withdrawals from gold therapy over 2–4 years of therapy. Toxicity does not correlate with the cumulative dose. The most frequent side effects include pruritus, rash, dermatitis and mouth ulcers. They respond well to drug discontinuation. As aurothioglucose is less likely to cause skin reactions than aurothiomalate, the former drug should be considered for reintroduction in very small doses when the skin reaction or mouth ulcers have settled. Vasomotor reactions such as sweating, nausea and hypotension immediately after injection and proteinuria are frequently seen. Fortunately, major serious side effects such as thrombocytopenia, aplastic anaemia, pneumonitis and membranous glomerulonephritis are rare. Initially, gold tolerance should be assessed with a test dose of 1 mg. Injection of gold may be painful but can be alleviated by adding lignocaine.

Auranofin is associated with fewer but similar side effects to those of injectable gold complexes. The most frequent adverse effect is diarrhoea, which may recede with drug continuation. Dosage reduction is often sufficient to stop it.

Monitoring

Before starting intramuscular gold therapy, a baseline evaluation should include a complete blood cell count, a urine dipstick analysis for protein and plasma creatinine. A full blood cell count and a urine dipstick analysis every 1–2 weeks for the first 20 weeks for intramuscular gold, and from then on at the time of each injection, is suggested. Patients should be asked about skin itching and mouth ulcers before each administration. The 24-h output of protein should be measured if the the qualitative test for urinary protein is positive. Treatment should be ceased if the protein excretion is greater than 500 mg in 24 h but can be restarted when urinary protein is negligible.

For oral gold therapy, the recommended baseline assessment is the same as for injectable gold. The follow-up monitoring should include a full blood cell count and a urine dipstick analysis every 4–12 weeks.

D-penicillamine

D-Penicillamine has been used for patients with RA and systemic sclerosis for nearly 30 years. It is a structural analogue of cysteine and a component of the penicillin molecule.

Mechanism of action

D-Penicillamine is a thiol drug that was introduced in RA because of its ability to dissociate the disulphide bonds of immunoglobulin M (IgM) RA *in vitro*. It now seems probable that improvement in rheumatoid arthritis is unrelated to its effects on rheumatoid factor, and the mechanism of action of D-penicillamine and other thiol drugs (bucillamine, tiopronine, thiopyridoxine) is unknown. It has long been noted that D-penicillamine and gold(I) thiolates have similar clinical properties in the treatment of RA, leading some authors to suggest that they have a similar mechanism of action through their reactivities with endogenous thiols.

D-Penicillamine inhibits AP-1 DNA binding in nuclear extracts in the presence of free radicals, presumably by forming disulphide bonds with the cysteine residues in the DNA binding domains of Jun and Fos [38]. Mutagenesis again confirms the necessity of cysteine residues in the DNA binding domains for this to occur [38]. Conversely, some authors have sought to explain the mode of action of thiol drugs according to their reducing properties, whereas the argument put forward here, based on their oxidising action, is the exact opposite. Whatever the details of molecular interactions, it is considered that cysteine residues within the DNA binding domains of proinflammatory transcription factors are therefore potential targets for gold and D-penicillamine.

AP-1

Pharmacokinetics

The drug is well absorbed orally but is subject to binding interactions in the gastrointestinal tract, particularly with iron salts and antacids. Administration on an empty stomach is therefore recommended. The elimination half-life of D-penicillamine is a few hours only. The main mechanism of clearance is via reactions with sulphydryl molecules, particularly those found in albumin. The disulphide-bonded products, including D-penicillamine-disulphide, and D-penicillamine cysteine disulphide, act as a "sink" for D-penicillamine. A good example is D-penicillamine albumin complexes, which have a half-life greatly in excess of the parent D-penicillamine [39].

D-penicillamine albumin

Efficacy

D-Penicillamine has been shown to improve clinical signs in RA patients as well as to correct abnormal laboratory parameters such as haemoglo-

joint destruction

bin, erythrocyte sedimentation rate, rheumatoid factor, immunoglobulins and circulating immune complexes. However, joint destruction as assessed by X-rays is not proven to be retarded by this DMARD. Otherwise, D-penicillamine seems to be as effective as gold and azathioprine [40]. Unfortunately, withdrawal rates from D-penicillamine are high (comparable to gold treatment) either due to inefficacy or side effects. An uncontrolled, open study with a 15 year follow-up in patients with

progressive systemic sclerosis

progressive systemic sclerosis treated with D-penicillamine suggested a reduction in the degree of diseased skin involvement. Treatment should be initiated with 125 mg daily for 4–8 weeks, then raising the dosage by the same increment until improvement is noticeable or a daily dose of 750 mg is achieved.

Toxicity

myelosuppression

Mild side effects such as rash, stomatitis and metallic taste are common with D-penicillamine, whereas serious toxicity such as myelosuppression, proteinuria, nephrotic syndrome and autoimmune syndromes are rare. Most adverse effects occur in the first 6 months after commencement of the drug, involving about 50% of patients and resulting in a significant dropout rate from treatment. A recent open study indicated that intermittent dosage of D-penicillamine may be as effective as daily treatment but caused fewer adverse effects.

Monitoring

The following baseline evaluations are recommended: complete blood cell count, creatinine and urine dipstick for protein. A complete blood cell count and test for urinary protein should be checked every 2 weeks until a stable dosage is achieved. After that, these evaluations may be performed every 1–3 months.

Cyclosporin A

nephrotoxicity

Cyclosporin A has recently become accepted as a DMARD. Cyclosporin A was discovered in 1972 while searching for antifungal agents. It is a mildly active fungal antimetabolite, but has profound effects on the immune response. This immunomodulatory agent is efficacious in patients with RA, but nephrotoxicity is a significant problem if doses are too high. Cyclosporine therapy in RA is reserved currently for patients with refractory disease or severe extraarticular complications. Cyclosporine should be initiated at doses of 2.5 mg/kg/day given in two divided doses every 12 h, increasing the dose 25–50% every 2–4 weeks until a maximum dose of 5 mg/kg/day is reached.

Mechanism of action

Cyclosporin A, along with rapamycin and tacrolimus (FK506), suppress the immune response by inhibiting key signal transduction pathways. This is achieved by intracellular binding to immunophillin receptors, the complexes thus formed inhibiting calcineurin. Blocking the actions of calcineurin leads to inhibition of the translocation to the nucleus of the cytosolic component of the nuclear factor of activated T-cells (NF-AT). Thus, genes dependent on this transcription factor such as IL-2 and IL-4 are not transcribed normally [41].

calcineurin

Pharmacokinetics

Cyclosporin A is difficult to formulate into a reliably absorbed product, and the drug is known to have very variable bioavailability. A capsule formulation containing the drug in solution which has recently been introduced has resulted in better and more predictable bioavailability, and it is likely that there will be less influence of meals on bioavailability. Cyclosporin A has a low therapeutic index, and kidney damage has been shown to be more likely to occur in RA patients at dosing rates greater than 5 mg/kg/day. The half-life of elimination is about 6 h but the drug is commonly administered twice daily. The drug is metabolised by the hepatic cytochrome P-450 oxidase system (3A4 isoenzyme in particular). Its metabolism is inhibited by a range of drugs including ketoconazole and diltiazem and induced by others such as carbamazepine and phenytoin (Table 3; for a more complete review of clinically significant drug interaction see Campara et al. [42]).

cytochrome P-450 oxidase system

Efficacy

Cyclosporine improves clinical signs and symptoms of RA. Patients treated with cyclosporin A doses between 2.5 and 5.0 mg/kg/day show significant improvements in the number of active joints, pain and functional

Table 3 Drug interactions with cyclosporine*

Agents which may increase cyclosporine blood concentrations	Drugs which may decrease cyclosporine blood concentrations	Drugs which may cause additive nephrotoxicity
allopurinol	carbamazepine	aminoglycosides
amiodarone	ciprofloxacin	amphotericin B
danazol	isoniazid	ciprofloxacin
diltiazem	octreotide	colchicine
doxycycline	phenobarbitone	enalapril
erythromycin	phenytoin	melphalan
fluconazole	rifampicin	nonsteroidal antiinflammatory drugs
glipizide	probucol	trimethoprim (including trimoxazole)
grapefruit juice	sulphadimidine +	
itraconazole	trimethoprim i.v.	
ketoconazole		
metoclopramide		
miconazole		
nicardipine		
oral contraceptives		
prednisolone		
tacrolimus		
verapamil		

* *Adapted from cyclosporine information brochure (Sandoz Aust. Pty Ltd; item no. 139535) and Compana et al. [42].*

joint damage

status compared with controls [43]. Doses of 10 mg/kg/day are more effective [44], but dose-dependent nephrotoxicity now limits dosage to 5 mg/kg/day. Low-dose cyclosporine is as effective as other DMARDs in controlling clinical symptoms. Further, this agent may be as effective as chloroquine in patients with early rheumatoid arthritis after 2 years of treatment [45]. There is evidence that low-dose cyclosporine retards further joint damage in previously involved joints, and decreases the rate of new joint erosions in previously uninvolved joints, in patients with early RA [46].

Toxicity

Nephrotoxicity is the principal adverse effect of cyclosporine. This agent should be avoided in patients with preexisting renal disease. Careful dosing is required when cyclosporine is used with other nephrotoxic agents (Table 3). If plasma creatinine increases by 30–50% above baseline, the dose should be reduced by 25–50%. Hypertension is another common side effect affecting up to one-third of cyclosporine-treated RA patients. Hypertension can usually be controlled with beta-blockers or angiotensin converting enzyme (ACE) inhibitors. The dose of cyclosporine should be reduced if the cyclosporine induced hypertension is not treated. Less serious side effects such as nausea, vomiting and loss of appetite are frequent. Elevated hepatic enzymes and bilirubin due to hepatotoxicity are usually associated with high doses of this agent. Other toxic side effects include anaemia, gum hyperplasia, transient hirsutism, tremor and parasthesias. Of concern are case reports of lymphoproliferative lesions and other malignancies developing in patients who have received cyclosporine therapy.

nephrotoxicity

hypertension

malignancy

Monitoring

A complete blood count, creatinine, uric acid and liver function tests as well as the measurement of blood pressure are recommended at baseline. For follow-up visits examination for oedema and measurement of blood pressure are suggested every 2 weeks until the cyclosporine dosage is stable and monthly from then on. Plasma creatinine should be checked every 2 weeks until the dosage is stable. Periodic complete blood counts, plasma potassium and liver function tests are suggested. Plasma concentrations of cyclosporine should be monitored on starting or discontinuing any of the drugs listed in Table 3. Patients should be made aware of the interaction with grapefruit juice.

Combination DMARD therapies

Despite the lack of knowledge on mechanisms of DMARD action, it seems likely that these drugs work in different ways. It is therefore possible that combining proven agents may allow a decreased dose of a particular agent (with concomitant decrease in its side effects) without diminished efficacy. There may also be an additive or synergistic effect from combinations.

A combination of an antimalarial and parenteral gold was first reported in the early 1960s, and combinations of hydroxychloroquine with methotrexate and sulphasalazine with methotrexate have been reported, but good trial data is lacking. A meta-analysis of five randomised controlled trials comparing single drug therapy versus combination therapy showed similar effectiveness. However, the results of a recent 2-year double-blind trial in 102 RA patients are encouraging. The combination of methotrexate, sulphasalazine and hydroxychloroquine was significantly more effective regarding clinical and laboratory parameters than methotrexate alone or the combination of sulphasalazine and hydroxychloroquine [47]. Also recently, the combination of methotrexate and cyclosporine has proven more efficacious than methotrexate alone [48].

Emerging therapies

Better understanding of the molecular pathogenesis of RA in the last few years has made the development of biological agents possible. To date, the clinical experience with them has been mixed, and their usage remains experimental. They involve the use of anti-T-cell agents, anti-cytokine antibodies and use of recombinant naturally occurring cytokine inhibitors.

cytokine inhibitor

Initially, beneficial effects were reported from open phase I trials with monoclonal antibodies against CD4, the T helper cell marker, but a recent randomised double-blind placebo-controlled study using humanised anti-CD4 "non-T-cell depleting" monoclonal antibodies in 30 patients with early RA did not show any therapeutic effect [49]. The importance of controlled studies is emphasized by this experience. IL-2 receptor antibodies have been shown to be effective in adjuvant arthritis in animal models, but open studies in humans report less favourable results with low response rates and a high incidence of side effects. Anticytokine treatment includes the administration of monoclonal antibodies or soluble receptors of IL-1 and TNFα. Results from randomised placebo-controlled trials using TNFα antibodies and soluble receptors in particular are very encouraging [50].

IL-2 receptor antibody

IL-1 and TNFα

Problems related to the immunogenicity of these biological agents and their toxicity, particularly that associated with cytokine therapy, were evident in most of the studies. Further well-conducted research using randomised controlled trials is required to decide the value of these biologic agents.

Another exciting potential area involves gene therapy, e.g. to introduce a gene for a natural inhibitor of the destructive matrix metalloproteinases and prevent joint destruction, and human clinical trials have commenced. Combinations of biological agents and conventional DMARDs such as methotrexate are now appearing and results are promising.

Acknowledgements

Dr. C. Bachmeier was supported by the Ciba-Geigy-Jubiläumsstiftung, Karger Fonds, Schweizerische Gesellschaft für Rheumatologie and Schweizerische Akademie der Wissenschaften in Basel, Switzerland.

D   Immunotoxicology

Immunotoxicology

Joseph G. Vos, Eric J. De Waal, Henk van Loveren, Ruud Albers and Raymond H.H. Pieters

Introduction

Pharmaceuticals for human use comprise a very wide variety of product types. These include traditional products (i.e. chemically synthesized or plant-derived pharmaceuticals) as well as biological products (such as vaccines and blood products isolated from biological sources) and biotechnology-derived pharmaceuticals (such as peptide products manufactured by recombinant DNA techniques, monoclonal antibodies and gene therapy products). In the interest of the public, these medicinal products are subject to worldwide regulatory control by government authorities. The major objective of this regulation is to ensure that the benefit of the products to the patients are not outweighed by their adverse effects. To achieve this goal, the authorities carefully assess the balance between efficacy and safety. If this balance is positive, they allow marketing. To support applications for marketing authorisation, the pharmaceutical industry therefore has to submit scientific data which prove that their products are efficacious and acceptably safe in the proposed therapeutic indication. Furthermore, the pharmaceutical quality of the products applied for has to meet high standards.

adverse effects

Chemicals used for a variety of purposes can have adverse effects on the immune system of both animals and humans. In the case of drugs, this can be the result of pharmacological interference with the immune system, or an undesired reaction. One form of immunotoxicity is the direct toxicity of the compound to components of the immune system, which often leads to suppressed function. This may result in decreased resistance to infection, the development of certain types of tumors or immune dysregulation and stimulation, thereby promoting allergy or autoimmunity. Other types or manifestations of immunotoxicity include allergy or autoimmunity in which the compound causes the immune system to respond as if the compound were an antigen or to respond to self-antigens that have been altered by the chemical.

undesired reaction

immunotoxicity

autoimmunity

immuno-suppression

immuno-stimulation

hypersensitivity

Except for cancer patients on chemotherapy and organ transplant patients on long-term immunosuppressive therapy, there is little evidence that drugs are associated with undesired, clinically significant immunosuppression. However, only a few valid epidemiological studies of immunologically based diseases have been carried out [1], probably due to the complication of such studies by confounding factors such as (disease-associated) stress, nutritional status, lifestyle, (co)medication and genetics. Few conventional drugs have been shown to induce unexpected enhancement of immune competence. Unwanted immunostimulation has gained attention primarily through the introduction of new biotechnologically manufactured drugs such as cytokines. Drug-induced hypersensitivity reactions and autoimmune disorders are a major concern, and often the reason for withdrawing drugs from the market or restricting their use.

For the detection of chemical-induced direct immunotoxicity animal models have been developed, and a number of these methods have been validated. Several compounds, including certain drugs, have been shown in this way to cause immunosuppression. Methods are also available for the detection of skin allergic responses, whereas no validated test is available to predict potential induction of autoimmunity.

In this chapter, the various mechanisms of immunotoxicity are introduced and discussed by which pharmaceuticals affect different cell types and interfere with immune responses, ultimately leading to immunotoxicity. Further, procedures for preclinical testing of drugs are covered, comprising direct immunotoxicity as well as sensitizing capacity. This section is followed by consideration of procedures for clinical and epidemiological testing of drugs. Finally, regulatory aspects of immunotoxicity are discussed, including current guidelines and new developments in immunotoxicity assessment.

Mechanisms of immunotoxicity by pharmaceuticals

Effects on precursor stem cells

stem cell
leucocytes

Precursor stem cells that are responsible for replenishing peripheral leukocytes reside in the bone marrow making it an organ that harbors many highly proliferating cells. All leukocyte lineages originate from these stem cells, but once distinct subsets of leukocytes are established, their dependence on replenishment from the bone marrow differs vastly. The short-lived neutrophils rely heavily on proliferation and new formation in the bone marrow, as each day more than 10^8 neutrophils enter and leave the circulation in a normal adult. In contrast, macrophages are long-lived and have little dependence on new formation of precursor cells [2]. The adaptive immune system, comprising antigen-specific T- and B-lymphocytes, is almost completely established around puberty and is therefore essentially bone marrow-independent in the adult.

neutrophils

macrophages

As a consequence of their high proliferation rate, stem cells in the bone marrow are extremely vulnerable to antiproliferative cytostatic drugs such as the antineoplastic drugs cyclophosphamide (CY), and methotrexate (MTX), and the antirheumatic azathioprine (AZA) [1, 3] (Fig. 1). This is particularly the case at high doses of these drugs, and lineages like neutrophils that are extremely bone marrow-dependent will be most vulnerable and are affected first by treatment with these drugs. After prolonged exposure, macrophages and T- or B-cells of the adaptive immune system are also suppressed.

adaptive immune system

Effects on maturation of lymphocytes

After leaving the bone marrow, cells of both the T-cell and the B-cell lineages mature into antigen-specific lymphocytes. T-lymphocytes mature in the thymus during a process referred to as thymocyte differentiation, which is a very complex selection process that takes place under the influence of the thymic microenvironment and ultimately generates an antigen-specific, host-tolerant population of mature T-cells (see Chapters A2 and A3). Because this process involves cellular proliferation, gene rearrangement, apoptotic cell death, receptor up- and downregulation and antigen-presentation processes, it is very vulnerable to a number of chemicals, including pharmaceuticals (Fig. 1). Drugs may target different stages of T-cell differentiation: bone marrow precursors (AZA); proliferating and differentiating thymocytes (AZA); antigen-presenting thymic epithelial cells and dendritic cells (cyclosporin A, CsA) [4]; cell death processes (corticosteroids) [5] (Fig. 2).

T-lymphocytes

cellular proliferation gene rearrangement antigen-presentation

In general, immunosuppressive drugs that affect the thymus cause a depletion of peripheral T-cells, particularly after prolonged treatment and during early stages of life when thymus activity is high and important in establishing a mature T-cell population.

thymus

After the bone marrow stage, B-cells mature in the spleen. With the exception of certain monoclonal antibodies, there are no drugs that specifically affect B-cell development, although some studies claim a

B-cells

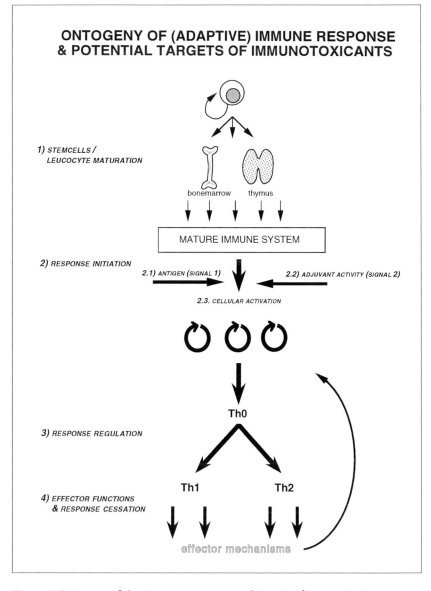

**ONTOGENY OF (ADAPTIVE) IMMUNE RESPONSE
& POTENTIAL TARGETS OF IMMUNOTOXICANTS**

*1) STEMCELLS /
LEUCOCYTE MATURATION*

bonemarrow   thymus

MATURE IMMUNE SYSTEM

2) RESPONSE INITIATION

2.1) ANTIGEN (SIGNAL 1)   *2.2) ADJUVANT ACTIVITY (SIGNAL 2)*

2.3. CELLULAR ACTIVATION

Th0

3) RESPONSE REGULATION

Th1   Th2

*4) EFFECTOR FUNCTIONS
& RESPONSE CESSATION*

effector mechanisms

*Figure 1 Ontogeny of the immune response and targets of immunotoxic
pharmaceuticals*

*This figure represents the different steps in the ontogeny of adaptive immune respons-
es from stem cell to response cessation. It forms our conceptual framework for identifying potential mechanisms of immunotoxicity. Indicated are effects of pharmaceuticals on
stem cells and leucocyte maturation, on the two signals that are essential for lymphocyte
activation, and the resulting cellular activation. Also indicated are the regulation and cessation of immune responses as potential targets for immunotoxic pharmaceuticals.*

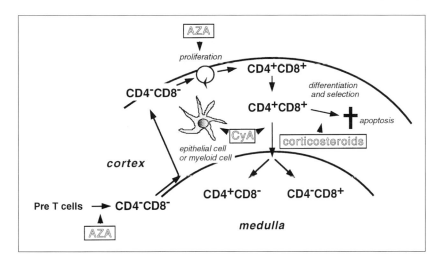

Figure 2 Schematic view of the thymus showing the cortical and medullary region
Immature pre-T-cells (CD4⁻CD8⁻) enter the thymus at the corticomedullary region and migrate to the subcapsular region, where they show high proliferative activity and differentiate into CD4⁺CD8⁺ thymocytes. In the cortex, most thymocytes are CD4⁺CD8⁺, and at this stage thymoctes are selected under the influence of thymic epithelial cells and are prone to apoptotic cell death. After the CD4⁺CD8⁺ stage, cells differentiate either to CD4⁺ or to CD8⁺ cells. Stages sensitive to pharmaceutical attack are indicated: AZA inhibits formation of pre-T-cells and may inhibit immature thymocyte proliferation; CyA interferes with thymocyte selection, possibly through an effect on thymic dendritic cells; and corticosteroids stimulate apoptosis.

more or less B-cell-specific effect of CY and MTX. In general, suppression of the adaptive immune system at the antibody level is the result of an effect on T-cells or their development.

Effects on initiation of immune responses

Once a mature immune system has been established, the native and adaptive immune systems cooperate to eliminate invading pathogens. Ideally, T-cells tailor the responses to neutralise invaders with minimal damage to the host. After elimination of T-cells with high affinity for self-antigens in the thymus, tolerance for autoantigens is further maintained in the periphery by the two distinct signals that govern lymphocyte activation. Signal 1 is the specific recognition of antigen via clonally distributed antigen receptors. Signal 2 consists of antigen nonspecific costimulation or "help" and involves interactions of various adhesive and sig-

pathogens

tolerance

costimulation

naling molecules [6]. It is imperative that lymphocytes receive both signals, as antigen recognition without costimulation induces tolerance, and lymphocytes are unresponsive to costimulation without an antigen-specific signal. The molecules transmitting signal 2 are mainly expressed in response to tissue damage, linking initiation of immune responses to situations of acute "danger" for the host [7]. This helps to aim immune responses at potentially dangerous microorganisms (non-self), while minimizing deleterious reactions to innocuous antigens and to the host (self) (Chapter A1). Certain pharmaceuticals and other xenobiotics, however, can interfere with the initiation of immune responses if they induce signal 1 by functioning as antigen, by forming haptens or by releasing previously hidden self-antigens. They may also induce signal 2 by triggering an inflammatory response, or by disturbing T-B-cell cooperation. Finally, pharmaceuticals may directly affect cellular activation following occupation of the receptors involved in the two activation signals (Fig. 1).

haptens

Interference with antigen recognition (signal 1)

Large (protein) pharmaceuticals can be antigens

Large molecular weight pharmaceuticals (>4000 Da) can function as antigens and become targets of specific immune responses themselves. This is particularly relevant for foreign protein pharmaceuticals, as these can activate both T- and B-lymphocytes. The resulting drug-specific immune responses may lead to formation of antibodies, and induce specific memory which can lead to allergic responses to the drug. For example, passive immunization to tetanus toxin or snake venoms with serum from immunized horses causes the temporary formation of immune complexes with symptoms of fever, joint tenderness and proteinuria (serum sickness). Because serum proteins are given in large amounts and have a long half-life, sensitization and allergic reactions take place after a single dose. Similar immunotoxic effects due to immunogenicity may occur after repeated treatment with pharmaceuticals like porcine insulin, murine antibodies and biotechnologically engineered "novel proteins". In patients developing neutralizing antibodies, absence of response or reversal of clinical efficacy has been described [8]. The danger of immunotoxic effects due to immunogenicity is much lower when homologous recombinant human or "humanized" proteins are used as pharmaceuticals.

memory

Reactive pharmaceuticals can form haptens

Low molecular weight pharmaceuticals cannot function as antigens, because they are too small to be detected by T-cells. Reactive drugs that bind to proteins, however, can function as haptens and become immunogenic if epitopes derived from the carrier protein prime T-cells, which in turn provide costimulation for hapten-specific B-cells. This effect is responsible for allergic responses to many new (neo) epitopes formed by chemical haptens including pharmaceuticals (penicillin, penicillamine, cephalosporin, aspirin and many others), occupational contact sensitizers and respiratory sensitizers (Fig. 3). Other compounds require metabolic activation to form reactive metabolites that bind to proteins. The anesthetic halothane, for instance, is metabolized to alkyl halides by cytochrome P-450 in the liver. The alkyl halides bind to microsomal proteins including P-450, and the bound haptens induce an immune response that causes so-called halothane hepatitis. Other compounds can be activated by extrahepatic metabolism, in particular by the myeloperoxidase system in phagocytic cells. For instance, activated macrophages and granulocytes can metabolize the antiarrhythmic procainamide to reactive metabolites that can bind to proteins, and immune responses to these haptens seem to be responsible for procainamide-related agranulocytosis and lupus [9].

epitopes

contact sensitizers respiratory sensitizers

Responses to haptens can spread to autoreactive responses

Modification of autoantigens can also lead to autoreactive responses to unmodified self-epitopes. Antigens composed of neo- and self-epitopes (i.e. haptenated autoantigens) can be recognized and internalized by B-cells specific to either the hapten or to unmodified B-cell epitopes on the autoantigen. These cells subsequently present a mixture of neo- and self-epitopes complexed to distinct class II major histocompatibility (MHC-II) molecules on their surface (Fig. 4). Since T-cell tolerance is obviously not established for the neoepitopes, neospecific Th cells provide signal 2 for the B-cell. This leads to production of either antihapten or anti-self antibodies depending on the exact specificity of the B-cell. Moreover, once these B-cells are activated, they can stimulate autoreactive Th cells recognizing unmodified self-epitopes. The underlying process is called epitope (determinant) spreading and causes the diversification of adaptive immune responses. Responses induced by injection of mercury salts, for instance, are initially directed only to unidentified chemically created neoepitopes, but after 3–4 weeks include reactivity to unmodified self-epitopes [10]. The distinction between allergic and autoimmune responses induced by haptens may therefore only be gradual, reflecting the relative antigenicity of the neo- and self-epitopes involved [11].

neoepitopes

anti-self antibodies

413

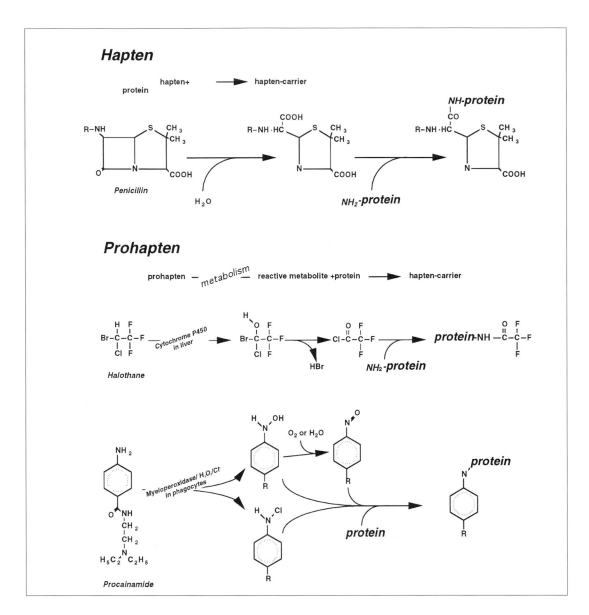

Figure 3 Haptens and prohaptens

Pharmaceuticals that are too small to attract a T-cell response can become antigenic when they bind as hapten to a protein carrier. In this case, T-cells responding to chemically induced neoepitopes on the carrier provide costimulation for B-cells responding to the hapten. Prohaptens require metabolic activation to a reactive metabolite that can function as a hapten. Penicillin is a well-known example of a pharmaceutical that can form haptens by direct binding to proteins. In contrast, halothane itself does not form haptens, but cytochrome P450-mediated metabolism in the liver results in reactive metabolites that do bind to proteins. Procainamide can be metabolized by the myeloperoxidase/H_2O_2/Cl^- system of phagocytes. These metabolites are very reactive and can bind covalently to nucleophilic thiol and amino groups of proteins.

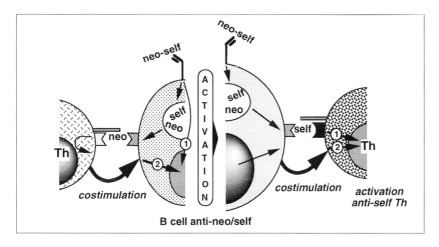

Figure 4 Determinant spreading

Immune responses to haptens can spread to autoreactive responses to the carrier protein. Haptenated autoantigens are recognized and internalized by specific B-cells. After uptake and processing, the B-cells present a mixture of the neo- and self-epitopes complexed to distinct MHC-II molecules. Naive T-cells do not respond to the self-epitopes, but neospecific T-cells provide costimulation for such B-cells. This leads to activation of the B-cell and production of antibodies. Moreover, when the B-cells are activated, they can provide costimulation for naive T-cells that recognize unmodified self-epitopes, leading to their activation and breaking of T-cell tolerance. 1, the antigen-specific or first signal; 2, the costimulatory or second signal; neo, neoepitope.

Pharmaceuticals can expose (epitopes of) autoantigens

Induction of self-tolerance involves specific recognition of autoantigen leading to selective inactivation of autoreactive lymphocytes, and tolerance is therefore not established for (epitopes of) autoantigens that are normally not available for immune recognition. Pharmaceuticals can expose such sequestered (epitopes of) autoantigens by disrupting barriers between the antigen and the immune system (i.e. blood-brain barrier, blood-testis barrier, cell membranes). Tissue damage, cell death and protein denaturation induced or enhanced by pharmaceuticals can largely increase the availability of such (epitopes of) autoantigens for immune recognition (Fig. 5). Moreover, altered antigen processing that augments presentation of epitopes that were previously not expressed increases the availability of these so-called subdominant or cryptic epitopes for recognition by T-cells [12, 13]. It has been shown, for instance, that mice immunized with antigen in adjuvant respond exclusively to dominant epitopes, whereas preincubation with Au(III), the oxidized metabolite of the antirheumatic auranofin, elicits additional T-cell responses to cryptic epitopes [11].

autoantigen

adjuvant

415

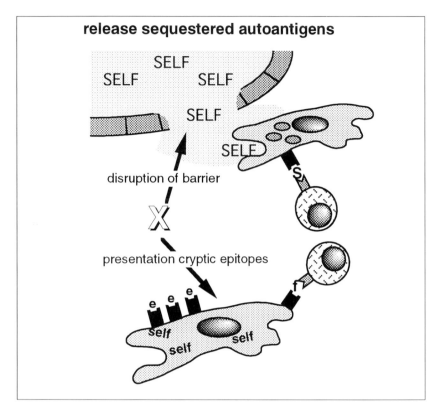

Figure 5 Release of sequestered self-epitopes

Pharmaceuticals can expose previously sequestered (epitopes of) self-antigens by disrupting barriers between the antigen and the immune system (i.e. blood-brain barrier, blood-testis barrier, cell membranes). Similarly, augmented presentation of cryptic epitopes by altered antigen processing increases the availability of these epitopes for recognition by T-cells.

Interference with costimulation (signal 2)

It is important to realize that antigen recognition by itself does not lead to activation of lymphocytes (above and Chapter A3). In addition, costimulation (i.e. signal 2) is required in the initiation of immune responses [14–16]. Many xenobiotics have the inherent capacity to induce this costimulation; they have intrinsic adjuvant activity. The underlying mechanisms are not always understood, but several nonexclusive possibilities have been described.

Induction of inflammation

Cytotoxic pharmaceuticals or their reactive metabolites can induce tissue damage which leads to accumulation of tissue debris, release of proinflammatory cytokines like tumor necrosis factor α (TNFα), interleukin-1 (IL-1), and IL-6, and attracts inflammatory cells like granulocytes and macrophages. Cytokines produced during this inflammatory response activate antigen-presenting cells. These present selected epitopes of antigens from the debris, and provide costimulation for Th cells, which leads to the initiation of an adaptive immune response [16]. Conceivably, all reactive and cytotoxic pharmaceuticals can have this effect to some extent. Side effects reported after the therapeutic use of cytokines have provided evidence that activation of the immune response may sometimes have deleterious consequences, such as flulike reactions, vascular leak syndrome and cytokine release syndrome. Cytokine-induced exacerbation of underlying autoimmune or inflammatory diseases may be other complications of concern [8]. The occurrence of cytokine release syndrome has also been reported as a serious consequence of the administration of certain therapeutic monoclonal antibodies [17].

cytokines

Noncognate T-B cooperation

Reactive xenobiotics may also stimulate adaptive immune responses by disturbing the normal cooperation of Th- and B-cells. Normally, B-cells receive costimulation from Th cells that cognately recognize (epitopes of) the same antigen. As such, B-cell tolerance for autoantigens is a corollary of the T-cell tolerance for such antigens. However, when Th cells respond to nonself epitopes on B-cells, such B-cells may be noncognately stimulated by the Th cell. This occurs during graft-versus-host responses following bone marrow transplantation, when Th cells of the host recognize nonself epitopes on B-cells of the graft and *vice versa*. This leads to T- and B-cell activation and results in production of autoantibodies to distinct autoantigens like DNA, nucleoli, nuclear proteins, erythrocytes and basal membranes. Drug-related lupus is characterized by a similar spectrum of autoantibodies, and it has therefore been suggested that noncognate – graft-versus-host-like – T-B cooperation caused by T-cell reactivity to haptens on (autoreactive) B-cells is one of the underlying mechanisms (Fig. 6) [18]. Chlorpromazine, hydralazine, phenytoine, isoniazid, α-methyldopa and procainamide are just a few of the pharmaceuticals that are associated with drug-related lupus [19].

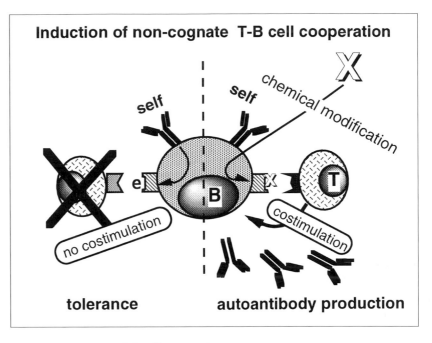

Figure 6 Non-cognate T-B-cell cooperation

Normally, activation of B-cells requires costimulation from activated T-cells that cognately recognize epitopes of the same antigen. B-cells with specificity for autoantigens do not receive this signal, because T-cells have learned to ignore autoantigens. However, certain pharmaceuticals can bind to B-cell proteins, and Th cells activated by the neoepitopes created can noncognately provide costimulation for the (e-specific) B-cell (e, a part of self for which tolerance exists). This can bypass tolerance in the T-cell compartment and can lead to activation of autoreactive B-cells and production of autoantibodies. This resembles stimulation of host B-cells by graft T-cells responding to the MHC molecules on the B-cells during graft-versus-host reactions, and leads to a similar spectrum of autoantibodies.

Interference with cellular activation

Occupation of various lymphocyte receptors results in a cascade of molecular processes that eventually lead to production of growth factors and cellular proliferation and/or activation. Its complexity makes this cascade vulnerable to pharmaceuticals at numerous stages, although most of these chemicals target very crucial processes like purine metabolism as in the case of AZA. Most drugs that interfere with cellular activation are not cell type-selective at higher doses, as all living cells depend on the same basic molecular processes. At low doses, however, drugs like AZA, CY and MTX appear to have a more selective effect. AZA, for instance, is claimed to selectively suppress T-lymphocyte function at low doses, whereas CY or MTX preferentially affect B-cells [1].

Suppressive effects of CsA and FK506, both interfering with the activation of the T-cell-specific transcription factor NF-ATc, and rapamycin, preventing IL-2 receptor activation, are obviously more specific to the T-lymphocyte.

Regulation of the immune response

Ongoing immune responses have to be carefully regulated in order to mount the most suited defense (Fig. 1). Elimination of (intra)cellular targets like virally infected or neoplastic cells is most efficient by Th1-driven cellular responses using cytotoxic T-cells and macrophages as effector mechanisms. Soluble targets, like extracellular bacteria and proteins, on the other hand, are most effectively eliminated by Th2-driven humoral responses, which rely on the formation of specific antibodies. The regulation of the type of immune response elicited and of the effector mechanisms activated is the result of a complex interplay of cytokines produced by macrophages, dendritic cells, mast cells, granulocytes and lymphocytes (Chapter A4) and is influenced by a number of endo- and exogenous factors. Genetic make-up, in particular genes encoding for MHC molecules, but also gender (estrogens) are among the endogenous factors, whereas the type and dose of antigen, the route of exposure but also the type of (ongoing) costimulatory adjuvant activity are among the exogenous factors [20]. The role of the genetic makeup is illustrated by the model compound $HgCl_2$. This chemical is capable of inducing a Th1-dependent immunosuppressive state in an $H2^d$ strain of mice or an $RT1^l$ strain of rat, whereas it induces an autoreactive Th2-dependent response in an $H2^s$ strain of mice or $RT1^n$ strain of rat [21, 22].

Within the same congeneic strain, however, different xenobiotics can skew the response to opposing directions: $HgCl_2$ induces a Th2-like response in BALB/c mice, whereas the diabetogenic antitumor compound streptozotocin (STZ) induces a Th1 response in the same mouse strain [23]. Other examples are the adjuvants complete Freund's adjuvant (CFA) and alum, stimulating the formation of immunoglobulin (Ig)G2a and IgG1/IgG2a isotypes of antibodies, respectively [20].

How chemicals exactly modulate the immune response is as yet unknown, but modulation of epitope selection by MHC molecules, selective activation of the innate immune system (e.g. mast cells in the case of $HgCl_2$) and chemical-specific factors (e.g. NO release by STZ) may be important factors.

MHC molecules

Effector functions and response cessation

To avoid unnecessary damage, the immune system has several feedback mechanisms to stop ineffective and obsolete responses (Fig. 1). The simplest feedback is the antigen itself, and complete degradation of the response-inducing antigen leads to response cessation. Pharmaceuticals that impair the activity of effector mechanisms delay antigen degradation and lead to accumulation of debris. It has been demonstrated, for instance, that several drugs, including D-penicillamine and procainamide, inhibit complement factor C4. This hampers the clearance of immune complexes and may therefore lead to their deposition and excessive tissue damage (reviewed in [24]).

Clinical consequences of immunotoxicity of pharmaceuticals

In general, pharmaceuticals that inhibit cellular replication or activation induce immunosuppression which is dose-dependent. Particularly, impaired activity of the first line of defense formed by the natural immune system can have disastrous consequences. These are generally not influenced by the genetic predisposition of the exposed individual, but actual outbreak of (opportunistic) infections or increased frequency of neoplasms may depend on the general immune status prior to exposition. This explains why immunosuppressive pharmaceuticals are most likely to have clinical consequences in immunocompromised individuals such as young children, the elderly and transplant recipients.

Immunotoxic pharmaceuticals that somehow activate the immune system can lead to autoimmune or allergic diseases. Actual development of clinical symptoms is influenced by the route and duration of exposure, the dosage of the pharmaceutical, and by immunogenetic (MHC haplotype, Th1-type versus Th2-type responders) and pharmacogenetic (acetylator phenotype, sulfoxidizer, Ah receptor etc.) predisposition of the exposed individual. From an immunological point of view it is clear that the polymorphic MHC molecules select the epitopes that are presented to T-cells, and therefore influence all immune responses, including allergic and autoimmune responses induced by pharmaceuticals. Moreover, **atopic individuals** that tend to mount Th2 immune responses are more susceptible to anaphylaxis triggered by an IgE response to chemical haptens than typical Th1 responders. Genetic variation in metabolism of pharmaceuticals is important as it determines the formation and clearance of immunotoxic metabolites. The slow acetylating phenotype for instance, predisposes for drug-related lupus because reactive intermediates of phase I metabolism have an increased opportunity to bind proteins as they are only slowly conjugated.

Drugs known to interfere with the immune system are normally prescribed by well-trained physicians and are taken under more or less controlled conditions. As a result, adverse effects should be recognized as soon as they become apparent and measures can be taken before permanent harm is done. However, in the case of allergenic drugs, the immune system is sensitized, which may hamper future treatments with the same or a structurally related chemical (penicillin). Severe immunosuppression may cause permanent detrimental effects when neoplasms are formed, but also (opportunistic) infections may have serious consequences.

neoplasms

As the clinical consequence of exposure to immunotoxic pharmaceuticals ranges from immunodepressed conditions on the one hand to allergic and autoimmune diseases on the other hand, preclinical testing of pharmaceuticals in laboratory animals requires different approaches. In the following sections, procedures are covered comprising direct immunotoxicity as well as sensitizing capacity.

Procedures for preclinical testing of direct immunotoxicity

Testing in rodents by tiered approach

Several laboratories have developed and validated a variety of methods to determine the effects of chemicals on the immune system of rats and mice [25]. Most employ a tier-testing system, whereas some investigators have advocated multiple testing in a single animal. The tier-testing approaches are similar in design in that the first tier is a screen for immunotoxicity with the second tier consisting of more specific or confirmatory studies, host resistance studies or in-depth mechanistic studies. At present, most information regarding these models comes from the model developed at the National Institute of Public Health and the Environment (RIVM) in Bilthoven, the Netherlands, and the model developed at the U.S. National Institute of Environmental Health Sciences National Toxicology Program (NIEHS-NTP). The RIVM tiered system [26, 27] is based on the guideline 407 of the Organization for Economic Cooperation and Development (OECD), and performed in the rat using at least three dose levels, i.e. one resulting in overt toxicity, one aimed at producing no toxicity and one intermediate level. There is no immu-

tier-testing system

**flow cytometric
analysis**

**OECD
guideline 407**

**immmune
function testing**

nization or challenge with an infectious agent. The first tier comprises general parameters including conventional hematology, serum immunoglobulin concentrations, bone marrow cellularity, weight and histology of lymphoid organs [thymus, spleen, lymph nodes, mucosa-associated lymphoid tissue (MALT)], flow cytometric analysis of spleen cells and possibly immunophenotyping of tissue sections (Table 1). This approach has been used for the immunotoxic evaluation of pesticides [28] and pharmaceuticals [29].

In the OECD guideline 407 (adopted in 1981), the only parameters for the immune system were hematology, including differential cell counting, in addition to histopathology of the spleen. In an evaluation that we made, it appeared that this protocol was insufficient for identification of direct toxicity for the immune system [30]. Also, results of an international collaborative immunotoxicity study carried out by the International Programme on Chemical Safety (IPCS) with the support of the Commission of the European Communities (CEC) showed that basic pathological investigations in the rat, specified in OECD guideline 407, did not reveal the immunological effects of AZA and CsA [31]. The immunotoxic actions of these drugs could be detected provided the test was extended to include additional pathology parameters. The OECD guideline has been updated and now includes weight of spleen and thymus, and histopathology of these organs, in addition to lymph nodes, Peyer's patches and bone marrow [32]. This update certainly appears to be an improvement over the earlier guideline, although even with this updated version, some immunotoxic compounds may not be identified as such [33], for instance this concerned the opiate analgesic buprenorphine [34] and the long-acting b2-adrenoreceptor agonist salmeterol [35], which affected serum immunoglobulins in rats. It should be borne in mind that in the recently adopted OECD guideline 407 for testing toxicants, the immune system is not evaluated functionally. The inclusion of an *in vivo* antigen challenge test, e.g. with sheep red blood cells (SRBC), is currently considered to improve the sensitivity of the toxicity test. Results of a recent study [36] indicate that intravenous injection with SRBC during a 30- and 90-day toxicity study did not alter hematological and clinical chemistry parameters. With the expected exception of the spleen, administration of SRBC did not significantly alter the weights or morphology of routinely analysed tissues.

It should be noted that the array of tests currently included in the updated OECD guideline 407 is aimed at detecting potential immunotoxicity. Once immunotoxicity has been identified, further testing is required to confirm and extend the earlier findings. Further testing should include immune function testing (Table 1). In addition to confirming functional

Table 1

Parameters	Procedures
TIER 1	
Non-functional	– Routine hematology, including differential cell counting
	– Serum IgM, G, A, and E determination
	– Lymphoid organ weights (thymus, spleen, local and distant lymph nodes)
	– Histopathology of thymus, spleen, lymph nodes and mucosa-associated lymphoid tissue
	– bone marrow cellularity
	– Analysis of lymphocyte subpopulations in spleen by flow cytometry.
TIER 2 PANEL	
Cell-mediated immunity	– Sensitization to T-cell dependent antigens (e.g. ovalbumin, tuberculin, *Listeria*), and skin test challenge
	– Lymphoproliferative responses to specific antigens (*Listeria*); mitogen responses (Con-A, PHA)
Humoral immunity	– Serum titration of IgM, IgG, IgA, IgE responses to T-dependent antigens (ovalbumin, tetanus toxoid, *Trichinella spiralis, sheep red blood cells*) with ELISA;
	– Serum titration of T-cell independent IgM response to LPS with ELISA
	– Mitogen response to LPS
Macrophage function	– *In vitro* phagocytosis and killing of *Listeria monocytogenes* by adherent spleen and peritoneal cells
	– Cytolysis of YAC-1 lymphoma cells by adherent spleen and peritoneal cells
NK cell function	– Cytolysis of YAC-1 lymphoma cells by non-adherent spleen and peritoneal cells
Host-resistance	– *Trichinella spiralis* challenge (muscle larvae counts and worm expulsion)
	– *Listeria monocytogenes* challenge (spleen clearance)
	– Rat cytomegalovirus challenge (clearance from salivary gland)
	– Endotoxin hypersensitivity
	– Autoimmune models (adjuvant arthritis, experimental allergic encephalomyelitis)

Panel of the Dutch National Institute of Public Health and the Environmental for detecting immunotoxic alterations in the rat

no-adverse-effect levels

host resistance model

implications of the immunotoxicity identified, functional tests will likely provide information on no-adverse-effect levels, and are therefore valuable for the process of risk assessment. Caution is needed in determining the relevance of slight effects on immune parameters in view of the functional reserve capacity of the immune system. In those cases, infection models can be very helpful for risk assessment, as they are tools to elucidate the actual consequences of disturbances of immune function; effects observed using such infection models have surpassed the reserve capacity of the immune system. The fate of the pathogen, and the associated host pathology, may serve as indicators of the health implications of the immunotoxicity of the test chemical. Pathogens used in these host resistance models are chosen so that they are good models for human disease [25]. With some compounds, induction of immunotoxicity occurs, especially during prenatal exposure.

The U.S. NTP has developed a tiered approach in mice that is linked closely to the standard protocol for subchronic oral toxicity and carcinogenicity studies [37]. Routinely, exposure periods of 14–30 days have been used at dose levels that have no effect on body weight or other toxicological end-points. In this way, compounds are identified for which the immune system represents the most sensitive target organ system. Tier 1 includes conventional hematology, lymphoid organ weight, cellularity and histology of the spleen, thymus and lymph nodes, *ex vivo* splenic IgM-antibody plaque-forming cell assay following SRBC immunization, *in vitro* lymphocyte proliferation after stimulation with mitogens and allogeneic cells, and an *in vitro* assay for natural killer (NK) cell activity. In an adapted form of this approach, 51 different chemicals were evaluated, selected on the basis of structural relationships with previously identified immunotoxic chemicals [38]. The splenic SRBC IgM plaque-forming cell response and cell surface marker analyses showed the highest accuracy for identification of potential immunotoxicity.

Immunotoxicity testing in nonrodent species

NK-cell activity lymphocyte

Various nonhuman primates, including *Macaca mulatta* (rhesus macaque), *Macaca nemestrina* (pig-tailed macaque), *Macaca fascicularis* (cynomolgus monkey) and the marmoset have been used in immunotoxicological studies. Virtually all of the immunotoxicology assays which are carried out in the mouse or rat can be and have been adapted for use with the nonhuman primates [39]. Phenotypic markers and functional assays in three different species of nonhuman primates were evaluated [40]. Functional assays included NK-cell activity, lymphocyte transformation and antigen presentation. The extensive phenotypic marker studies included the evaluation of over 20 markers or combination of markers for each of the three monkey species. Otherwise, strategies and methods applied in studies in humans have been introduced in studies on nonhuman primates (see Table 2).

transformation
antigen
presentation

Table 2 Assays recommended for immunotoxicity assessment in man

1. Complete blood count with differential count
2. Antibody-mediated immunity (one or more of following):
   - Primary antibody response to protein antigen (e.g. epitope labelled influenza vaccine)
   - Immunoglobulin concentrations in serum (IgM, IgG, IgA, IgE)
   - Secondary antibody response to protein antigen (diphtheria, tetanus or polio)
   - Natural immunity to bloodgroup antigens (e.g. anti-A, anti-B)
3. Phenotypic analysis of lymphocytes by flow cytometry:
   - Surface analysis of CD3, CD4, CD8, CD20
4. Cellular Immunity:
   - Delayed-type hypersensitivity (DTH) skin testing
   - Primary DTH reaction to protein (KLH)
   - Proliferation to recall antigens
5. Autoantibodies and Inflammation:
   - C-reactive protein
   - Autoantibody titers to nuclei (ANA), DNA, mitochondria and IgG (rheumatoid factor)
   - IgE to allergens
6. Measure of nonspecific immunity:
   - NK cell enumerations (CD56 or CD60) or cytolytic activity against K562 tumor cell line
   - Phagocytosis (NBT or chemiluminesce)
7. Clinical chemistry screen
   - Proposal for all persons exposed to immunotoxicants

From [25].

Also, other mammalian species have been used. While dogs are not the species of choice for immunotoxicological studies, they are one of the species predominantly used in toxicological safety assessments. Virtually all of the assays used for assessing immunotoxic potential have been adapted for use in the dog [25]. Among these are assay evaluation of basal immunoglobulin levels for IgA, IgG and IgM, allergen-specific serum IgE, mononuclear phagocyte function, NK-cell activity, cytotoxic T-cell activity, and mitogen and cell-mediated immune responses.

Procedures for preclinical testing of sensitizing capacity

Structure-activity relationships

structure-activity relationships

The intrinsic capacity of chemicals to exert adverse effects is linked to the structure of the compound. Structure-activity relationships with respect to direct toxicity of compounds to components of the immune system have received little attention. More attention has been given to structure-activity relationships with respect to the induction of allergy. Here, structure-activity relationship models are directed towards a fuller understanding of the relationship between chemical structure and physicochemical properties and skin-sensitizing activity, in order ideally to derive quantitative structure-activity relationships (QSAR), linked perhaps to the development of expert, rule-based systems. In this context, parameters that appear to be of particular importance are protein reactivity and lipophilicity associated with the capacity to penetrate into the viable epidermis [41]. The correlation of the protein reactivity of chemicals with their skin sensitization potential is well established [42], so that it is now accepted that if a chemical is capable of reacting with a protein either directly or after appropriate (bio)chemical transformation, it has the potential to be a contact allergen, assuming of course that it can accumulate in the appropriate epidermal compartment. Each of the existing structure-activity relationship (SAR) models proposes structural alerts, i.e. moieties associated with sensitizing activity. In all cases, the structural alerts comprise electrophilic moieties, or moieties which can be metabolized into electrophilic fragments (proelectrophiles).

structural alerts

Testing for skin allergy

Guinea-pig models

Buehler test
guinea-pig maximization test
guinea-pig optimization test

The guinea pig was for many years the animal of choice for experimental studies of contact sensitization and several test methods were developed in this species (reviewed in [43]). The best-known and most widely applied are the *Buehler test*, the *guinea-pig maximization test*, and the *guinea-pig optimization test*, and have formed the basis of hazard assessment for many years. Both the guinea-pig maximization test and the Buehler test are now recommended according to an OECD guideline, accepted in 1992. While these tests differ with respect to procedural details, they are similar in principle. Guinea pigs are exposed to the test material, or to the relevant vehicle. In the Buehler test, both induction and challenge exposures are done topically. The Buehler test is sensitive, but false negatives are frequently observed. The test was improved by occluded application of the test compound. In the guinea-pig maximization test, induction involves intradermal and occluded epidermal exposure, and in the optimization test induction is done by intradermal, and challenge by intradermal and occluded epidermal exposure. Adjuvant is employed in the guinea-pig maximization test and the optimization test to augment induced immune responses. Challenge-induced inflammatory reactions, measured as a function of erythema and/or edema, are recorded 24 and 48 h later. Classification of sensitizing activity in the guinea-pig tests is qualitative and not quantitative. It is based usually upon the percentage of test animals that display macroscopically detectable challenge reactions. Any compound inducing at least 30% positive animals in an adjuvant test is labeled as a sensitizer; in the case of a nonadjuvant test, 15% positivity is sufficient to classify the compound as a sensitizer.

Mouse models

In recent years, increased understanding of the cellular and molecular mechanisms associated with contact allergy have derived largely from experimental investigations in the mouse [44, 45]. Two different types of tests to predict the capacity of chemicals to induce skin allergy have been developed. One is the *mouse ear swelling test* (MEST) which, like the **mouse ear swelling test** guinea-pig methods described above, is based upon the evaluation of challenge-induced reactions in previously sensitized animals [46]. Sensitizing potential is evaluated by consideration of both the degree of edema (ear swelling) induced and the percentage of animals displaying a reaction.

The second test developed in mice is the *local lymph node assay* (LLNA) [47]. In contrast to the MEST and guinea-pig assays, activity in the **local lymph node assay** LLNA is measured by the primary T-cell response in the draining lymph node following topical application to the mouse ear. Mice are treated daily, for 3 consecutive days, on the dorsum of both ears with the test material or with an equal volume of vehicle alone. Proliferative activity in draining lymph nodes (measured by the incorporation *in situ* of radiolabeled thymidine) is evaluated 5 days following the initiation of exposure. Currently, chemicals are classified as possessing sensitizing potential if with one test concentration a stimulation index, relative to vehicle-treated controls, of 3 or greater is induced. The method has the advantages of short duration and objective measurement of proliferation and minimal animal treatment. In contrast to the MEST and guinea-pig assays, activity is measured as a function of events occurring during the induction, rather than elicitation phase of contact sensitization.

The LLNA has been developed further to discriminate skin sensitizers from respiratory sensitizers based on the induction of CD4+ T helper subsets (Th1- versus Th2-mediated responses) by the analysis of cytokine profiles in draining lymph node cells [48]. Chemicals differ with respect to the types of hypersensitivity they induce. Compounds that induce Th1 cells and mediate type IV delayed hypersensitivity are skin sensitizers. Such responses are associated with the production by draining lymph node cells of interferon-γ (IFNγ). Compounds that induce Th2 cells and mediate type I immediate hypersensitivity by the production of IgE and IgG1 are respiratory sensitizers, and are associated with the production by draining lymph node cells of high levels of IL-4. However, this is not true in all cases, as skin sensitization with some low molecular compounds such as picrylchloride [49] and toluene diisocyanate (TDI) [50] can induce respiratory hypersensitivity with features of type IV hypersensitivity in mice. Also, in humans, specific IgE is only detected in a minority of patients suffering from respiratory allergy induced by TDI.

Testing for respiratory allergy

Most of the animal models that are used for studying specific respiratory tract hypersensitivity were developed using high molecular weight allergens, notably proteins. Very few animal models have been developed as predictive tests for hazard identification and risk assessment in the area of chemical-induced respiratory allergy [51]. The majority of these models are based upon antibody-mediated events. The models differ with regard to the following aspects: the animal species utilized, the route of administration of the agent, the protocol for both induction and elicitation of responses, type of response measured and judgment of significant response.

Guinea-pig models

The guinea pig has been used for decades for the study of anaphylactic shock and pulmonary hypersensitivity. The guinea pig is similar to humans in that the lung is a major shock organ for anaphylactic responses to antigens. The guinea pig responds to histamine and can experience both immediate-onset and late-onset responses. Airway hyperreactivity and eosinophil influx and inflammation can also be demonstrated in this animal species. Mechanistic studies have been hampered by the lack of reagents needed to identify cells and mediators in respiratory allergy. In addition, the major anaphylactic antibody is IgG1, whereas it is IgE in humans and other rodent species.

airway hyperreactivity

IgG1, IgE

The guinea-pig model developed by Karol et al. [52] has proven to be valuable for low molecular weight chemical allergens. Guinea pigs sensitized by inhalation of free or protein-bound chemical allergens, such as TDI, will exhibit symptoms of pulmonary hypersensitivity following subsequent inhalation challenge. Hypersensitivity reactions are measured usually as a function of challenge-induced changes in respiratory rate or alterations in other breathing parameters such as tidal volume. Changes in breathing patterns can also be provoked in dermally sensitized guinea pigs by inhalation challenge with the free chemical. In this approach it is not necessary to use hapten-protein conjugates.

A tiered approach to hazard assessment in guinea pigs proposed by Sarlo and Clark [53] comprises sequential analyses of physicochemical similarities with known allergens, the potential to associate covalently with protein, the ability to stimulate antibody responses and finally activity in a model of respiratory hypersensitivity in which animals sensitized by subcutaneous injection are challenged by intratracheal instillation.

Mouse models

Models to investigate airway responses to sensitizing compounds have been developed in the mouse and comprise responses mediated by IgE [54] and non-IgE-mediated reactions [49, 50]. These models have not been used so far for predictive purposes.

As discussed earlier, analysis of the cytokine profile in the LLNA in the mouse may provide information on whether a compound is a respiratory allergen. In the same series of investigations, it was found that topical administration to mice of chemical respiratory allergens stimulated a substantial increase in the serum concentration of total IgE, a response not seen with contact allergens considered to lack the ability to cause sensitization of the respiratory tract [48]. These observations suggested that it might be possible to identify chemical respiratory sensitizers as a function of induced changes in serum IgE concentration. The advantage of this approach, which forms the basis of the mouse IgE test, is that measurement of a serum protein is required, rather than of hapten-specific antibody.

cytokine profile

Investigations suggest that the mouse IgE test may provide a useful method for the prospective identification of chemical respiratory allergens [52]. It must be emphasized, however, that to date the assay has been evaluated only with a limited number of chemicals and that most of the analyses have been performed in a single laboratory. Difficulties arise from the assumption of IgE mediation of respiratory hypersensitivity response in mice. As mentioned earlier, respiratory allergic responses, associated with increased reactivity of airways, may occur by a delayed type IV immune response-inducing compound [49]. For this reason, actual testing of lung functions *in vivo* seems prudent for those chemicals that are known to sensitize, but are unable to produce IgE responses.

Testing for autoimmunity

Autoimmune disease occurs when an individual's immune system attacks its own tissues or organs, resulting in functional impairment, inflammation and sometimes permanent damage. Diseases with multifactorial etiologies result from the loss of immune tolerance to self-antigens.

Induced and genetic models

For the detection of the potential of compounds to exacerbate induced or genetically predisposed autoimmunity, animal models are available [55]. In induced models, a susceptible animal strain is immunized with a mixture of an adjuvant and an autoantigen isolated from the target organ. Examples are *adjuvant arthritis*, *experimental encephalomyelitis* and *experimental uveitis* in the Lewis strain rat. Examples of spontaneous models of autoimmune disease are the BB-rat and the NOD-mouse that develop autoimmune *pancreatitis* and subsequently *diabetes*, and the (NZBxNZW)F$_1$ mouse or MRL/*lpr* mouse that develop pathology that resembles human *systemic lupus erythematosus*. These models are mainly used in the study of the pathogenesis of autoimmunity and the preclinical evaluation of immunosuppressive drugs. Very few studies have addressed the potential of these models for assessment of whether a xenobiotic exacerbates induced or congenital autoimmunity.

adjuvant arthritis
experimental
encephalomyelitis
experimental
uveitis
systemic lupus
erythematosus

Popliteal lymph node assay

Although currently no predictive assays have been developed and validated to identify, in the early phases of toxicity testing, the potential of drugs to induce systemic hypersensitivity or autoimmune responses, it should be noted that available assays to identify contact sensitizers might also be helpful to identify systemic sensitizers. Clinical signs of systemic adverse immune-mediated effects usually become manifest only during advanced clinical development of drugs. The conditions used in routine preclinical toxicological screening are obviously not optimal for the detection of the immune-dysregulating potential of drugs and chemicals (e.g. small animal number, use of outbred animal strains, dynamics of disease development versus snapshot determinations, lack of predictive parameters).

Autoimmunity often results from the association of the compound with normal tisssue components, thereby rendering them immunogenic. A variety of chemicals and drugs, in particular the latter, have been found to induce autoimmune-like responses [56]. For the detection of chemicals that produce this type of reaction, the popliteal lymph node assay (PLNA) in mice is a promising tool. The PLNA [57] is based upon the hyperplasia (increase in weight) of lymph nodes in graft-versus-host reactions or pseudo-graft-versus-host reactions, and has been modified to assess the immunomodulatory potential of drugs. The test substance is injected subcutaneously into one hind footpad, and the contralateral side is either untreated or inoculated with vehicle alone. Comparison of popliteal lymph nodes from both sides allows the effect of the test drug to be measured. Apart from differences in weight, histologic evidence of *in vivo* immunostimulatory activity can be discerned. These pseudo-graft-versus-host reactions with follicular hyperplasia have been documented in mice for drugs such as diphenylhydantoin, D-penicillamine and streptozotocin. The assay appears to be appropriate to recognize sensitizing, i.e. allergenic and autoimmunogenic chemicals, as well as non-sensitizing immunostimulating compounds, and has important advantages as it is a simple model based on local reactions that indicate direct immunostimulation with less interference of immunoregulatory mechanisms. So far, over 60 compounds with documented adverse immune effects in humans have been found to be positive in the PLNA in the mouse, i.e. caused an increase in PLN weight and cell numbers as compared with PLN of vehicle-injected controls [12]. Precaution has to be taken in the case of autoimmunogenic drugs, such as procainamide, that act as a prohapten. They are false-negative in the PLNA as such and require coinjection of metabolizing systems (S9 mix of granulocytes) to become pos-

popliteal lymph node assay

pseudo-graft-versus-host reaction

itive. Results of a preliminary interlaboratory validation study indicate the potential predictive value of the PLNA in the rat as well [58]. Thus, the direct PLNA seems to be a versatile tool to recognize T-cell activating drugs and chemicals, including autoimmunogenic chemicals, keeping in mind possible false-negative results with prohaptens. With the adoptive transfer PLNA, sensitized cells are used as probes to detect the formation *in vivo* of immunogenic metabolites of low molecular weight chemicals [12]. However, further interlaboratory validation is required before the direct PLNA assay, in particular, can be recommended for routine use in preclinical toxicity screening.

Procedures for immunotoxicity testing in humans

Epidemiology design

It is obvious that many of the compounds causing direct immunotoxicity have been identified in rodent studies, as the database in humans is less complete and often inconclusive. The most common design used in immunotoxicity research in humans is the cross-sectional study, in which exposure parameters and effect parameters are assessed at the same time point [59]. The immune function of "exposed" subjects is compared with the immune function of "nonexposed" subjects by the measurement of various immunological parameters. For this reason, proper definition of exposure criteria in the exposed group is necessary. This group should include subjects at the upper end of exposure. Where possible, the study should incorporate individual estimates of exposure or actual measurements of the compound. In the broadest sense, biomarkers are measurements on biological specimens that will elucidate the relationship between environmental exposure and human diseases, so that exposure and diseases can be prevented. In clinical medicine, biomarkers are valued as a tool for the presence or absence of diseases or the course of the disease during therapeutic intervention. As such indicators are available for *exposure, effect* or *susceptibility* [60].

cross-sectional study

biomarkers

Markers of exposure

A biological marker of exposure is a xenobiotic compound or its metabolite or the product of an interaction between the compound and some target cell or biomolecule. The most common markers of exposure are the concentration of the compound in urine, blood or target organ or tissue. Immune-specific biomarkers of exposure are antibodies or positive skin tests to the particular compound.

Markers of effect

A biomarker of effect is a measurable cellular or biochemical alteration within an organism that, depending on magnitude, can be recognized as an established or potential health impairment or disease. These range from markers of slight structural or functional changes to markers that are indicators of a subclinical stage of a disease or the manifestation of the disease itself. Functional changes in cells of the immune system by an immunotoxic chemical may be the first step in the process towards disease. For instance, longitudinal studies on asymptomatic individuals with low NK activity showed that they had an increased risk for upper respiratory infection and morbidity [61]. Immunosuppression may lead to more subtle changes in resistance to infections, such as influenza or common cold, rather than opportunistic infection. Data in experimental animals also indicate that small changes in immune function could increase the likelihood of disease [38].

Markers of susceptibility

Markers of susceptibility, also called effect modifiers, can act at any point along the exposure-disease continuum. Important sources of variability are genetic, endocrine, age-related and environmental factors. Over the last 2 decades it has become clear that many immunological disorders are linked to alleles of the major histocompatibility gene complex (MHC). The products of MHC alleles in humans [human lymphocyte antigens (HLA)] have aroused interest at a clinical level as potential biomarkers of disease susceptibility. In some instances, there is a remarkable increase in relative risk of disease in individuals possessing particular alleles. Similar associations have been described in drug-induced immunological disorders. However, it should be noted that other genetic factors as well as environmental factors are also of importance. Stress of various types can also affect the immune system and influence the susceptibility to and recovery from infectious, autoimmune and neoplastic diseases. Age-related variability is shown by the developing fetus, which is more susceptible to immunotoxic effects than is the adult.

Assays for assessment of immune status

There is a plethora of tests developed to assess immunity in humans [62, 63], as described in laboratory manuals [64, 65, 66]. Many of these tests are nowadays commercially available as kits. A systematic approach to the evaluation of immune function, which is based on simple screening procedures followed by appropriate specialized tests of immune function, usually permits the definition of the immune alteration. This should include evaluation of the B-cell system, of the T-cell system and of non-specific resistance (polymorphonuclear leukocytes, monocytes and macrophages, NK cells, the complement system).

Testing schemes for evaluation of individuals exposed to immunotoxicants are proposed, among others, by the Subcommittee on Immunotoxicology of the U.S. National Research Council [60] and by a task group of the World Health Organization (WHO) [25]. The panel proposed by the WHO is listed in Table 2, and is composed of assays that cover all major aspects of the immune system. Included are function assays to test for humoral immunity, i.e. specific antibodies to tetanus or diphtheria (for which vaccination programs exist), and for cellular immunity using recall antigens. It should be mentioned that these tests were all developed for diagnostic purposes, but that in the context of immunotoxicity testing in humans they are to be used in an epidemiological setting. This means that distinctions found in parameters between an exposed group and a control group may have a different biological significance than an altered value in an individual. Whereas a decrease in a single immune parameter in an individual may not indicate increased susceptibility to disease, a subtle alteration in an immune biomarker in a population may indicate immunotoxicity.

Establishing immune changes in humans is considerably more complex than in animals, considering that noninvasive tests are limited, exposure levels to the agent (i.e. dose) are difficult to establish and responses in the population are extremely heterogeneous. Also, the normal population exhibits a wide range of immunological responses with no apparent health impact. In addition to this underlying population variability, certain host characteristics or common exposures may be associated with significant, predictable alterations in immunological parameters. If not recognized and effectively addressed in the study design or statistical analysis, these confounding factors may severely alter the results of population studies. Examples of factors associated with measurable alterations in immunological parameters include age, race, gender, pregnancy, acute stress and the behavioral ability to cope with stress, coexistent diseases or infections, nutritional status, lifestyle, tobacco smoking and some medications. Besides these variables, periodic (ranging from daily to seasonal) influences also exist. Some of these effects are relatively minor; other differences may be sufficiently large to exceed the expected effect from a low level of immunotoxic exposure. They are therefore of primary concern in large epidemiological studies.

Predictive testing for allergy in humans

There are a variety of skin test procedures for the diagnosis of several types of allergic reactions, dealt with above. Basically, predictive tests in humans for skin allergy are similar to diagnostic tests, but the aims are different. For diagnostic tests, the aim is to determine sensitization to chemicals to which there has been a prior exposure, whereas sensitization as a result of the procedure should be avoided. For predictive testing in humans, the aim is to show sensitizing capacity in individuals who have not been exposed previously to the compound.

For obvious reasons, predictive testing for respiratory sensitization is not done in humans. Occasionally, case reports may serve as an adequate hazard identification, but not as a risk estimate, because data on route and extent of exposure, and on the "population at risk" are usually missing. In the absence of case reports, it cannot be concluded that no potential for sensitization exists.

hazard identification

Immunotoxicity regulations

Regulatory guidance

There is great variation in the approaches adopted by regulatory agencies throughout the world in the control of human pharmaceuticals. Whereas regulatory controls are negligible in some developing countries, all major regions in the world authorize medicinal products only after in-depth assessment. Leading agencies involved in the regulation of pharmaceuticals for human use are the U.S. Food and Drug Administration (FDA), the Committee on Proprietary Medicinal Products (CPMP) in the European Union (EU), and the Ministry of Health and Wellfare (MHW) in Japan. The requirements the industry has to meet in order to gain marketing approval for its products have been laid down in official documents called guidelines. These guidelines inform the industry about the data needed to demonstrate to the authorities the pharmaceutical quality of new pharmaceuticals to be marketed as well as their benefit and safety for the patient. The guidance given has a major impact on the research programmes adopted by the industry.

The regulations administered by government agencies are quite complex. Often they are greatly influenced by the history, culture and legislations of the countries concerned. This still accounts for many national differences [67]. However, worldwide harmonization of regulatory requirements is ongoing. In the 1990s, the International Conference on Harmonization of Technical Requirements for Registration of Pharmaceuticals for Human Use (ICH) has proved to be a success. In this international forum, government regulators and industry representatives of the three major regions of the world participated (i.e. United States, the EU, and Japan). A number of harmonized guidelines have been developed by the ICH. Some of these have already been adopted officially by the regulatory authorities mentioned, whereas others will soon come into operation. Existing national guidelines thus have been or will be replaced by new ones based on the ICH consensus.

Regulatory aspects of laboratory animal immunotoxicology

genotoxicity carcinogenicity reproductive toxicity

To identify potential target organs of toxicity in humans, the industry must screen the toxicity of pharmaceuticals in laboratory animals before their first administration to humans. The animal data are also used to set a safe starting dose in humans. During subsequent clinical development, additional animal studies are performed to further characterize the toxicity profile. Many guidelines address the various types of toxicity studies to be performed, such as genotoxicity, carcinogenicity and reproductive toxicity. In addition, adverse effects on the immune system need to be assessed. As a rule, the regulatory authorities do not dictate how specific tests have to be conducted. The detailed technical requirements defined by OECD may or may not be followed. This approach allows deviations from routine protocol toxicity testing whenever justified. The study protocols may be adjusted in such a way that they provide the most relevant information depending on the nature and therapeutic indication of the pharmaceutical to be tested. Because immunotoxicology is a rather new discipline, however, no guidelines are currently available in the United States, the EU, and Japan which focus particularly on immunotoxicological issues regarding pharmaceuticals.

Consequently, immunotoxicity testing is not a standard procedure. The animal toxicity tests that are routinely performed by the pharmaceutical industry provide little possibility to reveal immunotoxic effects.

However, some data relevant to immunotoxicity assessment may be generated in fulfilling requirements present in other guidelines. For instance, the current EU guideline on "Repeated Dose Toxicity" testing with pharmaceuticals in laboratory animals requires the macroscopic and microscopic examination of the spleen, thymus and some lymph nodes, together with the determination of organ weights and routine hematology. In addition to these traditional methods, the EU recognizes the need for further tests relying on the rationale and proposed use of the product at hand, and the current state of scientific knowledge. The additional tests which may actually prove beneficial in this regard, however, have not been described (Council Directive 91/507/EU) (see Insert 1). This is in accordance with the European philosophy that the applicant (and not the regulatory authority) is responsible for a "state-of-the-art" research programme on a given pharmaceutical for which marketing authorization is requested.

Insert 1 EU guideline on Repeated Dose Toxicity (Council Directive 91/507/EU)

Immunointerference:

The expansive growth of immunology and the recognition of its importance has made it necessary to pay attention to interference with the immunologic system by substances even when this does not belong to their intended activity. Such interference may cause undesired adverse reactions (interference with infection; carcinoma). Therefore, it is particularly important to examine the spleen, the thymus and some lymph nodes macroscopically and microscopically at the termination of the toxicity study. These should indicate any effect on the immune system and thus the need for further tests.

Since our present knowledge of the field is rapidly increasing, any test used to investigate the immunological effects of a substance should rely on the state of the scientific knowledge at

---

Nowadays good experience has been gained with tiered approaches to immunotoxicity testing in rodents which focus on immunosuppression; new methods are or will be available in the near future to test pharmaceuticals for hypersensitivity and autoimmunity [25, 33, 68–71]. This scientific progress provides room for improvement of existing animal toxicity guidelines to include more detailed assessment of pharmaceutical-induced effects on the immune system.

New developments

Recently, ICH issued a guideline on "Preclinical Safety Assessment of Biotechnology-Derived Pharmaceuticals". This guideline will soon come into force in the United States, the EU and Japan. This document contains guidance on the assessment of immunogenicity (see Insert 2). Little specific information is present on general immunotoxicity (see Insert 3) and developmental immunotoxicity (see Insert 4). The lack of detailed instructions is due to the fact that all three regions concerned have adopted a flexible, case-by-case, science-based approach to animal toxicity studies in this rapidly evolving scientific area. Consequently, the three regions involved in ICH are reluctant to formulate in-depth re-

---

Insert 2 ICH guideline on Preclinical Evaluation of Biotechnology-derived Pharmaceuticals

Immunogenicity:

Many biotechnology-derived pharmaceuticals intended for human use are immunogenic in animals. Therefore, measurement of antibodies associated with administration of these types of products should be performed when conducting repeated dose toxicity studies in order to aid in the interpretation of these studies. Antibody responses should be characterised (e.g. titer, number of responding animals, neutralising or non-neutralising), and their appearance should be correlated with any pharmacological and/or toxicological changes. Specifically, the effects of antibody formation on pharmacokinetics/pharmacodynamic parameters, incidence and/or severity of adverse effects, complement activation, or the emergence of new toxic effects should be considered when interpreting the data. Attention should also be paid to the evaluation of possible pathological changes related to immune complex formation and deposition. The detection of antibodies should not be the sole criterion for the early termination of a preclinical safety study or modification in the duration of the study design unless the immune response neutralises the pharmacological and/or toxicological effects of the biopharmaceutical in a large proportion of the animals. In most cases, the immune response to biopharmaceuticals is variable, like that observed in humans. If the interpretation of the data from the safety study is not compromised by these issues, then no special significance should be ascribed to the antibody response.

The induction of antibody formation in animals is not predictive of a potential for antibody formation in humans. Humans may develop serum antibodies against humanised proteins, and frequently the therapeutic response persists in their presence. The occurrence of severe anaphylactic responses to recombinant proteins is rare in humans. In this regard, the results of guinea pig anaphylaxis tests, which are generally positive for protein products, are not predictive for reactions in humans; therefore, such studies are considered to be of little value for the routine evaluation of these types of products.

quirements which may turn out to be too strict. Such guidance might be valid for some biotechnology-derived products, but not for others.

In addition to the ICH effort on biotechnology-derived products, important initiatives are being undertaken in the field of conventional pharmaceuticals as well. For instance, the Immunotoxicity Committee in the FDA Center for Drug Evaluation and Research has begun formulating a guidance document on animal immunotoxicity testing for investigational new drugs (INDs) before their first entry into humans. Of course, this will also have an impact on the toxicity package required by the FDA at later stages of drug development, particularly when marketing approval is asked for so-called new drug applications (NDAs). The basis of the document will be that the determination of a new product's potential to

---

Insert 3 ICH guideline on Preclinical Evaluation of Biotechnology-derived Pharmaceuticals

Immunotoxicity studies:

Many biotechnology-derived pharmaceuticals are intended to stimulate or suppress the immune system and therefore may affect not only humoral but also cell-mediated immunity. Inflammatory reactions at the injection site may be indicative of a stimulatory response. It is important, however, to recognise that simple injection trauma and/or specific toxic effects caused by the formulation vehicle may also result in toxic changes at the injection site. In addition, the expression of surface antigens on target cells may be altered, which has implications for autoimmune potential. Immunotoxicological testing strategies may require screening studies followed by mechanistic studies to clarify such issues. Routine tiered testing approaches or standard testing batteries, however, are not recommended for biotechnology-derived pharmaceuticals.

Insert 4 ICH guideline on Preclinical Evaluation of Biotechnology-derived Pharmaceuticals

Reproductive performance and developmental toxicity studies:

The need for reproductive/developmental toxicity studies is dependent upon the product, clinical indication and intended patient population. The specific study design and dosing schedule may be modified on issues related to species specificity, immunogenicity, biological activity and/or a long elimination half-life. For example, concerns regarding potential developmental immunotoxicity, which may apply particularly to certain monoclonal antibodies with prolonged immunological effects, could be addressed in a study design modified to assess immune function of the neonate.

adversely affect immune function should be a standard component of animal toxicity studies. However, the document will advocate a science-based approach stressing that specialized toxicity assessment should be done case by case based on what is known already about the pharmacology and toxicology of the pharmaceutical as well as its proposed therapeutic use. Consequently, the FDA will not require standard testing as there are many immunoassays, and in individual situations a particular test might be valuable whereas in other instances it might not [72]. The document has not yet been released outside the FDA. In the EU, the CPMP is considering the necessity for specific guidance. In Japan, no official immunotoxicity guideline for pharmaceuticals has been prepared either. The Japanese *Guidelines for Nonclinical Studies of Drugs*, however, do require antigenicity studies to be conducted on a case-by-case basis. They do not contain specific information on other types of immunotoxicity testing. However, the need for further requirements is also growing in Japan [73].

Conclusions

Preclinical testing of pharmaceuticals in laboratory animals requires different approaches through direct immunotoxicity, resulting in unwanted immunosuppression or immunostimulation, or drug-induced hypersensitivity and autoimmunity. Tiered immunotoxicity-testing procedures have been developed and validated in the rat and mouse, and are being used successfully to detect drug-induced direct immunotoxicity.

Drug-induced hypersensitivity and autoimmune reactions are of great clinical concern. For contact allergy, routine contact sensitization testing in guinea pigs of topically applied pharmaceuticals should be extended by LLNA in the mouse as an initial screen. An important issue in contact allergy is the development of quantitative measurements of the potency of allergens. No validated models are yet available to investigate the ability of drugs to induce respiratory sensitization. LLNA or skin sensitization testing in guinea pigs should be recommended as a first screen.

Animal models are currently available to detect the potential of compounds to exacerbate induced or genetically predisposed autoimmunity, but are seldomly used in immunotoxicity studies. Models to investigate the ability of chemicals to induce autoimmunity, as a result of an immune response to self-proteins modified by the chemical, are virtually limited to PLNA. As human data show that chemical agents, in particular drugs, can cause autoimmune diseases, new models should be developed.

In conclusion, immunotoxicology is a rapidly evolving field in the regulation of pharmaceuticals. This warrants updates of the guidelines available to date. The standard use of a large immunotoxicological test battery should not be recommended. Instead, a flexible approach on a case-by-case basis is needed, taking into account that some classes of drugs and some indications may be a greater cause of concern than others.

References

Chapter A1

Introductory Texts

Roitt IM (1996) *Essential immunology*, 8th ed., Blackwell Science, Oxford

Weir DM, Stewart J (1997) *Immunology*, 8th ed., Churchill Livingstone, Edinburgh

Advanced Text

Herzenberg L, Weir DM, Herzenberg L, Blackwell CC (eds) (1997) *Weir's handbook of experimental immunology*, 5th ed., Vol. 1, *Immunochemistry and molecular immunology*, Blackwell Science, Cambridge, MA

Journal papers

Bjorkman PJ, Parham P, (1990) Structure function and diversity of class 1 major histocompatibility complex molecules. *Annu Rev Biochem* 59: 253–288

Davenport MP, Smith KJ, Hill AS (1996) Evolution of allorecognition? *Immunol Today* 17: 589–590

Davis MM (1990) T-cell receptor gene diversity and selection. *Annu Rev Biochem* 59: 475–496

Garcia KCDegano M, Stanfield RL et al (1996) An α β T-cell receptor structure at 2.5 A and its orientation in the TCR-MHC complex. *Science* 274: 209–219

Strober W, Kelsall IF, Marth T, Ludviksson B, Ehrhardt R, Neurath M (1997) Reciprocal IFNγ and TGFβ responses regulate the occurrence of mucosal inflammation. *Immunol Today* 18; 61–64

Chapter A2

1   Kincade PW, Gimble JM (1993) B-lymphocytes. *In*: Paul WE (ed.): *Fundamental immunology*. Raven Press, New York, 43–73

2   Storb U, Kruisbeek A (1996) Lymphocyte development (editorial overview). *Curr Opin Immunol* 8: 155–159

3 Clevers HC, Grosschedl R (1996) Transcriptional control of lymphoid development: lessons from gene targeting. *Immunol Today* 17: 336–343

4 Anderson G, Moore NC, Owen JJT, Jenkinson EJ (1996) Cellular interactions in thymocyte development. *Annu Rev Immunol* 14: 73–99

5 Frearson JA, Alexander DR (1996) Protein tyrosine phosphatases in T-cell development, apoptosis and signalling. *Immunol Today* 17: 385–390

6 Zlotnik A, Moore TA (1995) Cytokine production and requirements during T-cell development. *Curr Opin Immunol* 7: 206–213

7 Sprent J (1993) Lymphocytes and the thymus. *In*: Paul WE (ed.): *Fundamental immunology*. Raven Press, New York, 75–109

8 Hosseinzadeh H, Goldschneider I (1993) Recent thymic emigrants in the rat express a unique antigenic phenotype and undergo post-thymic maturation in peripheral lymphoid tissues. *J Immunol* 150: 1670–1679

9 Griebel PJ, Hein WR (1996) Expanding the role of Peyer's patches in B-cell ontogeny. *Immunol Today* 17: 30–39

10 Melchers F, Rolink A, Grawunder U, Winkler TH, Karasuyama H, Ghia P, Andersson L (1995) Positive and negative selection events during B lymphopoiesis. *Curr Opin Immunol* 7: 214–227

11 Borell MA, Phipps RP (1996) The B/macrophage cell: an elusive link between CD5$^+$ B-lymphocytes and macrophages. *Immunol Today* 17: 471–475

12 Cornall RJ, Goodnow CC, Cyster JG (1995) The regulation of self-reactive B-cells. *Curr Opin Immunol* 7: 804–811

13 Weill J-C, Reynaud CA (1996) Rearrangement/hypermutation/gene conversion: when, where and why? *Immunol Today* 17: 92–97

14 MacLennan ICM (1994) Germinal Centres. *Annu Rev Immunol* 12: 117–139

15 Sykes M (1996) Chimerism and central tolerance. *Curr Opin Immunol* 8: 694–703

16 Hess AD (1993) Autologous graft-versus-host disease: mechanisms and potential therapeutic effect. *Bone marrow Transplant* 12 (Suppl 3): S65–S69

Chapter A3

Paul WE (ed.) (1993) *Fundamental immunology*, 3rd ed., Raven Press, New York

Janeway CA Jr, Travers P (1996) *Immunobiology: the immune system in health and disease*, 2d ed., Current Biology Ltd.

Mosmann T, R, Sad S (1996) The expanding universe of T-cell subsets: Th1, Th2 and more. *Immunol Today* 17(3): 138–146

Möller G (ed.) (1996) *Accessory molecules in the immune response*, Immunoogical reviews, vol. 153, Munksgaard, Copenhagen

Chapter A4

1   Callard R, Gearing A (1994) *The cytokine facts book*. London: Academic Press, London

2   Ibelgaufts H (1995) *Dictionary of cytokines*. CH, Weinheim

3   Nicola NA (ed.): (1994) *Guidebook to cytokines and their receptors*. Oxford University Press, Oxford

4   Silvernnoinen O, Ihle JN (1996) *Signalling by the hematopoietic cytokine receptors*. Springer Verlag, Heidelberg

5   Moore MAS (1991) The clinical use of colony stimulating factors. *Annu Rev Immunol* 9: 159

6   Jelkmann W (1992) Erythropoietin. Structure, control of production and function. *Physiol Rev* 72: 449–489

7   de Sauvage FJ, Hass PE et al (1994) Stimulation of megacaryocytopoieses and thrombopoiesis by the c-Mpl ligand. *Nature* 369: 533–538

8   von Boehmer H (1993) The developmental biology of T-lymphocytes. *Annu Rev Immunol* 6: 309–326

9   Paul WE, Seder RA (1994) Lymphocyte responses and cytokines. *Cell* 76: 241–251

10 Zurawski G, de Vries JE (1994) IL-13, an IL-4 like cytokine that acts on monocytes and B-cells, but not on T-cells. *Immunol Today* 15: 19–26

11 Stuart-Harris R, Penny R (1996) *Clinical applications of the interferons*. Chapmann and Hall, London

12 Vasalli P (1992) The pathophysiology of tumor necrosis factor. *Annu Rev Immunol* 10: 411–452

13 Dinarello CA (1996) Biological basis for interleukin-1 in disease. *Blood* 87: 2095–2147

14 Holmlund JT (1993) Cytokines. *Cancer Chemotherapy and Biological Response Modifiers Annual* 14: 150–206

15 Gutterman JU (1994) Cytokine therapeutics: lessons from interferon α. *Proc Natl Acad Sci USA* 91: 1198–1205

16 Pardoll DM (1995) Paracrine cytokine adjuvants in cancer immunotherapy. *Annu Rev Immunol* 13: 399–415

17 Romagnani S (1993) Induction of Th1 and Th2 responses: a key role for the "natural" immune response? *Immunol Today* 13: 379–381

18 Mosmann TR, Sad S (1996) The expanding universe of T-cell subsets: Th1, Th2 and more. *Immunol Today* 17: 138–146

19 Springer TA (1994) Traffic signals for lymphocyte recirculation and leukocyte emigration: the multistep paradigm. *Cell* 76: 301–314

20 Baggiolini M, Dewald B, Moser B (1991) Human chemokines: an update. *Annu Rev Immunol* 15: 675–705

21 Lee JC, Laydon JT et al (1994) A protein kinase involved in the regulation of

inflammatory cytokine biosynthesis. *Nature* 372: 739–746

22 Schattner A (1994) Lymphokines in autoimmunity – a critical review. *Clin Immunol Immunopathol* 70: 177–189

23 Elliott MJ, Maini RN et al (1993) Treatment of rheumatoid arthritis with chimeric monoclonal antibodies to tumor necrosis factor alpha. *Arthritis Rheum* 36: 1681–1690

24 Colombo MC, Forni G (1994) Cytokine gene transfer in tumor inhibition and tumor therapy: Where are we now? *Immunol Today* 15: 48–51

Chapter A5

Cambier JC, Pleiman CM, Clark MR (1994) Signal transduction by the B-cell antigen receptor and its coreceptors. *Annu Rev Immunol* 12: 457–486

Clark EA, Ledbetter JA (1994) How B- and T-cells talk to each other. *Nature* 367: 425–428

Fearon DT, Carter RH (1995) The CD19/CR2/TAPA-1 complex of B-lymphocytes: linking natural to acquired immunity. *Annu Rev Immunol* 13: 127–149

Gray D, Siepmann K, van Essen D, Poudrier J, Wykes M, Jainandunsing S, Bergthorsdottir S, Dullforce P (1996) B-T-lymphocyte interactions in the generation and survival of memory cells. *Immunol Rev* 150: 45–61

Reth M, Wienands J (1997) Initiation and processing of signals from the B-cell antigen receptor. *Annu Rev Immunol* 15: 453–479

Rijkers GT, Sanders EAM, Breukels MA, Zegers BJM (1996) Responsivenss of infants to capsular polysaccharides: implications for vaccine development. *Rev Med Microbiol* 7: 3–12

Chapter A6

1 Kuijpers TW, Roos D (1993) Extravasation of leukocytes. *Behring Inst Mitt* 92: 107–137

2 Henson PM, Henson JE, Fittschen C, Bratton DL, Riches DWH (1992) Degranulation, secretion by phagocytic cells. *In*: JI Gallin, IM Goldstein, R Synderman (eds): *Inflammation: basic principles and clinical correlates.* 2nd ed., Raven Press, New York, 511–539

3 Gallin JI (1992) Disorders of phagocytic cells (1992) *In*: JI Gallin, IM Goldstein, R Synderman (eds): *Inflammation: basic principles and clinical correlates.* 2nd ed., Raven Press, New York, 859–874

4 Weiss SJ (1989) Tissue destruction by neutrophils. *N Engl J Med* 320: 365–376

5   Spits H, Lanier LL, Phillips JH (1995) Development of human T and natural killer cells. *Blood* 85: 2654–2670

6   Scott P, Trinchieri G (1995) The role of natural killer cells in host-parasite interactions. *Curr Opin Immunol* 7: 34–40

7   Biron CA (1997) Activation and function of natural killer cell responses during viral infections. *Curr Opin Immunol* 9: 24–34

8   Kärre K (1997) NK cells, MHC class I antigens and missing self. *Immunol Rev* 155: 5–10

9   Trinchieri G (1997) Cytokines acting on or secreted by macrophages during intracellular infection (IL-10, IL 12, IFNγ). *Curr Opin Immunol* 9: 17–23

10 Bancroft GJ, Schreiber RD, Unanue ER (1991) Natural immunity: a T-cell-independent pathway of macrophage activation, defined in the scid mouse. *Immunol Rev* 124: 5–24

11 Unanue E (1997) Inter-relationship among macrophages, natural killer cells and neutrophils in early stages of *Listeria* resistance. *Curr Opin Immunol* 9: 35–43

12 Kagi D, Ledermann B, Burki K, Seiler P, Odermatt B, Olsen KJ, Podack ER, Zinkernagel RM, Hengartner H (1994) Cytotoxicity mediated by T-cells and natural killer cells is greatly impaired in perforin-deficient mice. *Nature* 369: 31–37

13 Oshimi Y, Oda S, Honda Y, Nagata S, Miyazaki S (1996) Involvement of Fas ligand and Fas-mediated pathway in the cytotoxicity of human natural killer cells. *J Immunol* 157: 2909–2915

14 Lanier LL (1997) Natural killer cell receptors and MHC class I interactions. *Curr Opin Immunol* 9: 126–31

15 Lanier LL, Corliss B, Phillips JH (1997) Arousal and inhibition of human NK cells. *Immunol Rev* 155: 145–54

16 Müller-Eberhard HJ (1992) Complement: chemistry and pathways. *In*: JI Gallin, IM Goldstein, R Synderman (eds): *Inflammation: basic principles and clinical correlates*. 2nd ed., Raven Press, New York, 33–61

17 Turner MW (1996) Mannose-binding lectin: the pluripotent molecule of the innate immune system. *Immunol Today* 17: 532–540

18 Goldstein IM (1992) Complement: biologically active products. *In*: JI Gallin, IM Goldstein, R Synderman (eds): *Inflammation: basic principles and clinical correlates*. 2nd ed., Raven Press, New York, 63–80

19 Vogt W (1986) Anaphylatoxins: possible roles in disease. *Complement* 3: 177–188

Chapter A7

1   Bunting S, Gryglewski RJ, Moncada S, Vane JR (1976) Arterial walls generate

from prostaglandin endoperoxides a substance (prostaglandin X) which relaxes strips of mesenteric and coeliac arteries and inhibits platelet aggregation. *Prostaglandins* 12: 897–913

2 Coleman RA, Grix SP, Head SA, Louttit JB, Mallett A, Sheldrick RLG (1994) A novel inhibitory prostanoid receptor in piglet saphenous vein. *Prostaglandins* 47: 151–166

3 Toh H, Ichikawa A, Naruyima S (1995) Molecular evolution of receptors for eicosanoids. *FEBS Lett* 361: 17–21

4 Raychowdhury MK, Yukawa M, Collins LJ, McGrail SJ, Kent KC, Ware AJ (1994) Alternative splicing produces a divergent cytoplasmic tail in the human endothelial thromboxane A_2 receptor. *J Biol Chem* 269: 19256–19261

5 Sigal E (1991) The molecular biology of mammalian arachidonic acid metabolism. *Am J Physiol* 260: L13–L28

6 Sala A, Aliev GM, Rossoni G, Berti F, Buccellati C, Burnstock G, Folco G, Maclouf J (1996) Morphological and functional changes of coronary vasculature caused by transcellular biosynthesis of sulfidopeptide leukotrienes in isolated heart of rabbit. *Blood* 87: 1824–1832

7 Feldberg W, Kellaway CH (1938) Liberation of histamine and formation of lysocithin-like substances by cobra venom. *J Physiol* 94: 187–226

8 McGiff JC, Carroll M, Escalante B, Ferreri NR (1995) Pieces in the puzzle: novel arachidonate metabolites. *Ad. Prostaglandin Thromboxane Leukot Res* 23: 187–192

9 Morrow JD, Hill KE, Burk RF, Nammour TM, Badr K, Roberts LJ (1990) II. A series of prostaglandin F_2-like compounds are produced *in vivo* in humans by a non-cyclooxygenase, free radical-catalyzed mechanism. *Proc Natl Acad Sci USA* 87: 9383–9387

10 Gryglewski RJ, Panczenko B, Korbut R, Grodzińska L, Ocetkiewicz A (1975) Corticosteroids inhibit prostaglandin release from perfused mesenteric blood vessels of rabbit and from perfused lungs of sensitized guinea pig. *Prostaglandins* 10: 343–355

11 Chilton FH, Ellis JM, Olson SC, Wykle RL (1984) 1-0-alkyl-2-arachidonoyl-*sn*-glycero-3-phosphocholine. *J Biol Chem* 259: 12014–12019

12 Chilton FH, O'Flaherty JT, Ellis JM, Swendsen CL, Wykle RL (1983) Metabolic fate of platelet-activating factor in neutrophils. *J Biol Chem* 258: 6357–6361

13 McIntyre TM, Zimmerman GA, Prescott SM (1986) Leukotrienes C_4 and D_4 stimulate human endothelial cells to synthesize platelet-activating factor and bind neutrophils. *Proc Natl Acad Sci USA* 83: 2204–2208

14 Chao W, Olson MS (1993) Platelet-activating factor: receptors and signal transduction. *Biochemistry* 292: 617–629

15 Koltai M, Hosford D, Guinot P, Esanu A, Braquet P (1991) Platelet-activating

factor (PAF): a review of its effects, antagonists and future clinical implications. *Drugs* 42: 9–29: 174–204

16 Dale MM, Foreman JC, Fan TP (1994) *Textbook of immunopharmacology.* Blackwell Scientific Publications, Oxford

17 Maggi CA, Patacchini R, Rovero P, Giachetti A (1993) Tachykinin receptors and tachykinin receptor antagonists. *J Auton Pharmacol* 13: 23–93

18 Regoli D, Rhaleb NE, Dion S, Drapeau G (1990) New selective bradykinin receptor antagonists and bradykinin B2 receptor characterization. *Trends Pharmacol Sci* 11: 156–161

19 Pellacani A, Brunner HR, Nussberger J (1992) Antagonizing and measurement: approaches to understanding of hemodynamic effects of kinins. *J Cardiovasc Pharmacol* 20 (Suppl 9): S28–S34

20 Dray A, Perkins M (1993) Bradykinin and inflammatory pain. *Trends Neurosci* 16: 99–104

21 Otterbein L, Lowe VC, Kyle DJ, Noronha-Blob L (1993) Additive effects of a bradykinin antagonists, NPC 17761, and a keumedin, NPC 15669, on survival in animal models of sepsis. *Agents Actions* 39: C125–C127

22 Griesbacher T, Tiran B, Lembeck F (1993) The pathological events in experimental acute pancreatitis prevented by the bradykinin antagonist, HOE 140. *Brit J Pharmacol* 108: 404–411

23 Furchgott RF, Zawadzki JV (1980) The obligatory role of endothelial cells in the relaxation of arterial smooth muscle by acetylcholine. *Nature* 288: 373–376

24 Korbut R, Trabka-Janik E, Gryglewski RJ (1989) Cytoprotection of human polymorphonuclear leukocytes by stimulators of adenylate and guanylate cyclases. *Eur. J. Pharmacol* 165: 171–172

25 Zifa E, Fillon G (1992) 5-hydroxytryptamine receptors. *Pharmcol Rev* 44: 401–458

26 Madden KS, Sanders VM, Felten DL (1995) Catecholamine influences and sympathetic neural modulation of immune responsiveness. *Annu Rev Pharmacol Toxicol* 35: 417–448

Chapter A8

Jawetz E, Melnick JL, Adelberg EA, Brooks GF, Butel JS, Ornston LN (eds) (1995) *Medical microbiology.* Prentice-Hall International, London

Mims CA, Playfair JHL, Roitt IM, Wakelin D, Williams R, Anderson RM (eds) (1993) *Medical microbiology.* Mosby, London

Roit I, Brostoff J, Male D (eds) (1989) *Immunology.* Gower Medical Publishing, London

Silverstein AM (ed.) (1988) *A history of immunology.* Academic Press, San

Diego

Snippe H, Willers JMN (1992) Attack and Defence. *In*: JJ van Everdingen (ed.): *The beast in man: microbes and macrobes as intimate enemies. Part II. The battle of bugs*. Belvedere, Overveen, The Netherlands

Verhoef J, Mattson E (1995) The role of cytokines in gram-positive bacterial shock. *Trends Microbiol* 3: 136–140

Chapter A9

1   Church MK, Levi-Schaffer (1997) The human mast cell. *J Allerg Clin Immunol* 99: 155–160

2   Teran LM, Davies DE (1996) The chemokines: their potential in allergic inflammation. *Clin Exp Allergy* 26: 1005–1019

3   Kroegel C, Virchow JC Jr, Luttmann W, Walker C, Warner JA (1994) Pulmonary immune cells in health and disease: the eosinophil leucocyte (Part 1) *Eur Resp J* 7: 519–543

4   Kroegel C, Warner JA, Virchow JC Jr, Matthys H (1994) Pulmonary immune cells in health and disease: the eosinophil leucocyte (Part 2) *Eur Resp J* 7: 743–760

Chapter A10

1   Bach FH, Sachs DH (1987) Current concepts: immunology. Transplantation immunology. *N Engl J Med* 317: 489–492

2   Lindhal KF, Wilson DB (1977) Histocompatibility antigen-activated cytotoxic T-lymphocytes. I. Estimates of the absolute frequency of killer cells generated *in vitro*. *J Exp Med* 145: 508–522

3   Ashwell JD, Chen C, Schwartz RH (1986) High frequency and nonrandom distribution of alloreactivity in T-cell clones selected for recognition of foreign antigen in association with self class II molecules. *J Immunol* 136: 389–395

4   Rotzschke O, Falk K, Faath S, Rammensee HG (1991) On the nature of peptides involved in T-cell alloreactivity. *J Exp Med* 174: 1059–1071

5   Sayegh MH, Watschinger B, Carpenter C (1994) Mechanisms of T-cell recognition of antigen. *Transplantation* 57: 1295–1302

6   Lee RS, Grusby MJ, Glimcher LH, Winn HJ, Auchincloss HJr, (1994) Indirect recognition by helper cells can induce donor-specific cytotoxic T-lymphocytes *in vivo*. *J Exp Med* 179: 865–872

7   Dalloul AA, Chmouzis E, Ngo K, Fung-Leung WP (1996) Adoptively transferred CD4[+] lymphocytes from CD8–/– mice are sufficient to mediate the rejection of MHC class II or class I disparate skin grafts. *J Immunol* 156: 4114–4119

8 Oluwole SF, Chowdhury NC, Jin MT, Hardy MA (1993) Induction of transplantation tolerance in rat cardiac allograft by intrathymic inoculation of allogeneic soluble peptides. *Transplantation* 56: 1523–1527

9 Russell ME, Hancock WW, Akalin E, Wallace AF, Glysin-Jensen T, Willett TA, Sayegh MH (1996) Chronic cardiac rejection in the LEW to F344 rat model. Blockade of CD28-B7 costimulation by CTLA4Ig modulate T-cell and macrophage activation and attenuates arteriosclerosis. *J Clin Invest* 97: 833–838

10 Larsen C, Elwood E, Alexander D, Ritchie S, Hendrix R, Tucker-Burden C, Cho H, Aruffo A, Hollenbaugh D, Linsley P et al (1996) Long-term acceptance of skin and cardiac allografts after blocking CD40 and CD28 pathways. *Nature* 381: 434–438

11 Kissmeyer-Nielsen F, Olsen S, Petersen VP, Fjeldborg O (1966) Hyperacute rejection of kidney allografts, associated with pre-existing humoral antibodies against donor cells. *Lancet* 2: 662–670

12 Rosenberg AS, Singer A (1992) Cellular basis of skin allograft rejection: an *in vivo* model of immune-mediated tissue destruction. *Annu Rev Immunol* 10: 333–358

13 Manning DD, Reed ND, Shaffer CF (1973) Maintenance of skin xenografts of widely divergent phylogenetic origin on congenitally athymic (nude) mice. *J Exp Med* 138: 488–494

14 Sprent J, Schaefer M, Lo D, Korngold R (1986) Properties of purified T-cell subsets. II. *In vivo* responses to class I vs. class II H-2 differences. *J Exp Med* 163: 998–1011

15 Mosmann TR, Coffman RL (1989) Th1 and Th2 cells: different patterns of lymphokine secretion lead to different functional properties. *Annu Rev Immunol* 7: 145–173

16 Ridge JP, Fuchs EJ, Matzinger P (1996) Neonatal tolerance revisited: turning on newborn T-cells with dendritic cells. *Science* 271: 1723–1726

17 Sarzotti M, Robbins DS, Hoffman PM (1996) Induction of protective CTL responses in newborn mice by a murine retrovirus. *Science* 271: 1726–1728

18 Forsthuber T, Yip HC, Lehmann PV (1996) Induction of T_H1 and T_H2 immunity in neonatal mice. *Science* 271: 1728–1730

19 Lehmann PV, Matesic D, Benichou G, Heeger PS (1997) Induction of T helper 2 immunity to an immunodominant allopeptide. *Transplantation* 64 (2): 292–296

20 Chen W, Murphy B, Waaga AM, Willett TA, Russell ME, Khoury SJ, Sayegh MH (1996) Mechanisms of indirect allorecognition in graft rejection: class II MHC allopeptide-specific T-cell clones transfer delayed-type hypersensitivity responses *in vivo*. *Transplantation* 62: 705–710

21 Chen N, Field E (1995) Enhanced type 2 and diminished type 1 cytokines in neonatal tolerance. *Transplantation* 59: 933–941

22 Sayegh MH, Akalin E, Hancock WW, Russel ME, Carpenter CB, Linsley PS,

Turka LA (1995) CD28-B7 blockade after alloantigenic challenge *in vivo* inhibits Th1 cytokines but spares Th2. *J Exp Med* 181: 1869–1874

23 Nickerson P, Steurer W, Steiger J, Zheng X, Steele AW, Strom TB (1994) Cytokines and the Th1/Th2 paradigm in transplantation. *Curr Opin Immunol* 6: 757–764

24 VanBuskirk AM, Wakely ME, Orosz CG (1996) Transfusion of polarized Th2-like cell populations into SCID mouse cardiac allograft recipients results in acute allograft rejection. *Transplantation* 62: 229–238

25 Dallman MJ (1995) Cytokines and transplantation: Th1/Th2 regulation of the immune response to solid organ transplants in the adult. *Curr Opin Immunol* 7: 632–638

26 Dupont E, Wybrom J, Toussaint C (1984) Glucocorticoids and organ transplantation. *Transplantation* 37: 331–335

27 Shevach EM (1985) The effect of cyclosporin A on the immune system. *Annu Rev Immunol* 3: 397–423

28 Brazelton TR, Morris RE (1996) Molecular mechanisms of action of new xenobiotic immunosuppressive drugs: tacrolimus (FK506), sirolimus (rapamycin), mycophenolate mofetil and leflunomide. *Curr Opin Immunol* 8: 710–720

29 Cosimi AB, Burton RC, Colvin RB, Goldstein G, Delmonico FL, LaQuaglia MP, Tolkoff-Rubin N, Rubin RH, Herrin JT, Russell PS (1981) Treatment of acute renal allograft rejection with OKT3 monoclonal antibody. *Transplantation* 32: 535–539

30 Sayegh MH, Carpenter CB (1997) Tolerance and chronic rejection. *Kid Int* 51:S11–S14

31 Sarzotti M (1997) Immunologic tolerance. *Curr Opin Hematol* 4: 48–52

32 Sykes M (1996) Chimerism and central tolerance. *Curr Opin Immunol* 8: 694–703

33 Naji A (1996) Induction of tolerance by intrathymic inoculation of alloantigen. *Curr Opin Immunol* 8: 704–709

34 Kirk AD, Harlan DM, Armstrong NN, Davis TA, Dong Y, Gray GS, Hong X, Thomas D, Fechner JHJr, Knechtle SJ (1997) CTLA-Ig and anti-CD40 ligand prevent renal allograft rejection in primates. *Proc Natl Acad Sci USA* 94: 8789–8794

Chapter A11

1 Schlom J (1995) Monoclonal antibodies in cancer therapy: basic principles. *In*: VT DeVita, S Hellman, SA Rosenberg (eds): *Biologic therapy of cancer.* J.B. Lippincott Company, Philadelphia, 507–521

2 Kast WM, Brandt RMP, Sidney J, Drijfhout JW, Kubo RT, Grey HM, Melief

CJM, Sette A (1994) Role of HLA-A motifs in identification of potential CTL epitopes in human papillomavirus type 16 E6 and E7 proteins. *J Immunol* 152: 3904–3912

3   Lee SP, Tierney RJ, Thomas WA, Brooks JM, Rickinson AB (1997) Conserved CTL epitopes within EBV latent membrane protein 2: a potential target for CTL-based tumor therapy. *J Immunol* 158: 3325–3334

4   Jung S, Schluesener HJ (1991) Human T-lymphocytes recognize a peptide of single point-mutated, oncogenic ras proteins. *J Exp Med* 173: 273–276

5   Ioannides CG, Fisk B, Fan D, Biddison WE, Wharton JT, O'Brian CA (1993) Cytotoxic T-cells isolated from ovarian malignant ascites recognize a peptide derived from the HER-2/*neu* proto-oncogene. *Cell Immunol* 151: 225–234

6   Houbiers JGA, Nijman HW, Van der Berg SH, Drijfhout JW, Kenemans P, Van de Velde CJH, Brand A, Momberg F, Kast WM, Melief CJM (1993) *In vitro* induction of human cytotoxic T-lymphocyte responses against peptides of mutant and wild-type p53. *Eur J Immunol* 23: 2072–2077

7   Traversari P, Van der Bruggen P, Luescher IF, Lurquin C, Chomez P, Van Pel A, De Plaen E, Amar-Costesec A, Boon T (1992) A nonapeptide encoded by human gene MAGE-1 is recognized on HLA-A1 by cytolytic T-lymphocytes directed against tumor antigen MZ2-E. *J Exp Med* 176: 1453–1457

8   Canevari S, Stoter G, Arienti F, Bolis G, Colnaghi MI, Di Re E, Eggermont AMM, Goey SH, Gratama JW, Lamers CHJ et al (1995) Regression of advanced ovarian carcinoma by intraperitoneal treatment with autologous T-lymphocytes retargeted by a bispecific monoclonal antibody. *J Nat Cancer Inst* 87: 1463–1469

9   Oosterwijk E, Debruyne FMJ, Schalken JA (1995) The use of monoclonal antibody G250 in the therapy of renal-cell carcinoma. *Semin Oncol* 22: 34–41

10 Rosenberg SA (1997) Cancer vaccines based on the identification of genes encoding cancer regression antigens. *Immunol Today* 18: 175–182

11 Darzynkiewicz Z, Juan G, Li X, Gorczyca W, Murakami T, Traganos F (1997) Cytometry in cell necrobiology: analysis of apoptosis and accidental cell death (necrosis). *Cytometry* 27: 1–20

12 Hannun YA (1997) Apoptosis and the dilemma of cancer chemotherapy. *Blood* 89: 1845–1853

Chapter A12

1   Ader R (1996) Historical perspectives on psychoneuroimmunology. *In*: H Friedman, TW Klein, AL Friedman (eds): *Psychoneuroimmunology, stress, and infection*. CRC Press, Boca Raton, 1–24

2   Besedovsky HO, delRey AE, Sorkin E, DaPrada M, Keller IIA (1979)

Immunoregulation mediated by the sympathetic nervous system. *Cell Immunol* 48: 346

3   Pierpaoli W, Baroni C, Fabris N, Sorkin E (1969) Hormones and immunological capacity. II. Reconstitution of antibody production in hormonally deficient mice by somatotropic hormone, thyrotropic hormone and thyroxin. *J Immunol* 16: 217–230

4   Besedovsky H, Sorkin E, Keller M, Miller J (1977) Hypothalamic changes during the immune response. *Eur J Immunol* 7: 323–325

5   Weigent DA, Blalock JE (1995) Associations between the neuroendocrine and immune systems. *J Leukocyte Biol* 58: 137–150

6   Blalock JE (1984) The immune system as a sensory organ. *J Immunol* 132: 1067–1070

7   Gala RR (1991) Prolactin and growth hormone in the regulation of the immune system. *Proc Soc Exp Biol Med* 198: 513–527

8   Kruger TE, Smith LR, Harbour DV, Blalock JE (1989) Thyrotropin: an endogenous regulator of the *in vitro* immune response. *J Immunol* 142: 744–747

9   Weigent DA, Blalock JE, LeBoeuf RD (1991) An antisense oligodeoxynucleotide to growth hormone messenger ribonucleic acid inhibits lymphocyte proliferation. *Endocrinology* 128: 2053–2057

10 Weigent DA, Baxter JB, Blalock JE (1992) The production of growth hormone and insulin-like growth factor-I by the same subpopulation of rat mononuclear leukocytes. *Brain Behav Immun* 6: 365–376

11 Smith EM, Meyer WJ, Blalock JE (1982) Virus-induced corticosterone in hypophysectomized mice: a possible lymphoid adrenal axis. *Science* 218: 1311–1312

12 Bayle JE, Guellati M, Ibos F, Roux J (1991) *Brucella abortus* antigen stimulates the pituitary-adrenal axis through the extra-pituitary B-lymphoid system. *Prog Neuro Endocrinol Immunol* 4: 99–105

13 Reynolds DG, Gurll NJ, Vargish T, Lechner RB, Faden AI, Holaday JW (1980) Blockade of opiate receptors with naloxone improves survival and cardiac performance in canine endotoxic shock. *Circulat Shock* 7: 39–48

14 Harbour DV, Smith EM, Blalock JE (1987) Splenic lymphocyte production of an endorphin during endotoxic shock. *Brain Behav Immun* 1: 123–133

15 Stein C, Hassan AHS, Przewlocki R, Gramsch C, Peter K, Herz A (1990) Opioids from immunocytes interact with receptors on sensory nerves to inhibit nociception in inflammation. *Proc Natl Acad Sci USA* 87: 5935–5939

16 Schafer M, Mousa SA, Zhang Q, Carter L, Stein C (1996) Expression of corticotropin-releasing factor in inflamed tissue is required for intrinsic peripheral opioid analgesia. *Proc Natl Acad Sci USA* 93: 6096–6100

Chapter B1

1 Köhler G, Milstein C (1975) Continous cultures of cells fused secreting antibody of predefined specificity. *Nature* 256: 495–497
2 Ring J (1981) Diagnostic methods in allergy. *Behring Inst Mitt* 68: 141–152
3 Ring J (ed.) (1988) *Angewandte Allergologie*. MMV Medizin Verlag, München
4 Wide L, Bennich H, Johansson SGO (1967) Diagnosis of allergy by an *in vitro* test for allergen antibodies. *Lancet* 2: 1105
5 Gleich GJ, Yunginger JW (1981) Variations of the radioallergosorbent test for measurement of IgE antibody levels, allergens and blocking antibody activity. *In*: J Ring, G Burg (eds): *New trends in allergy*. Heidelberg: Springer-Verlag, 98–107

Further reading
1 Tijssen P (1985) *Practice and theory of enzyme immunoassays*. Elsevier, Amsterdam
2 Abbas AK, Lichtman AH, Pober JS (eds) (1994) *Cellular and molecular immunology*. W.B. Saunders, Philadelphia
3 Crowther JR (ed.) (1995) *ELISA*. Humana Press, Totowa
4 Thomas L (ed.) (1988) *Labor und Diagnose*. Medizinische Verlagsgesellschaft, Marburg
5 Roitt IM, Brostoff J, Male DK (1986) *Immunology*. Mosby, St. Louis

Chapter B2

1 Jennings CD, Foon KA (1997) Recent advances in flow cytometry: application to the diagnosis of hematologic malignancy. *Blood* 90: 2863–2892
2 Catovsky D, Matutes E (1992) The classification of acute leukaemia. *Leukemia* 6 Suppl 2: 1–6
3 Cline MJ (1994) The molecular basis of leukemia. *N Engl J Med* 330: 328–336
4 Copelan EA, McGuire EA (1995) The biology and treatment of acute lymphoblastic leukemia in adults. *Blood* 85: 1151–1168
5 Pui CH, Behm FG, Crist WM (1993) Clinical and biologic relevance of immunologic marker studies in childhood acute lymphoblastic leukemia. *Blood* 82: 343–362
6 Coustan-Smith E, Behm FG, Sanchez J, Boyett JM, Hancock ML, Raimondi SC, Rubnitz JE, Rivera GK, Sandlund JT, Pui CH et al (1998) Immunological detection of minimal residual disease in children with acute lymphoblastic

leukaemia. *Lancet* 351: 550–554

7 San Miguel JF, Martinez A, Macedo A, Vidriales MB, Lopez-Berges C, Gonzalez M, Caballero D, Garcia-Marcos MA, Ramos F, Fernandez-Calvo J et al (1997) Immunophenotyping investigation of minimal residual disease is a useful approach for predicting relapse in acute myeloid leukemia patients. *Blood* 90: 2465–2470

8 O'Brien S, del Giglio A, Keating M (1995) Advances in the biology and treatment of B-cell chronic lymphocytic leukemia. *Blood* 85: 307–318

9 Harris NL, Jaffe ES, Stein H, Banks PM, Chan JK, Cleary ML, Delsol G, De Wolf-Peeters C, Falini B, Gatter KC et al (1994) Lymphoma classification proposal. *Blood* 84: 1361–139

10 Semenzato G, Zambello R, Starkebaum G, Oshimi K, Loughran TP Jr, (1997) The lymphoproliferative disease of granular lymphocytes: updated criteria for diagnosis. *Blood* 89: 256–260

11 van't Veer MB, Kluin-Nelemans JC, van der Schoot CE, van Putten WL, Adriaansen HJ, van Wering ER (1992) Quality assessment of immunological marker analysis and the immunological diagnosis in leukaemia and lymphoma: a multi-centre study. Dutch Cooperative Study Group on Immunophenotyping of Leukaemias and Lymphomas (SIHON). *Brit J Haematol* 80: 458–465

12 Kluin-Nelemans JC, van Wering ER, van'T Veer MB, van der Schoot CE, Adriaansen HJ, van der Burgh FJ, Gratama JW (1996) Pitfalls in the immunophenotyping of leukaemia and leukaemic lymphomas: survey of 9 years of quality control in The Netherlands. Dutch Cooperative Study Group on Immunophenotyping of Haematologica l Malignancies (SIHON). *Brit J Haematol* 9: 692–699

Chapter B3

1 Yalow RS, Berson SA (1959) Assay of plasma insulin in human subjects by immunologic methods. *Nature* 184: 1684–1649

2 Wild D (ed.) (1994) *The immunoassay handbook*. Stockton Press, New York

3 Baxendale PM (1990) Development of scintillation proximity assays for prostaglandins and related compounds. *Adv Prost Thromb Leuk Res* 21A: 303

4 O'Sullivan MJ, Marks V (1981) Methods for the preparation of enzyme-antibody-conjugates for use in enzyme immunoassay. *In*: JJ Langone, MV Vunakis (eds): *Methods in enzymology*, vol. 73, *Immunochemical techniques*, part B, Academic Press, New York, 147–166

5 Voller A, Bidwell DE, Huldt G, Engvell E (1978) A microtitre plate method of enzyme linked immunoassay and its application to malaria. *Bull WHO* 51: 209–216

6   O'Sullivan MJ, Bridges JW, Marks V (1979) Enzyme immunoassay: a review. *Annal Clin Biochem* 16: 221–239

Chapter C1

1   Plotkin SA, Mortimer EA (eds) (1994) *Vaccines*, 2nd ed. WB Saunders, Philadelphia
2   Woodrow GC, Levine MM (eds) (1990) *New generation vaccines*. Marcel Dekker, New York
3   Murdin AD, Barreto L, Plotkin S (1996) Inactivated poliovirus vaccine: past and present experience. *Vaccine* 14: 735–746
4   Rappuoli R (1994) Toxin inactivation and antigen stabilization: two different uses of formaldehyde. *Vaccine* 12: 579–581
5   Patel SS, Wagstaff AJ (1996) Acellular pertussis vaccine (Infanrix™-DTPa; SB-3): a review of its immunogenicity, protective efficacy and tolerability in the prevention of *Bordetella pertussis* infection. *Drugs* 52: 254–275
6   Madore DC (1996) Impact of immunization on *Haemophilus influenzae* type b disease. *Infect Agent Dis* 5: 8–20
7   Eskola J, Ölander R-M, Hovi T, Litmanen L, Peltola S, Käyhty H (1996) Randomised trial of the effect of co-administration with acellular pertussis DTP vaccine on immunogenicity of *Haemophilus influenzae* type b conjugate vaccine. *Lancet* 348: 1688–1692
8   Kaufmann SHE (ed.) (1996) *Concepts in vaccine development*. Walter de Gruyter, Berlin
9   Powell MF, Newman MJ (eds) (1995) *Vaccine design: the subunit and adjuvant approach*. Plenum Press, New York
10 Francis MJ (1991) Enhanced immunogenicity of recombinant and synthetic peptide vaccines. *In*: G Gregoriadis, AC Allison, G Poste (eds): *Vaccines: recent trends and progress*. Plenum Press, New York, 13–23
11 Hoogerhout P, Donders EMLM, Van Gaans-van den Brink JAM, Kuipers B, Brugghe HF, Van Unen LMA, Timmermans HAM, Ten Hove GJ, De Jong APJM, Peeters CCAM et al (1995) Conjugates of synthetic cyclic peptides elicit bactericidal antibodies against a conformational epitope on a class I outer membrane protein of *Neisseria meningitidis*. *Infect Immunity* 63: 3473–3478
12 Donnelly JJ, Ulmer JB, Liu MA (1997) DNA vaccines. *Life Sci* 60: 163–172
13 Walker RI (1994) New strategies for using mucosal vaccination to achieve more effective immunization. *Vaccine* 12: 387–400
14 Li Wan Po A, Rogers E, Sheppard M, Scott EM (1995) Delivery systems for non-parenteral vaccines. Adv. *Drug Deliv Rev* 18: 101–109
15 Shalaby WSW (1995) Development of oral vaccines to stimulate mucosal

and systemic immunity: barriers and novel strategies. *Clin Immunol Immunopathol* 74: 127–134

16 Almeida AJ, Alpar HO (1996) Nasal delivery of vaccines. *J Drug Targeting* 3: 455–467

Chapter C2

1 Behring EA, Kitasato S (1890) Über das Zustandekommen der Diphtherie-Immunität und der Tetanus-Immunität bei Thieren. *Dtsch Med Wochenschr* 49: 1113–1114

2 Gronski P, Seiler FR, Schwick HG (1991) Discovery of antitoxins and development of antibody preparations for clinical uses from 1890 to 1990. *Molec Immunol* 28(12): 1321–1332

3 Sedlacek HH, Gronski P, Hofstaetter T, Kanzy EJ, Schorlemmer HU, Seiler FR (1983) The biological properties of immunoglobulin G and its split products (F(ab')$_2$ and Fab). *Klin Wochenschr* 61: 723–736

4 Stokes J Jr, Maris EP, Gellis SS (1944) Chemical, clinical and immunological studies on the products of human plasma fractionation. XI. The use of concentrated normal human serum gamma globulin (human immune serum globulin) in the prophylaxis and treatment of measles. *J Clin Invest* 23: 531–540

5 Janeway CA (1948) The plasma proteins: their functions and uses. *Pediatrics* 2: 489–497

6 Moore GE, Sandberg A, Amos DB (1957) Experimental and clinical adventures with large doses of gamma and other globulins as anticancer agents. *Surgery* 41: 972–983

7 Schultze HE, Schwick G (1962) Über neue Möglichkeiten intravenöser Gammaglobulin-Applikation. *Dtsch Med Wochenschr* 87: 1643–1650

8 Römer J, Morgenthaler JJ, Scherz R, Skvaril F (1982) Characterization of various immunoglobulin preparations for intravenous application. I. Protein composition and antibody content. *Vox Sang* 42: 62–73

9 Römer J, Morgenthaler JJ, Scherz R, Skvaril F (1982) Characterization of various immunoglobulin preparations for intravenous application. II. Complement activation and binding to *Staphylococcus* protein A. *Vox Sang* 42: 74–80

10 Suez D (1995) Intravenous immunoglobulin therapy. Indications, potential side effects, and treatment guidelines. *J Intraven Nurs* 18: 178–190

11 Cohn EJ, Strong LE, Hughes WL, Mulford DJ, Ashworth JN, Melin N, Taylor HJ (1946) Preparation and properties of serum and plasma proteins. IV: A system for the separation into fractions of protein and lipoprotein components of biological tissues and fluids. *J Amer Chem Soc* 68: 459–475

12 Oncley JL, Melin M, Richert DA, Cameron JW, Gross PMJr, (1949) Preparation and properties of serum and plasma proteins. XIX. The separation of the antibodies, isoagglutinins, prothrombin, plasminogen, and X-proteins into subfractions of human plasma. *J Amer Chem Soc* 71: 541–550

13 Stephan W (1969) Beseitigung der Komplementfixierung von Gamma-Globulin durch chemische Modifizierung mit Beta-Propiolacton. *Z Klin Chem Klin Biochem* 7: 282–286

14 LoGrippo GA (1960) Investigations of the use of β-propiolactone in virus inactivation. *Ann N Y Acad Sci* 83: 587–594

15 Masuho Y, Tomibe K, Matsuzawa K, Ohtsu A (1977) Development of an intravenous γ-globulin with Fc-activities. I. Preparation and characterization of S-sulfonated human γ-globulin. *Vox Sang* 32: 175–181

16 Gronski P, Hofstaetter T, Kanzy EJ, Lüben G, Seiler FR (1983) S-sulfonation: a reversible chemical modification of human immunoglobulins permitting intravenous application. I. Physicochemical and binding properties of S-sulfonated and reconstituted IgG. *Vox Sang* 45: 144–154

17 Mobini N, Sarela A, Ahmed AR (1995) Intraveneous immunoglobulins in the therapy of autoimmune and systemic inflammatory disorders. *Ann Allerg Asth Immunol* 74: 119–128

18 Ronda N, Hurez V, Kazatchkine MD (1993) Intraveneous Immunoglobulin Therapy of Autoimmune and Systemic Inflammatory Diseases. *Vox Sang* 64: 65–72

19 Barandun S, Cottier H, Hässig A, Riva G (eds) (1959) *Das Antikörpermangelsyndrom*. Benno Schwabe and Co. Verlag, Basel/Stuttgart. Appeared as reprint of *Helv Med Acta* 26, Fasc. 2–4

20 Cunningham-Rundles C (1988) Intravenous immunoglobulin treatment in the primary immunodeficiency diseases. *Immunol Allergy Clin N Amer* 8(1): 17–28

21 Mobini N, Sarela A, Ahmed AR (1995) Intravenous immunoglobulins in the therapy of autoimmune and systemic inflammatory disorders. *Ann Allergy Asthma Immunol* 74: 119–128

22 Misbah SA, Chapel HM (1993) Adverse effects of intravenous immunoglobulin. *Drug Safety* 9 (4): 254–262

23 Köhler G, Milstein C (1975) Continuous cultures of fused cells secreting antibodies of predefined specificity. *Nature* 256: 495–497

Chapter C3

1 Nies AS, Spielberg SP (1996) Principles of therapeutics. *In*: JG Hardman, LE Limbird (eds): *Goodman and Gilman's the pharmacological basis of*

therapeutic (9th edn). Mc Graw-Hill, New York, 43–62

2   Pelikan Z (1996) *The late nasal response; its clinical and immunologic features, possible mechanism and pharmacologic modulation*. Thesis, Free University of Amsterdam

3   Pelikan Z (1990) Late nasal response – its clinical characteristics, features, and possible mechanisms. *In*: W Dorsch (ed.): *Late phase allergic reactions*. CRC Press, Boca Raton, 111–155

4   Pelikan Z (1990) Concept of pathogenesis and possible mechanism(s) underlying the late phase reactions, focused on the late asthmatic response (LAR). *In*: W Dorsch (ed.): *Late phase allergic reactions*. CRC Press, Boca Raton, 499–518

5   Foreman JC, Pearce FL (1993) Cromolyn and nedocromil. *In*: E Middleton, Ch Reed, EF Ellis, NF Adkinson, JW Yuninger, WW Busse (eds): *Allergy, principles and practice* (4th edn). Mosby-Year Book, St Louis 926–940

6   Brogden RN, Speight TM, Avery GS (1974) Sodium cromoglycate (cromolyn sodium): a review of its mode of action, pharmacology, therapeutic efficacy and use. *Drugs* 7: 188–282

7   Pearce FL, Al-Laith M, Bosman L, Brostoff J, Cunniffe TM, Flint KC, Hudspith BN, Jaffar ZH, Johnson NMI, Kassessinoff TA et al (1989) Effects of sodium cromoglycate and nedocromil sodium on histamine secretion from mast cells from various locations. *Drugs* 37 (Suppl 1): 37–43

8   Okayama Y, Church MK (1993) Drugs modifying the responses of mast cells and basophils. Foreman JC (ed.). *In*: JC Foreman (ed.): *Immunopharmacology of mast cells and basophils*. Academic Press, London, 139–152

9   Eady RP, Norris AA (1997) Nedocromil sodium and sodium cromoglycate: Pharmacology and putative modes of action. *In*: AB Kay (ed.): *Allergy and allergic diseases*. Blackwell, Oxford, 584–595

10 Norris AA (1996) Pharmacology of sodium cromoglycate. *Clin Exp Allergy* 26(Suppl 4): 5–7

11 Pelikan Z, Pelikan-Filipek M, Schoemaker MC, Berger MPF (1988) Effects of disodium cromoglycate and beclomethasone dipropionate on the asthmatic response to allergen challenge I. Immediate response (IAR). *Ann Allergy* 60: 211–216

12 Pelikan Z, Pelikan-Filipek M, Remeijer L (1988) Effects of disodium cromoglycate and beclomethasone dipropionate on the asthmatic response to allergen challenge II. Late response (LAR). *Ann Allergy* 60: 217–225

13 Pelikan Z, Pelikan-Filipek M (1989) Late asthmatic response to allergen challenge (LAR), its clinical feature and pharmacological modulation. *Agents Actions* 26: 57–59

14 Pelikan Z, Pelikan-Filipek M (1991) Pharmacological modulation of immediate (IAR) and late (LAR) asthmatic response to allergen challenge.

Eur Resp J 4(Suppl to no 13): 1628

15 Knottnerus I, Pelikan Z (1994) The effects of Cromolyn (DSCG), Nedocromil (NS) and Budesonide (BUD) on the early (EAR) and the late (LAR) asthmatic response, inhaled before and after allergen challenge. *J Allerg Clin Immunol* 93(no 1, part 2): 198

16 Pelikan Z, Pelikan-Filipek M, Oostenbrink JH (1997) Delayed asthmatic response (DYAR), its clinical feature and pharmacologic modulation. *J Allerg Clin Immunol* 99(no 1, part 2): S321

17 Pelikan Z, Fouchier SM, Pelikan HMP, Oosten v MCM (1997) Bronchial responsiveness to histamine. (2) Effects of topically administered Cromolyn (DSCG) and Nedocromil (NDS). *Allergy Clin Immunol Intern* Suppl no 4: 128

18 Pelikan-Filipek M, Pelikan Z (1991) Nasal secretions cytology (NS) during the immediate nasal response (INR), pretreated with Disodium cromoglycate (DSCG) and Budesonide (BSA). *J Allerg Clin Immunol* 87: 144

19 Pelikan Z, Pelikan-Filipek M (1991) Cytologic changes in nasal secretions (NS) during the late nasal response (LNR) pretreated with Disodium cromoglycate (DSCG), Beclomethasone dipropionate (BDA) or Budesonide (BSA). *J Allerg Clin Immunol* 87: 281

20 Pelikan Z, Pelikan-Filipek M (1991) Cytologic changes in nasal secretions (NS) during the delayed nasal response (DNR) pretreated with disodium cromoglycate (DSCG), beclomethasone dipropionate (BDA) or budesonide (BSA). *Allergy Clin Immunol News* Suppl 1: 334

21 Fouchier SM, Pelikan DMV, Stigt v HJ, Pelikan Z (1997) Pharmacologic modulation of the cytologic changes in the nasal secretions (NS) accompanying the immediate nasal response (INR) I. Topically administered drugs. *J Allerg Clin Immunol* 99: S443

22 Pelikan Z, Oers v JAH, Pelikan HMP (1997) Pharmacologic modulation of the cytologic changes in the nasal secretions (NS) accompanying the late nasal response (LNR). I. Topically administered drugs. *Allergy Clin Immunol Intern* Suppl 4: 260

23 Kingsley PJ, Cox JSG (1978) Cromolyn sodium (sodium cromoglycate) and drugs with similar activities. *In*: E Middleton, CHE Reed, EF Ellis (eds): *Allergy, principles and practice*, 1st ed. Mosby, Saint Louis, 481–498

24 Edwards AM (1995) Oral sodium cromoglycate: its use in the management of food allergy. *Clin Exp Allergy* 25 (Suppl 1): 31–33

25 Pelikan Z, Pelikan-Filipek M, Knikman G (1987) Immediate and late asthmatic response due to the food ingestion challenge and the protective effects of oral Disodium Cromoglycate (DSCG). *J Allerg Clin Immunol* 79: 244

26 Pelikan Z (1987) Rhinitis and Secretory Otitis Media: A Possible Role of Food Allergy, (Chapter 26), *In*: J Brostoff, SJ Challacombe (eds): *Food allergy and intolerance*, 1st ed. Bailliere Tindall, London, 467–485

27 Knottnerus I, Pelikan DMV, Pelikan Z (1996) The effects of oral disodium cromoglycate (DSCG) on the basic types of nasal response (NR) to food ingestion challenge (FICH) and accompanying cellular changes in nasal secretions (NS). *J Allerg Clin Immunol* 97 (No 1, Part 3): 337

28 Pelikan Z, Pelikan-Filipek M (1989) Effects of oral cromolyn on the nasal response due to foods. *Arch Otolaryngol Head Neck Surg* 115: 1238–1243

29 Pelikan Z (1996) The role of allergy in sinus disease. *In*: ME Gershwin, GA Incaudo (eds): *Diseases of the sinuses*. Humana Press, Totowa, 97–165

30 Church MK, Polosa R, Rimmer SJ (1991) Cromolyn sodium and nedocromil sodium. *In*: MA Kaliner, PJ Barnes, CGA Persson (eds): *Asthma, its pathology and treatment*. Marcel Dekker, New York, 561–593

31 Rainey DK (1992) Evidence for the anti-inflammatory activity of nedocromil sodium. *Clin Exp Allergy* 22: 976–979

32 Pelikan-Filipek M, Oostenbrink JH, Pelikan Z (1996) The protective effects of intranasal nedocromil sodium (NDS) on the Immediate (INR) and the late nasal response (LNR) to allergen challenge. *J Allerg Clin Immunol* 97 (no 1, part 3): 197

33 Schleimer RP, Claman HN, Oronsky A (1989) *Anti-inflammatory steroid action, basic and general aspects*. Academic Press, San Diego

34 Barnes PJ (1997) Glucocorticosteroids. *In*: kay AB (ed.): *Allergy and allergic diseases*, 1st edn. Blackwell, Oxford, 619–641

35 Parente L, Mugridge KG (1993) Glucocorticosteroids and gastrointestinal inflammation. *In*: JL Wallace (ed.): *The handbook of immunopharmacology – Immunopharmacology of the gastrointestinal system*. Academic Press, London 169–184

36 Woolcock AJ, Jenkins ChR (1991) Clinical responses to corticosteroids. *In*: MA Kaliner, PJ Barnes, CGA Persson (eds): *Asthma, its pathology and treatment*. Marcel Dekker, New York, 633–665

37 Lemanske RF, Kaliner MA (1993) Late phase allergic reactions. *In*: E Middleton, CE Reed, EF Ellis, NF Adkinson, JW Yuninger, WW Busse (eds): *Allergy, principles and practice*, 4th edn. Mosby, St. Louis, 320–361

38 Ellul-Micallef R (1992) Glucocorticosteroids. *In*: PJ Barnes, IW Rodger, NC Thompson (eds): *Asthma, basic mechanisms and clinical management*. Academic Press, London, 613–657

39 Kamada AK, Szelfer SJ (1995) Mechanisms of action of glucocorticosteroids in asthma and rhinitis. *In*: WW Busse, ST Holgate (eds): *Asthma and rhinitis*. Blackwell, Oxford, 1255–1266

40 Haaksma EEJ Leurs R, Timmerman H (1990) Histamine receptors:subclasses and specific ligands. *Pharmacol Ther* 47: 73–104

41 Leurs R, Van der Groot H, Timmerman H (1991) Histaminergic agonists and antagonists: recent developments. *In*: B Testa (ed.): *Advances in drug research*, (vol 20). Academic Press, London, 217–304

42 Ganellin CR (1992) Pharmacochemistry of H_1 and H_2 receptors. *In*: JC Schwartz, H Haas (eds): *The histamine receptor*. Wiley-Liss, New York, 1–56

43 Rimmer SJ, Church MK (1990) The pharmacology and mechanisms of action of histamine H1-antagonists. *Clin Exp Allergy* 20(Suppl 2): 3–17

44 Simons FER (1997) Histamine and antihistamines. *In*: kay AB (eds): *Allergy and allergic diseases*. Blackwell, Oxford, 421–438

45 Simons EFR (1992) Pharmacological characteristics of second-generation H_1-blockers. *In*: MK Church, J-P Rihoux (eds): *Therapeutic index of antihistamines*. Hogrefe and Huber, Lewiston, 1–16

46 Rocklin RE (1990) *Histamine and H_2-antagonists in inflammation and immuno-deficiency*. Marcel Dekker, New York

47 Gross NJ (1997) Cholinergic antagonists. *In*: AB Kay (ed.): *Allergy and allergic diseases*. Blackwell, Oxford, 596–608

48 Warner O (1986) Immunotherapy: yeasterday's treatment. *In*: CE Reed (ed.): *Proceedings of the 12th International Congress of Allergology and Clin Immunology*. Mosby, St. Louis, 323–326

49 Malling HJ (1997) Practical Immunotherapy. *In*: AB Kay (ed.): *Allergy and allergic diseases*. Blackwell, Oxford, 1243–1257

50 Hill DJ, Hoskins CS, Shelton MJ, Turner MW (1982) Failure of hyposensitisation in treatment of children with grass-pollen asthma. *Brit Med J* 248: 306–309

51 Greenberg MA, Kaufman CR, Gonzalez GE, Rosenblatt CD, Smith LJ, Summers RJ (1986) Late and immediate systemic reactions to inhalant allergen immunotherapy. *J Allerg Clin Immunol* 77: 865–870

52 Malling HJ (1993) European Academy of Allergology and Clinical Immunology, Immunotherapy position paper. *Allergy* 14(suppl): 3–35

53 Pelikan Z (1990) The value of desensibilization therapy. *Dutch J Med (Ned Tijdsch Geneeskd)* 134: 2518 2520

Chapter C4

1 Nelson HS (1995) Beta-adrenergic bronchodilators. *N Engl J Med* 333: 499–506

2 Barnes PJ (1995) Beta-adrenergic receptors and their regulation. *Amer J Respir Crit Care Med* 152: 838–860

3 Torphy TJ (1994) β-Adrenoceptors, cAMP and airway smooth muscle relaxation: challenges to the dogma. *Trends Pharmacol Sci* 15: 370–374

4 Grove A, BJ Lipworth (1995) Tolerance with β_2-adrenoceptor agonists: time for reappraisal. *Brit J Clin Pharmacol* 39: 109–118

5 Hall IP (1996) β_2-Adrenoceptor polymorphisms: are they clinically important? *Thorax* 51: 351–353

6 Boulet L (1994) Long versus short-acting β_2-agonists. *Drugs* 47: 207–222

7 Weinberger M, L Hendeles (1996) Theophylline in asthma. *N Engl J Med* 334: 1380–1388

8 Barnes PJ, RA Pauwels (1994) Theophylline in asthma: time for reappraisal? *Eur Resp J* 7: 579–591

9 Barnes PJ (1995) Inhaled glucocorticoids for asthma. *N Engl J Med* 332: 868–875

10 Barnes PJ (1996) Molecular mechanisms of steroid action in asthma. *J Allerg Clin Immunol* 97: 159–168

11 Barnes PJ, S Pedersen (1993) Efficacy and safety of inhaled steroids in asthma. *Amer Rev Respir Dis* 148:S1–S26

12 British Thoracic Society (1993) Guidelines on management of asthma. *Thorax* 48 (Suppl):S1–S24

13 Smith LJ (1996) Leukotrienes in asthma. The potential therapeutic role of antileukotriene agents. *Arch Intern Med* 156: 2181–2189

14 Hill SJ, AE Tattersfield (1995) Corticosteroid sparing agents in asthma. *Thorax* 50: 577–582

Chapter C5

1 Talmadge JE, Herberman RB (1986) The preclinical screening laboratory. Evaluation of immunomodulatory and therapeutic properties of biological response modifiers. *Cancer Treatment Res* 70: 171

2 Mihich E (1986) Future perspectives for biological response modifiers: a viewpoint. *Semin Oncol* 13: 234

3 Ellenberg SS (1993) Surrogate endpoints. *Brit J Cancer* 68: 457

4 Holden C (1993) Okays Surrogate Markers. *Science* 259: 32

5 Tomlinson E (1991) Site-specific proteins. *In*: RC Hider, D Barlow (eds): *Polypeptide and protein drugs: production, characterization and formulation.* Ellis Horwood, Chichester, 251

6 Talmadge JE, Tribble HR, Pennington RW, Phillips H, Wiltrout RH (1987) Immunomodulatory and immunotherapeutic properties of recombinant γ-interferon and recombinant tumor necrosis factor in mice. *Cancer Res* 47: 2563

7 Misset JL, Mathe G, Gastiaburu J, Goutner A, Dorval T, Gouveia J, Schwarzenberg L, Machover D, Ribaud P, de Vassal F (1982) Treatment of leukemias and lymphomas by interferons: II. Phase II of the trial treatment of chronic lymphoid leukemia by human interferon a+. *Biomed Pharmacother* 39: 112

8 Golomb HM, Fefer A, Golde DW, Ozer H, Portlock C, Silber R, Rappeport J, Ratain MJ, Thompson J, Bonnem E et al (1988) Report of a multi-

institutional study of 193 patients with hairy cell leukemia treated with interferon-a 2b. *Semin Oncol* 15: 7

9 Quesada JR, Reuben J, Manning JT, Hersh EM, Gutterman JU (1984) Alpha interferon for induction of remission in hairy-cell leukemia. *N Engl J Med* 310: 15

10 O'Connell MJ, Colgan JP, Oken MM, Ritts Jr, Kay NE, Itri LM (1986) Clinical trial of recombinant leukocyte A interferon as initial therapy for favorable histology non-Hodgkin's lymphomas and chronic lymphocytic leukemia. An Eastern Cooperative Oncology Group pilot study. *J Clin Oncol* 4: 128

11 Bunn PA, Foon KA, Ihde DC, Longo DL, Eddy J, Winkler CF, Veach SR, Zeffren J, Sherwin S, Oldham R (1984) Recombinant leukocyte A interferon: an active agent in advanced cutaneous T-cell lymphomas. *Ann Intern Med* 101: 484

12 Muss HB (1987) Interferon therapy for renal cell carcinoma. *Semin Oncol* 14: 36

13 Quesada JR, Rios A, Swanson D, Trown P, Gutterman JU (1985) Antitumor activity of recombinant-derived interferon alpha in metastatic renal cell carcinoma. *J Clin Oncol* 3: 1522

14 Lane HC, Feinberg J, Davey V, Deyton L, Baseler M, Manischewitz J, Masur H, Kovacs JA, Herpin B, Walker R (1988) Anti-retro-viral effects of interferon-a in AIDS-associated Kaposi's sarcoma. *Lancet* 2: 1218

15 Teichmann JV, Sieber G, Ludwig WD, Ruehl H (1988) Modulation of immune functions by long-term treatment with recombinant interferon-a2 in a patient with hairy-cell leukemia. *J Interferon Res* 8: 15

16 Smalley RV, Anderson SA, Tuttle RL, Connors J, Thurmond LM, Huang A, Castle K, Magers C, Whisnant JK (1991) A randomized comparison of two doses of human lymphoblastoid Interferon-a in hairy cell leukemia. *Blood* 78: 3133

17 Black PL, Phillips H, Tribble HR, Pennington RW, Schneider M, Talmadge JE (1993) Antitumor response to recombinant murine interferon γ correlates with enhanced immune function of organ-associated, but not recirculating cytolytic T-lymphocytes and macrophages. *Cancer Immunol Immunother* 37: 299

18 Maluish AE, Urba WJ, Longo DLO, Overton WR, Coggin D, Crisp ER, Williams R, Sherwin SA, Gordon K, Steis RG (1988) The determination of an immunologically active dose of interferon-gamma in patients with melanoma. *J Clin Oncol* 6: 434

19 Jaffe HS, Herberman RB (1988) Rationale for recombinant human IFNα adjuvant immunotherapy for cancer. Editorial *J Nat Cancer Inst* 314: 1065

20 The International Chronic Granulomatous Disease Cooperative Study Group (1991) A controlled trial of interferon gamma to prevent infection in chronic granulomatous disease. *N Engl J Med* 324: 509

21 Woodman RC, Richard W, Rae J, Jaffe HS, Curnutte JT (1992) Prolonged recombinant interferon-g therapy in chronic granulomatous disease: evidence against enhanced neutrophil oxidase activity. *Blood* 79: 1558

22 Rosenberg SA, Lotze MT, Yang JC, Topalian SL, Chang AE, Schwartzentruben DJ, Aebersold P, Leitman S, Linehan WM, Seipp CA (1993) Prospective randomized trial of high-dose interleukin-2 alone or in conjunction with lymphokine-activated killer cells for the treatment of patients with advanced cancer. *J Nat Cancer Inst* 85: 622

23 West WH, Tauer KW, Yannelli JR, Marshall GD, Orr DW, Thurman GB, Oldham RK (1987) Constant-infusion recombinant interleukin-2 in adoptive immunotherapy of advanced cancer. *N Engl J Med* 316: 898

24 Lotze MT, Chang AE, Seipp CA, Simpson C, Vetto SJ, Rosenberg SA (1986) High-dose recombinant interleukin 2 in the treatment of patients with disseminated cancer. Responses, treatment-related morbidity and histologic findings. *JAMA* 256: 3117

25 Heslop HE, Gottlieb DJ, Bianchi ACM, Meager A, Prentice HG, Mehta AB, Hoffbrand AV, Brenner MK (1989) *In vivo* induction of gamma interferon and tumor necrosis factor by interleukin-2 infusion following intensive chemotherapy or autologous marrow transplantation. *Blood* 74: 1374

26 Thompson JA, Shulman KL, Benyunes MC, Lindgren G, Collins C, Lange PH, Bush WH Jr, Benz LA, Fefer A (1992) Prolonged continuous intravenous infusion interleukin-2 and lymphokine-activated killer-cell therapy for metastatic renal cell carcinoma. *J Clin Oncol* 10: 960

27 Hladik F, Tratkiewicz JA, Tilg H, Vogel W, Schwulera U, Kronke M, Aulitzky WE, Huber C (1994) Biologic activity of low dosage IL-2 treatment *in vivo*. Molecular assessment of cytokine network interaction. *J Immunol* 153: 1449

28 Mier JW, Vachino G, Van Der Meet JWM (1988) Induction of circulating tumor necrosis factor (TNF-alpha) as the mechanism for the febrile response to interleukin-2 (IL-2) in cancer patients. *J Clin Immunol* 8: 426

29 Kovacs JA, Baseler M, Dewar RJ, Vogel S, Davey RT Jr, Falloon J, Polis MA, Walker RE, Stevens R, Salzman NP et al (1995) Increases in CD4 T-lymphocytes with intermittent courses of interleukin-2 in patients with human immunodeficiency virus infection. A preliminary study (see comments). *N Engl J Med* 332: 567

30 Jacobson EL, Pilaro F, Smith KA (1996) Rational interleukin 2 therapy for HIV positive individuals: daily low doses enhance immune function without toxicity. *Proc Natl Acad Sci USA* 93: 10405

31 Sleijfer DT, Janssen RA, Butler J et al (1992) Phase II study of subcutaneous interleukin-2 in unselected patients with advanced renal cell cancer on an outpatient basis. *J Clin Oncol* 10: 1119

32 Nauts HC (1975) *The bibilography of reports concerning the experimental clinical use of coley toxins.* Cancer Research Institute Publication, New York

33 Haaff EO, Dresner SM, Ratliff TL, Catalona WJ (1986) Two courses of intravesical Bacillus Calmette-Guerin for transitional cell carcinoma of the bladder. *J Urol* 136: 820

34 Pinsky CM, Camacho FJ, Kerr D, Geller NL, Klein FA, Herr HA, Whitmore WF, Oettgen HF (1985) Intravesical administration of Bacillus Calmette-Guerin in patients with recent recurrent superficial carcinoma of the urinary bladder: Report of a prospective, randomized trial. *Cancer Treat Rep* 69: 47

35 Lage JM, Bauer WC, Kelley DR, Ratliff TL, Catalona WJ (1986) Histological parameters and pitfalls in the interpretation of bladder biopsies in Bacillus Calmette-Guerin treatment of superficial bladder cancer. *J Urol* 135: 916

36 Haaff EO, Caralona WJ, Ratliff TL (1986) Detection of interleukin-2 in the urine of patients with superficial bladder tumors after treatment with intravesical BCG. *J Urol* 136: 970

37 Amery WKP, Bruynseels JPJM (1992) Levamisole, the story and the lessons. *Int J Immunopharmacol* 14(3): 481

38 Mutch RS, Hutson PR (1991) Levamisole in the adjuvant treatment of colon cancer. *Clin Pharm* 10(2): 95

39 Ellouz F, Adam A, Cirobaru R, Lederer E (1974) Minimal structural requirements for adjuvant activity of bacterial peptido-glycan derivatives. *Biochem Biophys Res Commun* 59: 1317

40 Wood DD, Staruch MJ, Durette PL, Melvin WV, Graham BK (1983) Role of interleukin-1 in the adjuvanticity of muramyl dipeptide *in vivo. In*: JJ Oppenheim, S Cohen (eds): *Interleukins, lymphokines and cytokines.* Raven Press, New York, 691

41 Kleinerman ES (1995) Biologic therapy for osteosarcoma using liposome-encapsulated muramyl tripeptide. *Hematol Oncol Clin N Amer* 9: 927

42 Kleinerman ES, Meyers PA, Raymond AK, Gano JB, Jia SF, Jaffe N (1995) Combination therapy with ifosfamide and liposome-encapsulated muramyl tripeptide: tolerability, toxicity, and immune stimulation. J Immunother Empahsis Tumor Immunol 17(3): 181–193

43 Aoyagi T, Suda H, Nagai M, Ogawa K, Suzuki J (1976) Aminopeptidase activities on the surface of mammalian cells. *Biochim Biophys Acta* 452: 131

44 Morahan PS, Edelson PJ, Gass K (1980) Changes in macrophage ectoenzymes associated with anti-tumor activity. *J Immunol* 125: 1312

45 Urabe A, Mutoh Y, Mizoguchi H, Takaku F, Ogawa N (1993) Ubenimex in the treatment of acute nonlymphocytic leukemia in adults. *Ann Hematol* 67: 63

46 Yasumitsu T, Ohshima S, Nakano N, Kotake Y, Tominaga S (1990) Bestatin in resected lung cancer. *Acta Oncol* 29: 827

47 Hiraoka A, Shibata H, Masaoka T (1992) *Study Group of Ubenimex for BMT: Immunopotentiation with ubenimex for prevention of leukemia relapse after allogeneic BMT. Transplant Proc* 24: 3047

48 Goldstein AL (1984) *Thymic hormones and lymphokines.* Plenum Press, New York

49 Maraninchi D, Gluckman E, Blaise D, Guyotat D, Rio B, Pico J, Leblond V, Michallet M, Dreyfus F, Ifrah N (1987) Impact of T-cell depletion on outcome of allogeneic bone marrow transplantation for standard-risk leukaemias. *Lancet* 2: 175

50 Weiden PL, Flournoy N, Thomas ED, Prentice R, Fefer A, Buckner CD, Storb R (1979) Antileukemic effect of graft-versus-host disease in human recipients of allogeneic-marrow grafts. *N Engl J Med* 300: 1068

51 Horowitz MM, Gale RP, Sondel PM, Goldman JM, Kersey J, Kolb HJ, Rimm AA, Ringden O, Rozman C, Speck B et al (1990) Graft-versus-leukemia reactions after bone marrow transplantation. *Blood* 75: 555

52 Mitsuyasu RT, Champlin RE, Gale RP, Ho WG, Lenarsky C, Winston D, Selch M, Elashoff R, Giorgi JV, Wells J et al (1986) Treatment of donor bone marrow with monoclonal anti-T-cell antibody and complement for the prevention of graft-versus-host disease. A prspective, randomized, double-blind trial. *Ann Intern Med* 105: 20

53 Hood AF, Vogelsang GB, Black LP, Farmer ER, Santos GW (1987) Acute graft-versus-host disease. Development following autologous and syngeneic bone marrow transplantation. *Arch Dermatol* 123: 745

54 Higuchi CM, Thompson JA, Petersen FB, Buckner CD, Fefer J (1991) Toxicity and immunomodulatory effects of interleukin-2 after autologous bone marrow transplantation for hematologic malignancies. *Blood* 77: 2561

55 Blaise D, Olive D, Stoppa AM, Viens P, Pourreau C, Lopez M, Attal M, Jasmin C, Monges G, Mawas C et al (1990) Hematologic and immunologic effects of the systemic administration of recombinant interleukin-2 after autologous bone marrow transplantation. *Blood* 76: 1092

56 Negrier S, Ranchere JY, Phillip I, Merrouche Y, Biron P, Blaise D, Attal M, Rebattu P, Clavel M, Pourreau C et al (1991) Intravenous interleukin-2 just after high dose BCNU and autologous bone marrow transplantation. Report of a multicentric French pilot study. *Bone Marrow Transplant* 8: 259

57 Soiffer RJ, Murray C, Cochran K, Cameron C, Wang E, Schow PW, Daley JF, Ritz J (1992) Clinical and immunologic effects of prolonged infusion of low-dose recombinant interleukin-2 after autologous and T-cell-depleted allogeneic bone marrow transplantation. *Blood* 79: 517

58 Klingemann HG, Grigg AP, Wilkie-Boyd K, Barnett MJ, Eaves AC, Reece DE, Shepherd JD, Phillips GL (1991) Treatment with recombinant interferon (alpha-2b) early after bone marrow transplantation in patients at high risk for relapse. *Blood* 78: 3306

59 Meyers JD, Flournoy N, Sanders JE, McGuffin RW, Newton BA, Fisher LD, Lum LG, Appelbaum FR, Doney K, Sullivan KM et al (1987) Prophylactic use of human leukocyte interferon after allogeneic marrow transplantation.

Ann Intern Med 107: 809

60 Ratanatharathorn V, Uberti J, Karanes C, Lum LG, Abella E, Dan ME, Hussein M, Sensenbrenner LL (1994) Phase I study of alpha-interferon augmentation of cyclosporine-induced graft versus host disease in recipients of autologous bone marrow transplantation. *Bone Marrow Transplant* 13: 625

61 Kennedy MJ, Vogelsang GB, Jones RJ, Farmer ER, Hess AD, Altomonte V, Huelskamp AM, Davidson NE (1994) Phase I trial of interferon gamma to potentiate cyclosporine-induced graft-versus-host disease in women undergoing autologous bone marrow transplantation for breast cancer. *J Clin Oncol* 12: 249

62 Gosse ME, Nelson TE (1997) Approval times for supplemental indications for recombinant proteins. *Nat Biotechnol* 15: 130

Chapter C6

1 Masihi KN (ed.) (1994) *Immunotherapy of infections.* Marcel Dekker, New York

2 Masihi KN, Lange W (eds) (1990*) Immunotherapeutic prospects of infectious diseases.* Springer-Verlag, Berlin

3 Masihi KN, Lange W (eds) (1988) *Immunomodulators and nonspecific host defence mechanisms against microbial infections.* Pergamon Press, Oxford

4 Friedman H, Klein T, Yamaguchi H (eds) (1992) *Microbial infections: role of biological response modifiers.* Plenum Press, New York

5 Masihi KN (1996) Immunotherapy of microbial diseases. *In*: JW Hadden, A Szentivanyi (eds): *Immunopharmacology reviews*, vol 2. Plenum Press, New York, 157–199

6 Goldstein G, Conant MA, Beall G, Grossman HA, Galpin JE, Blick G, Calabrese LH, Hirsch RL, Fisher A, Stampone P (1995) Safety and efficacy of thymopentin in zidovudine (AZT)-treated asymptomatic HIV-infected subjects with 200–500 CD4 cells/mm^3: a double-blind placebo-controlled trial. *J Acq Immun Defic Synd* 8: 279–288

7 Garaci E, Rocchi G, Perroni L, D'Agostini C, Soscia F, Grelli S, Mastino A, Favalli C (1994) Combination treatment with zidovudine, thymosin alpha 1 and interferon-alpha in human immunodeficiency virus infection. *Int J Clin Lab Res* 24: 23–28

8 Hadden JW, Ongradi J, Specter S, Nelson R, Sosa M, Monell C, Strand M, Giner-Sorolla A, Hadden EM (1992) Methyl inosine monophosphate: a potential immunotherapeutic for early human immunodeficiency virus (HIV) infection. *Int J Immunopharmacol* 14: 555–563

9 Caramia G, Clemente E, Solli R, Mei V, Cera R, Carnelli V, Venturoli V,

Corsini A (1994) Efficacy and safety of pidotimod in the treatment of recurrent respiratory infections in children. *Arzneim Forsch-Drug Res* 44(12A): 1480–1484

10 Azuma I, Otani T (1994) Potentiation of host defense mechanism against infection by a cytokine inducer, an acyl-MDP derivative, MDP-Lys(L18) (romurtide) in mice and humans. *Med Res Rev* 14: 401–414

11 Masihi KN, Lange W, Rohde-Schulz B, Chedid L (1990) Muramyl dipeptide inhibits replication of human immunodeficiency virus *in vitro*. *AIDS Res Hum Retrovirus* 6: 393–399

12 Masihi KN, Rohde-Schulz B, Masek K, Palache B (1992) Antiviral and adjuvant activity of immunomodulator adamantylamide dipeptide. *Adv Exp Med Biol* 319: 275–286

13 Maeda YY, Yonekawa H, Chihara G (1994) Application of lentinan as cytokine inducer and host defense potentiator in immunotherapy of infectious diseases. *In*: KN Masihi (ed.): *Immunotherapy of infections*. Marcel Dekker, New York, 261–279

14 Jagodzinski PP, Wiaderkiewicz R, Kurazawski G, Kloczewiak M, Nakashima H, Hyjek E, Yamamoto N, Uryu T, Kaneko Y, Posner MR et al (1994) Mechanism of the inhibitory effect of curdlan sulfate on HIV-1 infection *in vitro*. *Virology* 202: 735–745

15 Babineau TJ, Hackford A, Kenler A, Bistrian B, Forse RA, Fairchild PG, Heard S, Keroack M, Caushaj P, Benotti P (1994) A phase II multicenter, double-blind, randomized, placebo-controlled study of three dosages of an immunomodulator (PGG-glucan) in high-risk surgical patients. *Arch Surg* 129: 1204–1210

16 Masihi KN (1994) Cytokines and immunomodulators: promising therapeutic agents. *Parasitol Today* 10: 1–2

17 Todd B, Pope JH, Georghiou P (1991) Interleukin-2 enhances production in 24 h of infectious human immundeficiency virus type 1 *in vitro* by naturally infected mononuclear cells from seropositive donors. *Arch Virol* 121: 227–232

18 Doherty P, Allan JE, Clark IA, (1989) Tumor necrosis factor inhibits the development of viral meningitis or induces rapid death depending on the severity of inflammation at the time of administration. *J Immunol* 142: 3576–3580

Chapter C7

1 Leake CD (1975) *An histological account of pharmacology to the twentieth century*. C. C. Thomas, Springfield

2 Foster S (1991) *Echinacea. Nature's immune enhancer*. Healing Arts Press,

Rochester

3   Bauer R, Wagner H (1990) *Echinacea. Handbuch für Ärzte, Apotheker und andere Naturwissenschaftler.* Wissenschaftliche Verlagsgesellschaft, Stuttgart

4   Parnham MJ (1996) Benefit-risk assessment of the squeezed sap of the purple coneflower (*Echinacea purpurea*) for long-term oral immunostimulation. *Phytomedicine* 3: 95–102

5   Holtskog R, Sandvig K, Olsnes S (1988) Characterization of a toxic lectin in Iscador, a mistletoe preparation with alleged cancerostatic properties. *Oncology* 45: 171–179

6   Joller PW, Menrad JM, Schwarz T, Pfüller U, Parnham MJ, Weyhenmeyer R, Lentzen H (1996) Stimulation of cytokine production via a special standardized mistletoe preparation in an *in vitro* human skin bioassay. *Arzneim-Forsch-Drug Res* 46: 649–653

7   Beuth J, Ko HL, Gabius H-J, Burrichter H, Oette K, Pulverer (1992) Behavior of lymphocyte subsets and expression of activation markers in response to immunotherapy with galactoside-specific lectin from mistletoe in breast cancer patients. *Clin Invest* 70: 658–661

8   Bendich A (1990) Antioxidant vitamins and their functions in immune responses. *Adv Exp Med Biol* 262: 35–55

9   Wang YJ, Huang DS, Eskelson CD, Watson RR (1994) Long-term dietary vitamin-E retards development of retrovirus-induced disregulation in cytokine production. *Clin Immunol Immunopathol* 72: 70–75

10 Boxer LA, Oliver JM, Spielberg SP, Allen JM, Schulman JD (1979) Protection of granulocytes by vitamin E in glutathione synthesis deficiency. *N Engl J Med* 301: 901–905

11 Meydani M (1995) Vitamin E. *Lancet* 345: 170–175

12 Berry MJ, Banu L, Larsen PR (1991) Type I iodothyronine deiodinase is a selenocysteine-containing enzyme. *Nature* 349: 438–440

13 Finch JM, Turner RJ (1996) Effect of selenium and vitamin E on the immune response of domestic animals. *Res Vet Sci* 60: 97–106

14 Urban T, Jarstrand C (1986) Selenium effects on human neutrophilic granulocyte function *in vitro*. *Immunopharmacology* 12: 167–172

15 Reinhold U, Pawelec G, Enczmann J, Werner P (1989) Class-specific effects of selenium on PWM-driven human antibody synthesis *in vitro*. *Biol Trace Elem Res* 20: 45–58

16 Bonomini M, Forster S, De Risio F, Rychly J, Nebe B, Manfrini V, Klinkmann H, Albertazzi A (1995) Effects of selenium supplementation on immune parameters in chronic uraemic patients on hemodialysis. *Nephrol Dialysis Transplant* 10: 1654–1661

17 Peretz A, Nève J, Desmedt J, Duchateau J, Dramaix M, Famaey JP (1991) Lymphocyte response is enhanced by supplementation of elderly subjects

with selenium-enriched yeast. *Amer J Clin Nutr* 53: 1323–1328

18 Parnham MJ (1996) The pharmaceutical potential of seleno-organic compounds. *Expert Opin Invest Drugs* 5: 861–870

19 Inglot AD, Mlochowski J, Zielínska-Jenczylik J, Piasecki E, Ledwon TK, Kloc K (1996) Seleno-organic compounds as immunostimulants: an approach to the structure-activity relationship. *Arch Immunol Ther Exp* 44: 67–75

Chapter C8

1 Lieberman R, Mukherjee A (eds) (1996) *Principles of drug development in transplantation and autoimmunity*. Chapmann and Hall, New York

2 Thomson AW, Starzl TE (eds) (1994) *Immunosuppressive drugs: developments in anti-rejection therapy*. Edward Arnold, London

3 Allison AC, Lafferty KJ, Fliri H (eds) (1993) *Immunosuppressive and antiinflammatory drugs. Ann N Y Acad Sci* , New York, vol 696

4 Borel JF, Kis ZL, Beveridge T (1995) The history of the discovery and development of cyclosporine (Sandimmune). *In*: VJ Merluzzi, J Adams (eds): *The Search for anti-inflammatory drugs*. Birkhäuser, Boston, 27–63

5 Morris RE (1996) Mechanism of action of new immunosuppressive drugs. *Kidney Int* 49(Suppl): S26–S38

6 Brazelton TR, Morris RE (1996) Molecular mechanisms of action of new xenobiotic immunosuppressive drugs: tacrolimus (FK506), sirolimus (rapamycin), mycophenolate mofetil and leflunomide. *Curr Opin Immunol* 8: 710–720

7 Borel JF (1990) Pharmacology of cyclosporine (Sandimmune). IV. Pharmacological properties *in vivo*. *Pharmcol Rev* 41: 259–371

8 Schreier MH (1997) Mechanism of action of cyclosporin. *In*: T Anke (ed.): *Fungal biotechnology*. Chapmann and Hall, New York, 137–146

9 Silva HT, Morris RE (1997) Leflunomide and malononitriloamides. *Expert Opin Invest Drugs* 6: 51–64

10 Nashan B, Moore R, Amlot P, Schmidt AG, Abeywickrama K, Soulillou JP (1997) Randomised trial of basiliximab versus placebo for control of acute cellular rejection in renal allograft recipients. *Lancet* 350: 1193–1198

11 Vincenti F, Kirkman R, Light S, Bumgardner G, Pescovitz M, Halloran P, Neylan J, Wilkinson A, Ekberg H, Gaston R et al (1998) Interleukin-2-receptor blockade with daclizumab to prevent acute rejection in renal transplantation. *N Engl J Med* 338: 161–165

12 Akamine S, Katayama Y, Higewnbottam T, Lock T (1998) Developments in inhaled immunosuppressive therapy for the prevention of pulmonary graft rejection. *Biodrugs* 9: 49–59

13 Kirk AD, Harlan DM, Armstrong NN, Davis TA, Dong Y, Gray GS, Hong X,

Thomas D, Fechner JHJr, Knechtle SJ (1997) CTLA4-Ig and anti-CD40 ligand prevent renal allograft rejection in primates. *Proc Natl Acad Sci USA* 94: 8789–8794

14 Mani RN, Elliott M, Brennan FM, Williams RO, Feldman M (1997) TNF blockade in rheumatoid arthritis: implications for therapy and pathogenesis. *APMIS* 105: 257–263

15 Chiba K, Yanagawa Y, Masubuchi Y, Kataoka H, Kawaguchi T, Ohtsuki M, Hoshino Y (1988) FTY720, a novel immunosuppressant, induces sequestration of circulating mature lymphocytes by acceleration of lymphocyte homing in rats. I. FTY720 selectively decreases the number of circulating mature lymphocytes by acceleration of lymphocyte homing. *J Immunol* 160: 5037–5044

16 Knechtle SJ, Vargo D, Fechner J, Zhai Y, Wang J, Hanaway MJ, Scharf J, Hu HZ., Knapp L, Watkins D et al (1997) FN18-CRM9 immunotoxin promotes tolerance in primate renal allografts. *Transplantation* 63: 1–6

17 Nikolic B, Sykes M (1997) bone marrow chimerism and transplantation tolerance. *Curr Opin Immunol* 9: 634–640

Chapter C9

1 Addison T (1855) *On the constitutional and local effects of disease of the suprarenal capsules.* Samuel Highley, London

2 Munck A, Guyre PM, Holbrook NJ (1984) Physiological functions of glucocorticoids in stress and their relation to pharmacological actions. *Endocrine Rev* 5: 25–44

3 Perretti M, Becherucci C, Scapigliati G, Parente L (1989) The effect of adrenalectomy on interleukin 1 release *in vitro* and *in vivo*. *Brit J Pharmacol* 98: 1137–1142

4 Flower RJ, Parente L, Persico P, Salmon JA (1986) A comparison of the acute inflammatory response in adrenalectomised and sham operated rats. *Brit J Pharmacol* 87: 57–62

5 Dobbs CM, Vasquez M, Glaser R, Sheridan JF (1993) Mechanisms of stress-induced modulation of viral pathogenesis and immunity. *J Neuroimmunol* 48: 151–160

6 Sternberg EM, Hill JM, Chrousos GP, Kamilaris T, Listwak SJ, Gold PW, Wilder RL (1989) Inflammatory mediator-induced hypothalamic-pituitary-adrenal axis activation is defective in streptococcal cell wall arthritis-susceptible Lewis rats. *Proc Natl Acad Sci USA* 86: 2374–2378

7 Buckingham JC (1996) Stress and the neuroendocrine axis: the pivotal role of glucocorticoids and lipocortin 1. *Brit J Pharmacol* 118: 1–19

8 Buckingham JC, Loxley HD, Christian HC, Philip JG (1996) Activation of

the HPA axis by immune insults: roles and interactions of cytokines eicosanoids and glucorticoids. Pharmacol. Biochem. *Behaviour* 54: 285–298

9   Hammond GL (1990) Molecular properties of corticosteroid binding globulin and the sex-steroid binding proteins. *Endocrine Rev* 11: 65–79

10 Hollenberg SM, Weinberger MC, Ong ES, Cerelli G, Oro A, Lebo R, Thompson EB (1985) Primary structure and expression of a functional human glucocorticoid receptor cDNA. *Nature* 318: 635–641

11 Funder JW (1993) Mineralocorticoids, glucocorticoids, receptors and response elements. *Science* 259: 1132–1133

12 Diamond MI, Miner JN, Yoshinga SK, Yamamoto KR (1990) Transcription factor interactions: selectors of positive or negative regulation from a single DNA element. *Science* 249: 1266–1272

13 Ballard PL, Baxter JD, Higgins SJ, Rousseau GG, Tomkins GM (1974) General presence of glucocorticoid receptors in mammalian tissues. *Endocrinology* 94: 998–1002

14 Edwards CRW, Benediktsson R, Lindsay RS, Seckl JR (1996) 11-beta-hydroxysteroid dehydrogenases – key enzymes in determining tissue-specific glucocorticoid effects. *Steroids* 61: 263–269

15 Edwards CRW, Benediktsson R, Lindsay RS, Seckl JR (1993) Dysfunction of the placental glucocorticoid barrier: a line between the foetal environment and adult hypertension. *Lancet* 341: 355–357

16 Lew W, Oppenheim JJ, Matsushima K (1988) Analysis of the suppression of IL-1alpha and IL-1beta production in human peripheral blood mononuclear adherent cells by a glucocorticoid hormone. *J Immunol* 140: 1895–1902

17 Masferrer JL (1989) Endogenous glucocorticoids regulate an inducible cyclooxygenase enzyme. *Proc Natl Acad Sci USA* 89: 3917–3921

18 Moncada S, Palmer RMJ (1991) Inhibition of the induction of nitric oxide synthase by glucocorticoids; yet another explanation of their anti-inflammatory effects. *Trends Pharmacol Sci* 12: 130–131

19 Ahluwalia A, Buckingham JC, Croxtall JD, Flower RJ, Goulding NJ (1996) The biology of annexin 1. *In*: BA Seaton (ed.): *The annexins*. R. L. Landes, Austin, TX, 162–199

20 Goulding NJ, Flower RJ (1997) Glucocorticoids and the immune system. *In*: J Buckingham, G Gillies, AM Cowell (eds): *Stress, stress hormones and the immune system*. John Wiley, London, 199–223

21 Schleimer RP, Bochner BS (1994) The effects of glucocorticoids on human eosinophils. *J Allerg Clin Immunol* 94: 1202–1213

22 Finotto S, Mekori YA, Metcalfe DD (1997) Glucocorticoids decrease tissue mast cell number by reducing the production of the c-kit ligand, stem-cell factor, by resident cells – *in vitro* and *in vivo* evidence in murine systems. *J Clin Invest* 99: 1721–1728

23 Meagher LC, Cousin JM, Seckl JR, Haslett C (1996) Opposing effects of

glucocorticoids on the rate of apoptosis in neutrophilic and eosinophil granulocytes. *J Immunol* 156: 4422–4428

24 Raynal P, Pollard HB (1994) Annexins: the problem of assessing the biological role for a gene family of multifunctional calcium- and phospholipid-binding proteins *Biochim Biophys Acta* 1197: 63–93

25 Fava RA, McKanna J, Cohen S (1989) Lipocortin I [p35] is abundant in a restricted number of differentiated cell types in adult organs. *J Cell Physiol* 14: 284–293

26 Smith T, Flower RJ, Buckingham JC (1993) Lipocortins 1, 2 and 5 in the central nervous system and pituitary gland of the rat: elective induction by dexamethasone of lipocortin in the anterior pituitary gland. *Mol Neuropharmacol* 3: 45–55

27 Woods MD, Kiss JZ, Smith T, Buckingham JC, Flower RJ, Antoni FA (1990) Localisation of lipocortin 1 in rat hypothalamus and pituitary gland. *Biochem Soc Trans* 18: 1236–1237

28 Johnson MD, Gray ME, Pepinsky RB, Stahlman MT (1990) Lipocortin-1 immunoreactivity in the human pituitary gland. *J Histochem Cytochem* 38: 1841–1845

29 Browning JL, Ward MP, Wallner BP, Pepinsky RB (1990) Studies on the structural properties of lipocortin-1 and the regulation of its synthesis by steroids. *In*: M Melli and L Parente (eds): *Cytokines and lipocortins in inflammation and differentiation*. Wiley-Liss, New York, 27–45

30 Vishwanath BS, Frey FJ, Bradbury M, Dallman MF, Frey BM (1992) Adrenalectomy decreases lipocortin-I messenger ribonucleic acid and tissue protein content in rats. *Endocrinology* 130: 585–591

31 Perretti M, Flower RJ (1996) Measurement of lipocortin 1 levels in murine peripheral blood leukocytes by flow cytometry: modulation by glucocorticoids and inflammation. *Brit J Pharmacol* 118: 605–610

32 Flower RJ (1988) Eleventh Gaddum memorial lecture. Lipocortin and the mechanism of action of the glucocorticoids. *Brit J Pharmacol* 94: 987–1015

33 Davidson FF, Dennis EA, Powell M, Glenney JR (1987) Inhibition of phospholipase A2 by "lipocortins " and calpac*Trends Neurosci*. An effect of binding to substrate phospholipids. *J Biol Chem* 262: 1698–1705

34 Croxtall JD, Choudhury Q, Tokumoto H, Flower RJ (1995) Lipocortin 1 and the control of arachidonic acid release in *Cell Signal* ling. *Biochem Pharmacol* 50: 465–474

35 Goulding NJ, Guyre PM (1992) Regulation of Inflammation. A potential role for lipocortin [annexin-I] receptors on phagocytes. *Immunol Today* 13: 295–297

36 Perretti M (1994) Lipocortin-derived peptides. *Biochem Pharmacol* 47: 931–938

37 Cirino G, Peers SH, Browning JL, Flower RJ, Pepinsky RB (1989) Human

recombinant lipocortin 1 has acute local anti-inflammatory properties in the rat paw edema test. *Proc Natl Acad Sci USA* 86: 3428–3432

38 Carey F, Forder R, Edge MD, Greene AR, Horan MA, Strijbos PJ, Rothwell NJ (1990) Lipocortin 1 fragment modifies pyrogenic actions of cytokines in rats. *Amer J Physiol* 259: 266–269

39 Davidson J, Flower RJ, Milton AS, Peers SH, Rotondo D (1991) Antipyretic actions of human recombinant lipocortin-1. *Brit J Pharmacol* 102: 7–9

40 Perretti M, Flower RJ (1993) Modulation of IL-1-induced neutrophil migration by dexamethasone and lipocortin 1. *J Immunol* 150: 992–999

41 Relton K, Strijbos PJLM, O'Shaughnessy CT, Carey F, Forder RA, Tilders FJH, Rothwell NJ (1991) Lipocortin-1 is an endogenous inhibitor of ischemic damage in the rat brain. *J Exp Med* 174: 305–310

42 Croxtall JD, Flower RJ (1994) Antisense oligonucleotides to human lipocortin-1 inhibit glucocorticoid-induced inhibition of A549 cell growth and eicosanoid release. *Biochem Pharmacol* 48: 1729–1734

43 Hirata F, del Carmine R, Nelson CA, Axelrod J, Schiffman E (1981) Presence of autoantibody for phospholipase inhibitory protein, lipomodulin, in patients with rheumatic diseases. *Proc Natl Acad Sci USA* 78: 3190–3194

44 Goulding NJ, Podgorski MR, Hall ND, Flower RJ, Browning JL, Pepinsky RB, Maddison PJ (1989) Autoantibodies to recombinant lipocortin-1 in rheumatoid arthritis and systemic lupus erythematosus. *Ann Rheum Dis* 48: 843–850

45 Loxley HD, Cowell A-M, Flower RJ, Buckingham JC (1993) Modulation of the hypothalamo-pituitary adrenocortical responses to cytokines in the rat by lipocortin 1 and glucocorticoids: a role for lipocortin 1 in the feedback inhibition of CRF-41 release? *Neuroendocrinology* 57: 801–813

46 Taylor AD, Cowell A-M, Flower RJ, Buckingham JC (1993) Lipocortin 1 mediates an early inhibitory action of glucocorticoids on the secretion of ACTH by the rat anterior pituitary gland *in vitro*. *Neuroendocrinology* 58: 430–439

47 Taylor AD, Loxley HD, Flower RJ, Buckingham JC (1995) Immunoneutralization of lipocortin 1 reverses the acute inhibitory effects of dexamethasone on the hypothalamo-pituitary-adrenocortical responses to cytokines in the rat *in vitro* and *in vivo*. *Neuroendocrinology* 62: 19–31

48 Loxley HD, Cowell A-M, Flower RJ, Buckingham JC (1993) Effects of lipocortin 1 and dexamethasone on the secretion of corticotrophin releaseing factors in the rat: *in vitro* and *in vivo* studies. *J Neuroendocrinol* 5: 51–61

49 Taylor AD, Cowell A-M, Flower RJ, Buckingham JC (1995) Dexamethasone suppresses the release of prolactin from the rat anterior pituitary gland by lipocortin 1 dependent and independent mechanisms. *Neuroendocrinology* 62: 530–542

50 Taylor AD, Flower RJ, Buckingham JC (1997) Antisense and

immunoneutralisation strategies reveal a role for lipocortin 1 in the control of growth hormone *in vivo* and *in vitro*. *Brit J Pharmacol* 120,345P

51 Taylor AD, Flower RJ, Buckingham JC (1994) Dexamethasonc inhibits the release of TSH from the rat anterior pituitary gland *in vitro* by mechanisms dependent on *de novo* protein synthesis and lipocortin 1. *J Endocrinol* 14: 533–544

52 Philip JG, Flower RJ, Buckingham JC (1998) Blockade of the classical pathway of protein secretion does not affect the cellular exportation of lipocortin 1. *Regul Peptides* 73: 133–139

53 Taylor AD, Christian HC, Morris JF, Flower RJ, Buckingham JC (1997) An antisense oligodeoxynucleotide to lipocortin 1 reverses the inhibitory actions of dexamethasone on the release of adrenocoritcotrophin from rat anterior pituitary tissues *in vitro*. *Endocrinology* 138: 2909–2918

54 Christian HC, Taylor AD, Morris JF, Flower RJ, Buckingham JC (1997) Characterisation and localisation of lipocortin 1 binding sites on the anterior pituitary gland by fluorescence activated cell analysis/sorting. *Endocrinology* 138: 5341–5351

55 Croxtall JD, Flower RJ (1992) Lipocortin 1 mediates dexamethasone-induced growth arrest of the A549 lung adenocarcinoma cell line. *Proc Natl Acad Sci USA* 89: 3571–3575

56 Wu CC, Thiemermann C, Szabo C, Perretti MCroxtall JD, Flower RJ, Vane JR (1995) Lipocortin 1 mediates the inhibition by dexamethasone of the induction by endotoxin of nitric oxide synthase in the rat. *Proc Natl Acad Sci USA* 92: 3473–3477

57 Slotkin TA, Barnes GA, McCook EC, Seidler FJ (1996) Programming of brain-stem serotonin transporter development by prenatal glucocorticoids. *Dev Brain Res* 93: 155–161

Chapter C10

1 Kirwan JR (1995) The effect of glucocorticoids on joint destruction in rheumatoid arthritis. *N Engl J Med* 333: 142–146

2 Smith MD, Ahern MJ, Roberts-Thompson PJ (1990) Pulse methylprednisolone therapy in rheumatoid arthritis: unproved therapy, unjustified therapy or effective adjunctive treatment? *Ann Rheum Dis* 49: 265–267

3 Perretti M, Croxtall JD, Wheller SK, Goulding NJ, Hannon R, Flower RJ (1996) Mobilizing lipocortin 1 in adherent human leukocytes downregulates their transmigration. *Nat Med* 2: 1259–1262

4 Flower RJ, Rothwell NJ (1994) Lipocortin-1: cellular mechanisms and clinical relevance. *Trends Pharmacol Sci* 15: 71–76

5   Cato ACB, Wade E (1996) Molecular mechanisms of anti-inflammatory action of glucocorticoids. *Bioessays* 18: 371–378

6   Kamai Y, Xu L, Heinzel T, Tarchia J, Kurokawa R, Gloss B, Lin SC, Heyman RA, Rose DW, Glass CK et al (1996) A CBP integrator complex mediates transcriptional activation and AP-1 inhibition by nuclear receptors. *Cell* 85: 403–414

7   Ray A, Prefontaine KE (1994) Physical association and functional antagonism between the p65 subunit of transcription factor NF-κB and the glucocorticoid receptor. *Proc Natl Acad Sci USA* 91: 752–756

8   Auphan N, DiDonato JA, Rosette C, Helmberg A, Karin M (1995) Immunosuppression by glucocorticoids: Inhibiton of NF-κB activity through induction of IκB synthesis. *Science* 270: 286–290

9   Scheinman RI, Cogswell PC, Lofquist AK, Baldwin Jr, AS (1995) Role of transcriptional activation of IκBα in mediation of immunosuppression by glucocorticoids. *Science* 270: 283–286

10 Sambrook PN, Jones G (1995) Corticosteroid osteoporosis. *Brit J Rheumatol* 34: 8–12

11 Fries JF, Williams CA, Morfeld D, Singh G, Sibley J (1996) Reduction in long-term disability in patients with rheumatoid arthritis by disease-modifying antirheumatic drug-based treatment strategies. *Arthritis Rheum* 39: 616–622

12 American College of Rheumatology Ad Hoc Committee on Clinical Guidelines (1996) Guidelines for monitoring the management of rheumatoid arthritis. *Arthritis Rheum* 39: 713–722

13 American College of Rheumatology Ad Hoc Committee on Clinical Guidelines (1996) Guidelines for monitoring drug therapy in rheumatoid arthritis. *Arthritis Rheum* 39: 723–731

14 Buchbinder R, Hall S, Sambrook PN, Champion GD, Harkness A, Lewis D et al (1993) Methotrexate therapy in rheumatoid arthritis: a life table review of 587 patients treated in community practice. *J Rheumatol* 20: 639–644

15 Tugwell P, Bennett K, Gent M (1987) Methotrexate in rheumatoid arthritis. Indications, contraindications, efficacy, and safety. *Ann Intern Med* 107: 358–366

16 Lopez-Mendez A, Daniel WW, Reading JC, Ward JR, Alarcon GS (1993) Radiographic assessment of disease progression in rheumatoid arthritis patients enrolled in the cooperative systematic studies of the rheumatic diseases program: randomized clinical trial of methotrexate, auranofin, or a combination of the two. *Arthritis Rheum* 36: 1364–1369

17 Jeurissen MEC, Boerbooms AMT, van der Putte LBA, Doesburg WH, Lemmens AM (1993) Influence of methotrexate and azathioprine on radiologic progression of rheumatoid arthritis. *Arthritis Rheum* 36: 613–619

18 Cronstein BN (1996) Molecular Therapeutics. Methotrexate and its mechanism of action. *Arthritis Rheum* 39: 951–960

19 Seideman P, Beck O, Eksborg S, Wennberg M (1993) The pharmacokinetics of methotrexate and its 7-hydroxymetabolite in patients with rheumatoid arthritis. *Brit J Pharmacol* 35: 409–412

20 Conaghan PC, Brooks PM, Quinn DI, Day RO (1995) Hazards of low dose methotrexate. *Aust NZ J Med* 25: 670–673

21 Kremer JM, Alarcon GS, Lightfoot RWJr, Willkens RF, Furst DE, Williams HJ et al (1994) Methotrexate for rheumatoid arthritis: suggested guidelines for monitoring liver toxicity. *Arthritis Rheum* 37: 316–328

22 Day RO (1993) Sulphasalazine. *In*: WN Kelly, ED Harris, S Ruddy, CB Sledge (eds): *The Textbook of Rheumatology*, 4th edn., 692–699

23 Van der Heijde DM, van Riel PL, Nuver-Zwart IH, van der Putte LB (1990) Sulphasalazine versus hydroxychloroquine in rheumatoid arthritis: 3 year follow-up. *Lancet* 335: 539

24 Ferraz MB, Tugwell P, Goldsmith CH, Atra E (1990) Meta-analysis of sulfasalazine in ankylosing spondylitis. *J Rheumatol* 17: 1482–1486

25 Tett SE, Cutler D, Day RO (1991) Antimalarials in rheumatic diseases. *In*: P Brooks (ed.): *Balliere's clinical rheumatology, slow acting anti-rheumatic drugs and immunosuppressives*. Balliere, London, 4: 467–489

26 Esdaile JM, Suissa S, Shiroky JB, Lamping D, Tsakomas B, Anderson D et al (1995) A randomized trial of hydroxychloroquine in early rheumatoid arthritis: the HERA study. *Amer J Med* 98: 156–168

27 Van Der Heijde D, Van Riel P, Nuver-Zwart I, Gribnau F, Van de Putte L (1989) Effects of hydroxychloroquine and sulfasalazine on progression of joint damage in rheumatoid arthritis. *Lancet* 334: 1036–1038

28 Wiegmann K, Schutze S, Machleidt T, Witte D, Kronke M (1994) Functional dichotomy of neutral and acidic sphingomyelinases in tumour necrosis factor signaling. *Cell* 78: 1005–1015

29 McLachlan AJ, Tett SE, Cutler DJ, Day RO (1994) Bioavailability of hydroxychloroquine tablets in patients with rheumatoid arthritis. *Brit J Rheumatol* 33: 235–239

30 Tett SE, Day RO, Cutler DJ (1993) Concentration-effect relationship of hydroxychloroquine in rheumatoid arthritis-a cross sectional study. *J Rheumatol* 20: 1874–1879

31 Champion GD, Graham G, Ziegler J (1990) The gold complexes. *In*: Brooks P (ed.): *Balliere's clinical rheumatology, slow acting anti-rheumatic drugs and immunosuppressives*. Balliere, London, 4: 491–534

32 Buckland-Wright J, Graham S, Chikanza I, Grahame R (1993) Quantitative microfocal radiography detects changes in erosion area in patients with early rheumatoid arthritis treated with myocrisin. *J Rheumatol* 20: 243–247

33 Handel ML, Watts CKW, deFazio A, Day RO, Sutherland RL (1995) Inhibition of AP-1 binding and transcription by gold and selenium involving conserved cysteine residues in Jun and Fos. *Proc Natl Acad Sci USA* 92:

4497–4501

34 Yang JP, Merin JP, Nakano T, Kato T, Kitade Y, Okamoto T (1995) Inhibition of the DNA-binding activity of NF-kappa B by gold compounds *in vitro*. *FEBS Lett* 361: 89–96

35 Koike R, Miki I, Otoshi M, Totsuka T, Inoue H, Kase H, Saito I, Miyasaka N (1994) Gold sodium thiomalate downregulates intercellular adhesion molecule-1 and vascular cell adhesion molecule-1 expression on vascular endothelial cells. *Mol Pharmacol* 46: 599–604

36 Gerber RC, Paulus HE, Bluestone R, Lederer M (1972) Kinetics of aurothiomalate in serum and synovial fluid. *Arthritis Rheum* 15: 625–629

37 Graham GG, Champion GD, Ziegler JB (1994) The cellular metabolism and effects of gold complexes. *Metal Based Drugs* 1: 395–404

38 Handel ML, Watts CKW, Sivertsen S, Day RO, Sutherland RL (1996) D-Penicillamine causes free radical-dependent inactivation of activator protein-1 DNA binding. *Mol Pharmcol* 50: 501–505

39 Joyce DA, Day RO (1990) D-Penicillamine and D-penicillamine-protein disulphide in plasma and synovial fluid of patients with rheumatoid arthritis. *Brit J Clin Pharmacol* 30: 511–517

40 Day RO, Paulus HE (1987) D-Penicillamine. *In*: HE Paulus, DE Furst, SH Dromgoole (eds): *Drugs for rheumatic disease*. Churchill Livingstone, New York:, 85–112

41 Ho S, Clipstone N, Timmermann L, Northrop J, Graef I, Fiorentino D, Nourse J, Crabtree GR (1996) The mechanism of action of cyclosporin A and FK506. *Clin Immunol Immunopathol* 80: S40–45

42 Campana C, Regazzi MB, Buggia I, Molinaro M (1996) Clinically significant drug interactions with cyclosporin. *Clin Pharmacokinet* 30: 141–179

43 Tugwell P, Bombardier C, Gent M, Bennett KJ, Bensen WG, Carette S et al (1990) Low dose cyclosporin versus placebo in patients with rheumatoid arthritis. *Lancet* 335: 1051–1055

44 Yocum DE, Klippel JH, Wilder RL, Gerber NL, Austin HA, Wahl SM et al (1988) Cyclosporin A in severe, treatment-refractory rheumatoid arthritis. A randomized study. *Ann Intern Med* 109: 863–869

45 van den Borne BE, Landewe RB, The HS, Breedveld FC, Dijkmans BA (1996) Low dose cyclosporine in early rheumatoid arthritis: effective and safe after two years of therapy when compared with chloroquine. *Scand J Rheumatol* 25: 307–316

46 Pasero G, Priolo F, Marubini E, Fantini F, Ferracioli G, Magaro M et al (1996) Slow progression of joint damage in early rheumatoid arthritis treated with cyclosporin A. *Arthritis Rheum* 39: 1006–1015

47 O'Dell JR, Haire CE, Erikson N, Drymalski W, Palmer W, Eckhoff PJ et al (1996) Treatment of rheumatoid arthritis with methotrexate alone, sulfasalazine and hydroxychloroquine, or a combination of all three

medications. *N Engl J Med* 334: 1287–1291

48 Tugwell P, Pincus T, Yocum D, Stein M, Gluck O, Kraag G, McKendry R, Teser J, Baker P, Wells G (1995) Combination therapy with cyclosporine and methotrexate in severe rheumatoid arthritis. The methotrexate-cyclosporine combination study group. *N Engl J Med* 333: 137–141

49 van der Lubbe PA, Dijkmans BAC, Markusse HM, Nassander U, Breedveld FC (1995) A randomized, double-blind, placebo-controlled study of CD4 monoclonal antibody therapy in early rheumatoid arthrtitis. *Arthritis Rheum* 38: 1097–1106

50 Elliott MJ, Maini RN, Feldmann M, Calden JR, Antoni C, Smolen JS et al (1994) Randomised double-blind comparison of chimeric monoclonal antibody to tumor necrosis factor alpha (cA2) versus placebo in rheumatoid arthritis. *Lancet* 344: 1105–1110

Chapter D1

1   Descotes JG, Vial T (1994) Cytoreductive drugs. *In*: JH Dean, MI Luster, AE Munson, I Kimber (eds): *Immunotoxicology and immunopharmacology,* 2nd edn. Raven Press, New York, 293–301

2   Broide DH (1991) Inflammatory cells:structure and function. *In*: DP Stites, AI Terr (eds): *Basic and clinical immunology*. Prentice Hall International, London, 141–153

3   Ryffel B, Car BD, Eugster H-P, Woerly G (1994) Transplantation Agents. *In*: JH Dean, MI Luster, AE Munson, I Kimber (eds): *Immunotoxicology and immunopharmacology,* 2nd edn. Raven Press, New York, 267–292

4   Majoor GD, Wodzig WH, Vriesman PJCVB (1991) Cyclosporin-induced autoimmunity. *In*: MD Kendall, MA Ritter (eds): *Thymus update: thymus in immunotoxicology*. Harwood Academic Publishers, London, 179–200

5   Cohen JJ (1992) Glucocorticoid-induced apoptosis in the thymus. *Seminars in immunology* Academic Press, New York

6   Clark EA, Ledbetter JA (1994) How B- and T-cells talk to each other. *Nature* 367: 425–428

7   Matzinger P (1994) Tolerance, danger and the extended family. *Annu Rev Immunol* 12: 991–1045

8   Vial T, Descotes J (1995) Immune-mediated side effects of cytokines in humans. *Toxicology* 105: 31–57

9   Uetrecht J (1990) Drug metabolism by leukocytes and its role in drug-induced lupus and other idiosyncratic drug reactions. *Crit Rev Toxicol* 20: 213–235

10 Kubicka-Muranyi M, Kremer J, Rottmann N, Lübben B, Albers R, Bloksma N, Lührmann R, Gleichmann E (1996) Murine systemic autoimmune disease

induced by mercuric chloride: T helper cells reacting to self proteins. *Int Arch Allergy Immunol* 109: 11–20

11 Griem P, Panthel K, Kalbacher H, Gleichmann E (1996) Alteration of a model antigen by Au (III) leads to T-cell sensitization to cryptic peptides. *Eur J Immunol* 26: 279–287

12 Bloksma N, Kubicka-Muranyi M, Schuppe H-C, Gleichmann E, Gleichmann H (1995) Predictive immunotoxicological test systems: suitability of the popliteal lymph node assay in mice and rats. *Crit Rev Toxicol* 25: 369–396

13 Griem P, Gleichmann E (1995) Metal ion induced autoimmunity. *Curr Opin Immunol* 7: 831–838

14 Janeway CA (1992) The immune system evolved to discriminate infectious nonself from noninfectious self. *Immunol Today* 13: 11–16

15 Cohen IR (1992) The cognitive paradigm and the immunological homunculus. *Immunol Today* 13: 490–494

16 Ibrahim MAA, Chain BM, Katz DR (1995) The injured cell: the role of the dendritic cell system as a sentinel receptor pathway. *Immunol Today* 16: 181–186

17 Sgro C (1995) Side effects of a monoclonal antibody, muromonab CD3/orthoclone OKT3: bibliographic review. *Toxicology* 105: 23–29

18 Gleichmann E, Pals ST, Rolink AG, Radaszkiewicz T, Gleichmann H (1984) Graft-versus-host reactions: clues to the etiopathology of a spectrum of immunological diseases. *Immunol Today* 5: 324–332

19 Adams LE, Hess EV (1991) Drug-related lupus. Incidence, mechanisms and clinical implications. *Drug Safety* 6: 431–449

20 Janeway CA, Travers P (1994) *Immunobiology: the immune system in health and disease.* Current Biology, Oxford

21 Druet P, Pelletier L, Rossert J, Druet E, Hirsch F, Sapin C (1989) Autoimmune reactions induced by metals. *In*: ME Kammuller, N Bloksma, W Seinen (eds): *Autoimmunity and toxicology: immune disregulation induced by drugs and chemicals.* Elsevier, Amsterdam, 349–361

22 Van Vliet E, Uhrberg M, Stein C, Gleichmann E (1993) MHC control of IL-4-dependent enhancement of B-cell Ia expression and Ig class switching in mice treated with mercuric chloride. *Int Arch Allergy Immunol* 101: 392–401

23 Albers R (1996) Chemical-induced autoimmunity -Immune disregulation assessed with reporter antigens.Utrecht University, *PhD thesis*

24 Coleman JW, Sim E (1994) Autoallergic responses to drugs: mechanistic aspects. *In*: JH Dean, MI Luster, AE Munson, I Kimber (eds): *Immunotoxicology and immunopharmacology*, 2nd edn. Raven Press, New York, 553–572

25 IPCS (1996) International Programme for Chemical Safety, Environmental Health Criteria Document 160. *Principles and methods for assessing direct*

immunotoxicity associated with chemical exposure. Geneva: World Health Organization

26 Vos JG (1980) Immunotoxicity assessment: screening and function studies. *Arch Toxicol* Suppl 4: 95–108

27 Van Loveren H, Vos JG (1989) Immunotoxicological considerations: a practical approach to immunotoxicity testing in the rat. *In*: Dayan AD, Paine AJ (eds): *Advances in applied toxicology*. Taylor and Francis, London, 143–165

28 Vos JG, Krajnc EI (1983) Immunotoxicity of pesticides. *In*: AW Hayes, RC Schnell, TS Miya (eds): *Developments in the science and practice of toxicology*. Elsevier, Amsterdam, 229–240

29 De Waal EJ, Van Loveren H, Vos JG (1997) Practice of tiered testing for immunosuppression in rodents. *Drug Inf J* 31: 1317–1323

30 Van Loveren H, Vos JG (1992) *Evaluation of OECD guideline #407 for assessment of toxicity of chemicals with respect to potential adverse effects to the immune system*. RIVM Report , 158801001, Bilthoven

31 The ICISISGroup Investigators (1998) Report of interlaboratory validation study of assessment of direct immunotoxicity in the rat. *Toxicology* 125: 183–201

32 Koeter HBWM (1995) International harmonisation of immunotoxicity testing. *Hum Exp Toxicol* 14: 151–154

33 Van Loveren H, Vos JG, De Waal EJ (1996) Testing immunotoxicity of chemicals as a guide for testing approaches for pharmaceuticals. *Drug Inf J* 30: 275–279

34 Van Loveren H, Gianotten N, Hendriksen CFM, Schuurman H-J, Van Der Laan JW (1994) Assessment of immunotoxicity of buprenorphine. *Lab Animals* 28: 355–363

35 De Waal EJ, De Jong WH, Van Der Vliet H, Verlaan B, Van Loveren H (1996) *Int J Immunopharmacol* 18: 523–528

36 Ladics GS, Smith C, Heaps K, Ellioo GS, Slone TW, Loveless SE (1995) Possible incorporation of an immunotoxicological funtional assay for assessing humoral immunity for hazard identification purposes in rats on standard toxicology study. *Toxicology* 96: 225–238

37 Luster MI, Munson AE, Thomas PT, Holsapple MP, Fenters JD, White KL, Lauer LD, Germolec DR, Rosenthal GJ, Dean JH (1988) Development of a testing battery to assess chemical-induced immunotoxicity: National Toxicology Program's guidelines for immunotoxicity evaluation in mice. *Fund Appl Toxicol* 10: 2–19

38 Luster MI, Portier C, Pait DG, Rosenthal GJ, Germolec DR, Corsini E, Blaylock BL, Pollock P, Kouchi Y, Craig W et al (1993) Risk assessment in immunotoxicology. II. Relationship between immune and host resistance tests. *Fund Appl Toxicol* 21: 71–82

39 Bugelski PJ, Thiem PA, Solleveld HA, Morgan DG (1990) Effects of sensitization to dinitrochlorobenzene (DNCB) on clinical pathology parameters and mitogen-mediated blastogenesis in cynomolgus monkeys (*Macaca fascicularis*). *Toxicol Pathol* 18: 643–650

40 Ahmed-Ansari A, Brodie AR, Fultz PN, Anderson DC, Sell KW, McClure HM (1989) Flow microfluorometric analysis of peripheral blood mononuclear cells from nonhumam primates: Correlation of phenotype with immune function. *Amer J Primatol* 17: 107–131

41 Barratt MD, Basketter DA, Chamberlain M, Admans GD, Langowski JJ (1994) An expert system rulebase for identifying contact allergens. *Toxicol Vitro* 8: 1053–1060

42 Dupuis G, Benezra C (1982) *Contact dermatitis to simple chemicals: a molecular approach*. Marcel Dekker, New York

43 Maurer T (1996) Predictive testing for skin allergy. *In*: JG Vos, M Younes, E Smith (eds): *Allergic hypersensitivities induced by chemicals. recommendations for prevention*. CRC Press, Boca Raton, 237–259

44 Garssen J, Vandebriel RJ, Kimber I, Van Loveren H (1996) Hypersensitivity reactions: definitions, basic mechanisms, and localizations. *In*: JG Vos, M Younes, E Smith (eds): *Allergic hypersensitivities induced by chemicals. recommendations for prevention*. CRC Press, Boca Raton, 19–58

45 Kimber I, Dearman RJ (1996) Contact hypersensitivity: immunological mechanisms. *In*: I Kimber, T Maurer (eds): *Toxicology of contact hypersensitivity*. Taylor and Francis, London, 14–25

46 Gad SC, Dunn BJ, Dobbs DW, Reilly C, Walsh RD (1986) Development and validation of an alternative dermal sensitization test: the mouse ear swelling test (MEST). *Toxicol Appl Pharmacol* 84: 93–114

47 Kimber I, Mitchell JA, Griffin AC (1986) Development of a murine local lymph node assay for the determination of sensitizing potential. *Food Chem Toxicol* 24: 585–586

48 Dearman RJ, Mitchell JA, Basketter DA, Kimber I (1992) Differential ability of occupational chemical contact and respiratory allergens to cause immediate and delayed dermal hypersensitivity reactions in mice. *Int Arch Allergy Appl Immunol* 97: 315–321

49 Garssen J, Nijkamp FP, Van Der Vliet H, Van Loveren H (1991) T-cell mediated induction of airway hyperreactivity in mice. *Amer Rev Resp Dis* 144: 931–938

50 Scheerens H, Buckley TL, Davidse EM, Garssen J, Nijkamp FP, Van Loveren H (1996) Toluene diisocyanate-induced *in vitro* tracheal hyperreactivity in the mouse. *Amer J Respir Crit Care Med* 154: 858–865

51 Karol MH (1996) Predictive testing for respiratory allergy. *In*: JG Vos, M Younes, E Smith (eds): *Allergic hypersensitivities induced by chemicals. Recommendations for prevention*. CRC Press, Boca Raton, 125–137

52 Karol MH, Griffiths-Johnson DA, Skoner DP (1993) Chemically induced pulmonary hypersensitivity, airway hyperreactivity and asthma. *In*: D Gardner ct al (eds): *Toxicology of the lung*, 2nd edn. Raven Press, New York, 417–433

53 Sarlo K Clark ED (1992) A tier approach for evaluating the respiratory allergenicity of low molecular weight chemicals. *Fund Appl Toxicol* 85: 55–58

54 Hessel EM, Van Oosterhout AJM, Hofstra CL, De Bie JJ, Garssen J, Van Loveren H, Verheyen AKCP, Savelkoul HFJ, Nijkamp FP (1995) Bronchoconstriction and airway hyperresponsiveness after ovalbumin inhalation in sensitized mice. *Eur J Pharmacol Env Tox Pharmacol Sect* 293: 401–412

55 Kammüller ME, Bloksma N, Seinen W (eds) (1989*) Autoimmunity and toxicology: Immune dysregulation induced by drugs and chemicals*. Elsevier, Amsterdam

56 Gleichmann E, Vohr HW, Stringer C, Nuyens J, Gleichmann H (1989) Testing the sensitization of T-cells to chemicals. From murine graft-versus-host (GVH) reactions to chemical-induced GVH-like immunological diseases. *In*: ME Kammüller, N Bloksma, W Seinen (eds): *Autoimmunity and toxicology: immune dysregulation induced by drugs and chemicals*. Elsevier, Amsterdam, 364–390

57 Gleichmann E, Kind P, Schuppe HC, Merk H (1990) Tests for predicting sensitization to chemicals and their metabolites, with special reference to heavy metals. *In*: AD Dayan, RF Hertel, E Heseltine, G Kazantzis, EM Smith, Van Der Venne MT (eds): *Immunotoxicity of metals and immunotoxicology*. Plenum Press, New York, 139–152

58 Vial T, Carleer J, Legrain B, Verdier F, Descotes J (1997) The popliteal lymph node assay: results of a preliminary interlaboratory validation study. *Toxicology* 122: 213–218

59 Selgrade MJ, Cooper KD, Devlin RB, Van Loveren H, Biagini RE, Luster MI (1995) Immunotoxicity-Bridging the gap between animal research and human health effects. *Fund Appl Toxicol* 24: 13–21

60 National Research Council (1992) *Biological markers in immunotoxicology*. National Academiy Press, Washington

61 Levy SM, Herberman RB, Lee J, Whiteside T, Beadle M, Heiden L, Simons A (1991) Persistantly low natural killer activity, age, and environmental stress as predictors of infectious morbidity. *Nat Immun Cell Growth Regul* 10: 289–307

62 Bentwich Z, Bianco N, Jager L, Houba V, Lambert PH, Knaap W, Rose N, Seligman M, Thompson R, Torrigiani G et al (1982) Use and abuse of laboratory tests in clinical immunology: Critical considerations of eight widely used diagnostic procedures. Report of a Joint IUIS/WHO Meeting on

Assessment of Tests Used in Clinical Immunology. *Clin Immunol Immunopathol* 24: 122–138

63 Bentwich Z, Beverley PCL, Hammarstrom L, Kalden JR, Lambert PH, Rose NR, Thompson RA (1988) Laboratory investigations in clinical immunology: Methods, pitfalls, and clinical indications. *Clin Immunol Immunopathol* 49: 478–497

64 Coligan JE, Kruisbeek AM, Margulies DH, Shevach EM, Strober W (eds) (1994) *Current protocols in immunology*, vol. 1 and 2. John Wiley and Sons, New York

65 Lawlor GJ, Fischer TJ (eds) (1988) *Manual of allergy and immunology. Diagnosis and therapy*, 2nd edn. Little, Brown, Boston

66 Miller LE, Ludke HR, Peacock JE, Tomar RH (eds) (1991) *Manual of laboratory immunology*, 2nd edn. Lea and Fabiger, Philadelphia

67 Diggle GE (1993) Overview of regulatory agencies. *In*: B Ballantyne, T Marrs, P Turner (eds): *General and applied toxicology*. MacMillan, Basingstoke, 1071–1090

68 Vos JG, Younes M, Smith E (eds) (1996) *Allergic hypersensitivities induced by chemicals: recommendations for prevention*. CRC Press, Boca Raton

69 Dean J. (1997) Issues with introducing new immunotoxicology methods into the safety assessment of pharmaceuticals. *Toxicology* 119: 95–101

70 De Waal EJ, Van Der Laan JW, Van Loveren H. (1996) Immunotoxicity testing of pharmaceuticals: a regulatory perspective. *Toxicol Ecotoxicol News* 3: 165–172

71 Van Der Laan JW, Van Loveren H, Vos JG, Dean JH, Hastings KL (1997) Immunotoxicity of pharmaceuticals: current knowledge, testing strategies, risk evaluation and consequences for human health. *Drug Inf J.* 31: 1301–1305

72 Hastings KL, Chang-Ho A., Alam SN, Aszalos A, Young SC, Jessop JJ, Weaver JL (1997) Points to consider for assessment of the immunotoxic potential of investigational new drugs: FDA perspective. *Drug Inf J.* 31: 1357–1362

73 Maki E (1997) Practice of preclinical immunotoxity testing in Japan. *Drug Inf J.* 31: 1325–1330

Subject index